Surveillance, Prevention, and Control of Infectious Diseases

Muhammad E. H. Chowdhury • Serkan Kiranyaz
Editors

Surveillance, Prevention, and Control of Infectious Diseases

An AI Perspective

Springer

Editors
Muhammad E. H. Chowdhury
Department of Electrical Engineering
College of Engineering, Qatar University
Doha, Qatar

Serkan Kiranyaz
Department of Electrical Engineering
College of Engineering, Qatar University
Doha, Qatar

ISBN 978-3-031-59966-8 ISBN 978-3-031-59967-5 (eBook)
https://doi.org/10.1007/978-3-031-59967-5

This Springer imprint is published by the registered company Springer Nature Switzerland AG
The registered company address is: Gewerbestrasse 11, 6330 Cham, Switzerland

Preface

Infectious diseases pose a significant threat to public health worldwide, requiring constant vigilance, innovative strategies, and rapid responses to mitigate their impact. In recent years, Artificial Intelligence (AI) has emerged as a powerful tool in the fight against infectious diseases, revolutionizing the way we surveil, prevent, and control outbreaks. This book, *Surveillance, Prevention, and Control of Infectious Diseases: An AI Perspective*, explores the intersection of AI and infectious disease management, offering insights into the latest advancements, challenges, and opportunities in this rapidly evolving field.

The chapters in this book provide a comprehensive overview of various aspects of infectious disease management through the lens of AI. We begin with an exploration of the prospects and challenges of using AI for infectious disease detection, highlighting its potential to expedite outbreak identification and facilitate proactive public health interventions. We then delve into the development and application of AI algorithms for rapid pathogen detection and surveillance, discussing innovative approaches for identifying and monitoring infectious diseases in real-time. One of the key areas covered in this book is the use of wearable devices and continuous physiological signal monitoring for early disease detection. We examine how wearable sensors and AI algorithms can be utilized to analyze physiological data and identify early symptoms of infectious diseases, enabling timely intervention and improved patient outcomes. Additionally, we explore the development of low-cost, automated digital microscopes for detecting diseases such as malaria, showcasing the potential of AI-driven technologies to improve diagnostic capabilities in resource-limited settings. This book addresses the challenge of under-vaccination in developing countries, proposing a comprehensive framework to identify and support children who miss essential vaccinations. It reviews research on vaccine gaps, synthesizes effective intervention strategies, and explores the potential of advanced technologies like AI and blockchain. By offering a systematic approach, the framework aims to improve vaccination coverage and promote global health equity by ensuring equitable access to vaccines for all children. Another highlight of this book is the discussion on the interpretability of deep learning models for tuberculosis detection using X-ray images. We explore how lightweight parallel

CNN models can enhance diagnostic accuracy while providing insights into the prediction process, paving the way for more effective disease diagnosis and management. Furthermore, we investigate the use of AI in the surveillance of seasonal respiratory infections, showcasing its role in automating outbreak identification and reducing transmission rates through early detection and intervention.

Throughout this book, we emphasize the importance of collaboration between healthcare professionals, researchers, policymakers, and technologists in harnessing the full potential of AI for infectious disease management. We hope that the insights and findings presented in this book will inspire further research and innovation in this critical area, ultimately leading to more effective strategies for surveilling, preventing, and controlling infectious diseases on a global scale.

We are immensely grateful for the dedicated efforts of our contributors in shaping this comprehensive volume on *Surveillance, Prevention, and Control of Infectious Diseases: An AI Perspective*. Your expertise and commitment have ensured the quality and relevance of each chapter, enriching the book with diverse insights and innovative approaches. As we move forward with the editing process, we encourage thoroughness and attention to detail to maintain the book's excellence. We extend our heartfelt appreciation to our esteemed reviewers for their invaluable feedback and constructive criticism, which have been instrumental in refining the manuscript. Your thorough reviews have enhanced the rigor and clarity of the content, contributing significantly to the scholarly integrity of the book. We are deeply grateful for your time, expertise, and dedication to advancing knowledge in this critical field.

Doha, Qatar

Muhammad E. H. Chowdhury
Serkan Kiranyaz

About the Book

Surveillance, Prevention, and Control of Infectious Diseases: An AI Perspective is a cutting-edge book that explores the transformative role of Artificial Intelligence (AI) in managing infectious diseases. Through ten comprehensive chapters, the book delves into various facets of AI application, offering insights into disease surveillance, prevention, and control. Beginning with an introduction to the potential of AI in infectious disease detection, the book progresses to review AI algorithms for rapid pathogen detection and surveillance. It further examines the integration of big data into infectious disease surveillance and discusses the development of low-cost, automated digital microscopes for malaria detection. The book also explores innovations in tuberculosis screening, robust dengue patient detection, interpretable deep learning models for tuberculosis detection, and continuous physiological signal monitoring using wearables for early infectious disease detection. Additionally, it discusses AI's role in monitoring seasonal respiratory infections, highlighting its contributions to detection, forecasting, and management. By showcasing the efficacy of AI-driven approaches in disease identification, the book underscores their potential to revolutionize infectious disease management, making it an indispensable resource for healthcare professionals, researchers, and policymakers striving for more effective disease surveillance and control strategies.

Contents

Artificial Intelligence for Infectious Disease Detection: Prospects and Challenges

Md. Moradul Siddique, Md. Masrafi Bin Seraj, Md. Nasim Adnan, and Syed Md. Galib

1 Introduction

Infectious diseases are sicknesses brought on by pathogens like bacteria, viruses, fungi, or parasites that can spread from person to person or by transporters like mosquitoes. It poses a significant threat to global health, causing widespread morbidity, mortality, and socioeconomic disruption. Infectious diseases can range from common infections like the flu to more severe outbreaks like COVID-19 and historical pandemics like the Black Death [91]. From an AI perspective, infectious diseases present a complex challenge that can benefit from advanced technological solutions. AI offers the potential to enhance various aspects of infectious disease management, including early detection, accurate diagnosis, outbreak prediction, and treatment optimization [85]. By leveraging machine learning algorithms, deep neural networks, and data analytics, AI can process vast amounts of medical data, identify patterns, and provide insights that empower healthcare professionals and

M. M. Siddique
Department of Computer Science and Engineering, Jashore University of Science and Technology (JUST), Jashore, Bangladesh

Artificial Intelligence for Development Lab (AID Lab), Jashore University of Science and Technology, Jashore, Bangladesh

Department of Computer Science and Engineering, University of Information Technology & Sciences (UITS), Dhaka, Bangladesh

M. M. B. Seraj · M. N. Adnan · S. M. Galib (✉)
Department of Computer Science and Engineering, Jashore University of Science and Technology (JUST), Jashore, Bangladesh

Artificial Intelligence for Development Lab (AID Lab), Jashore University of Science and Technology, Jashore, Bangladesh
e-mail: galib.cse@just.edu.bd

M. E. H. Chowdhury, S. Kiranyaz (eds.), *Surveillance, Prevention, and Control of Infectious Diseases*, https://doi.org/10.1007/978-3-031-59967-5_1

public health authorities to respond effectively to outbreaks and minimize their impact on global health.

In terms of timely response, early detection allows for a rapid response to contain and mitigate the spread of the disease. Swift identification of cases enables health authorities to implement measures such as isolation, quarantine, and treatment, reducing the chances of widespread transmission [83]. Hospitals and healthcare facilities can prepare for potential surges in patient numbers, ensuring that sufficient medical supplies, personnel, and equipment are available to provide adequate care. Swift detection facilitates the identification of the source of the outbreak, helping to trace and isolate cases before they spread widely. This is particularly crucial in infectious diseases with high transmission rates. In addition, early detection contributes to robust disease surveillance systems. Monitoring the progression of an outbreak provides insights into its dynamics, allowing for adjustments to control strategies as needed [86].

However, the journey towards a harmonious integration of AI in infectious disease detection is not without its share of challenges. Data quality, availability, and privacy emerge as formidable hurdles, demanding innovative strategies to ensure a robust and representative dataset. Ethical considerations of patient confidentiality, consent, and transparency underscore the need for responsible AI deployment in a domain where human lives are at stake [89].

Certainly, there have been several successful applications of AI in various medical domains that demonstrate its potential for revolutionizing healthcare. These successes set the stage for AI's promising role in infectious disease detection and management. Remarkably, Medical Imaging Analysis, Drug Discovery and Development, Personalized Medicine, Patient Care and Management, Natural Language Processing (NLP) in healthcare, and Robot-Assisted Surgery are some of the successful and ongoing AI-based techniques currently in use in disease detection and management [84].

Interdisciplinary collaboration between AI researchers, healthcare professionals, and policymakers is paramount in harnessing the full potential of AI in healthcare. This collaboration brings together diverse expertise and perspectives to address complex challenges, drive innovation, and ensure the responsible and effective integration of AI technologies. Apart from the chapter navigates through the diverse terrain of AI applications in infectious diseases detection, spotlighting successful cases. Whereas AI's prowess has led to early warnings of outbreaks, accurate diagnostics through medical imaging analysis, and proactive management of disease spread. As we navigate the dynamic interplay between technology and medicine, the chapters to come will elucidate the path towards a future where AI and human expertise synergize to fortify our defenses against infectious diseases in an ever-evolving global landscape.

2 Background Study

Our aim is to shed light on major Artificial Intelligence approaches for infectious disease detection. Therefore, we will discuss some preliminaries in this section.

2.1 Artificial Intelligence

Artificial Intelligence comprises various technologies, including machine learning, deep learning, natural language processing, and data analytics. These tools empower computers to execute activities that traditionally demand human intelligence, like identifying patterns, forecasting, and gaining knowledge through experience. In healthcare, AI is being harnessed to tackle some of the most pressing challenges, including improving diagnostics, personalizing treatment plans, managing medical records, and even drug discovery [46]. Early detection and accurate diagnosis play a pivotal role in effectively controlling infectious disease outbreaks. Whereas AI systems can continuously learn from new data, improving their detection and diagnostic capabilities over time. This adaptability ensures that the AI remains effective even as pathogens evolve, or new infectious diseases emerge.

2.2 Machine Learning

Machine Learning (ML) constitutes a subset of AI that centers on creating algorithms and models to facilitate computers in acquiring knowledge from data, thereby enabling them to formulate forecasts and choices. The fundamental idea is that machines can automatically improve their performance on a task through experience. A graphical illustration of the disease detection framework using machine learning classification techniques is shown in Fig. 1.

ML algorithms require substantial amounts of data to learn patterns and relationships. This data can be labeled (with known outcomes) or unlabeled, and it serves as the foundation for training models. Later on, features are the attributes or characteristics extracted from the data that the model uses to make predictions.

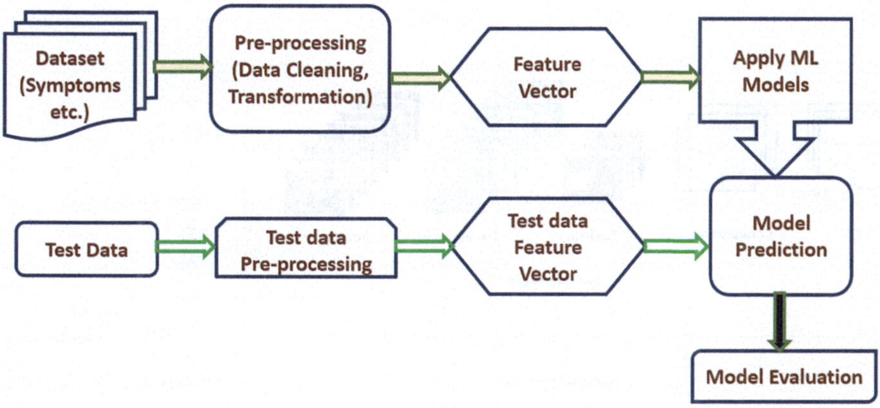

Fig. 1 A framework for disease detection method using Machine Learning

Effective feature selection and engineering are crucial for model performance. During training, the model learns patterns and relationships in the data by adjusting its parameters. The model is exposed to a dataset and learns to make predictions based on the input features [88]. The algorithms used in machine learning can be categorized into two major categories—supervised and unsupervised learning models. In a supervised learning model, the model learns from labeled data, where the input is paired with the correct output. It aims to learn the mapping between inputs and outputs to make predictions on new, unseen data [87]. On the other hand, unsupervised learning deals with unlabeled data. The goal is to uncover hidden patterns or structures within the data, such as clustering similar data points together [90].

2.3 *Deep Learning*

Deep Learning (DL) stands as a subdivision of machine learning, emphasizing the utilization of multi-layered neural networks to simulate and address intricate challenges. These neural networks draw inspiration from the human brain's architecture, composed of interconnected nodes (neurons) arranged in layers. Particularly, deep neural networks encompass numerous layers of interconnected nodes. Each layer extracts and transforms features from the input data [52]. Deep learning leverages hierarchical feature representations, with early layers detecting simple features and later layers combining them to detect more complex patterns. For instance, CNNs are particularly effective for image and visual data. They use convolutional layers to automatically learn relevant features from images [2]. Based on the image data, a conventional framework of a deep learning approach (CNN) is shown in Fig. 2. On the flip side, RNNs are suited for sequential data, like time series or natural language. They have connections that loop back, allowing them to capture temporal dependencies [50].

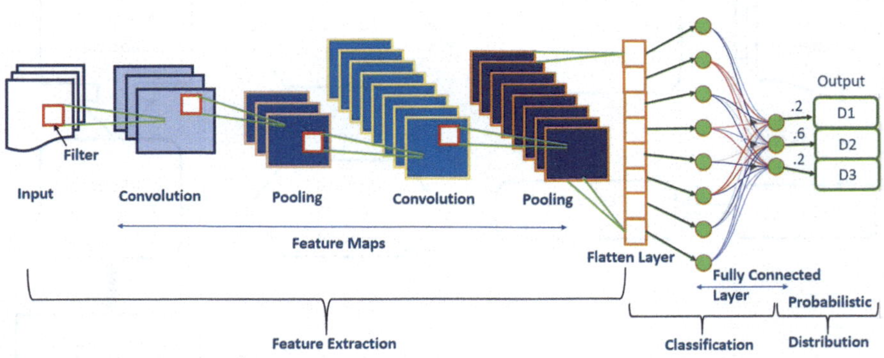

Fig. 2 A general framework of the Convolutional Neural Network (CNN)

In a deep neural network (e.g., a CNN in Fig. 2), the first few layers capture simple features like edges, textures, and basic shapes from the raw input data. As information propagates through subsequent layers, these simple features are combined to recognize more complex structures, such as object parts or specific characteristics. Each layer in the network performs a transformation on the input it receives, generating a new representation that highlights specific aspects of the data. This process is referred to as feature learning [43]. Deeper layers learn to represent high-level features that are combinations of the lower-level features learned by preceding layers. Furthermore, deep networks typically use non-linear activation functions (e.g., ReLU, sigmoid) between layers. These activation functions introduce non-linearity, enabling the network to capture intricate relationships in the data that linear models cannot easily handle [49]. As a result, deep networks allow end-to-end learning, where the entire system learns directly from raw input data to produce desired outputs. This eliminates the need for manual feature engineering and intermediate processing steps, making the modeling process more streamlined. One challenge of deep networks is the vanishing or exploding gradient problem, which can affect the stability of training [64]. Several techniques like skip connections and batch normalization have been introduced to mitigate these issues, enabling the training of very deep networks [31]. To sum up, DL focuses on learning feature representations directly from data, eliminating the need for manual feature engineering in many cases.

2.4 The Intersection of AI and Infectious Diseases

Artificial Intelligence (AI) can significantly complement traditional methods of infectious disease detection by providing enhanced speed, accuracy, and scalability [41]. AI algorithms can rapidly process large datasets, such as patient records, medical images, and genetic sequences. This speed enables quicker identification of patterns and anomalies associated with infectious diseases. As a consequence, AI algorithms are capable of identifying subtle patterns and correlations that may go unnoticed by human experts, leading to more accurate disease detection and diagnosis [48]. Besides, AI systems can handle an enormous volume of data simultaneously, making them well-suited for processing data from diverse sources and at different scales. In terms of genomic data, AI can swiftly analyze genomic data to identify specific genetic markers associated with infectious diseases, aiding in early detection and personalized treatment strategies [21]. Meanwhile, AI algorithms can uncover genetic variations and mutations that might contribute to disease transmission or resistance, guiding effective intervention measures [23]. AI accelerates drug discovery by analyzing molecular structures, identifying potential drug candidates, and predicting their interactions with pathogens [57]. By complementing traditional methods with AI-powered techniques, infectious disease detection can become more efficient, accurate, and scalable, ultimately leading to better preparedness and response in addressing health crises.

3 Related Work

In disease detection, several machine learning algorithms were used, each with strengths and effectiveness for particular types of data and disease identification tasks. In supervised learning, Support Vector Machine (SVM), Random Forests (RF), Naïve Bayes (NB), Decision Tree (DT), etc. can be used for early disease diagnosis by learning patterns from patient data and classifying new cases [8].

In order to forecast disease outbreaks, researchers utilize machine learning algorithms to assess epidemiological data, climate information, and population mobility. For instance, [67] used machine learning to forecast dengue fever outbreaks based on historical incidence and climate factors. AI-powered wearable devices and remote monitoring systems can track patient vital signs and symptoms, enabling healthcare providers to remotely monitor and manage infectious disease cases [7].

The pandemic of coronavirus disease 2019 (Covid-19) has demonstrated the ease of how quickly illnesses can spread and jeopardize the world [62, 63]. The primary focus on advancing neural network methods for COVID-19 detection resulted in the creation of numerous cutting-edge neural network models aimed at improving the accuracy of COVID-19 detection. Researchers developed deep learning models, including Convolutional Neural Networks (CNNs), Transfer Learning to analyze chest X-rays and CT scans for COVID-19 detection [37]. In essence, AI models assist radiologists in identifying COVID-19-related patterns in lung images, aiding in early diagnosis and monitoring disease progression [3, 59].

Parkinson's disease is a neurological condition that worsens over time and impairs movement control. Detecting Parkinson's disease through AI involves utilizing machine learning algorithms and data analysis techniques to analyze various data sources and identify patterns indicative of the disease. In Parkinson's disease (PD) detection, researchers used different types of data such as movement data, voice and speech data, imaging data (MRI or PET scans), and clinical data [82].

To detect red blood cells infected with malaria, machine learning algorithms were trained using microscopic blood smear images [54]. When compared to other diseases, heart disease (HD) affects the lives of the greatest number of people worldwide. With the advent of advanced machine learning techniques, researchers have been able to develop predictive models that aid in the early detection of heart disease, thereby potentially saving lives [16]. In order to predict the spread of the Zika virus, researchers developed machine learning models by analyzing factors like mosquito density, climate, and human mobility [35]. Due to the virus's highly rapid transmission and potential to infect people indiscriminately, researchers employed machine learning algorithms on the disease dataset to aid in predicting and preparing for the influenza pandemic [6, 38].

Diabetes has become a growing worry due to its elevated morbidity rates, and the age range of those impacted by this condition has now shifted to the early twenties. Numerous researchers and medical professionals have currently devised methods of detection utilizing artificial intelligence, aiming to address issues that may go unnoticed due to human mistakes [18, 70].

The recent occurrence of monkeypox (MPX) infection has evolved into a worldwide issue of significant interest over the previous year. Epidemiological studies employing artificial intelligence for managing the ongoing MPX outbreak need to account for the origin of the infection and assess all avenues of transmission [15].

Every year, dengue's notable increase constitutes 10% of fevers in youth within endemic nations. Given similar symptoms to other viruses, early diagnosis challenges persist, potentially exacerbated by inadequate sensitive tools. In upcoming diagnostic approaches, a combination of viral and clinical indicators will be essential, sequentially analyzed using artificial intelligence technology. This will enable a more comprehensive assessment of illness onset, severity determination, and treatment management [11, 77].

Pneumonia is a prevalent respiratory infection that poses a potential threat to lives, impacting millions of individuals worldwide. Recently, the incorporation of AI methods has displayed encouraging outcomes in improving the identification of pneumonia [75].

Even with the progress achieved in expanding HIV treatment initiatives, there still exists a significant unfulfilled need for monitoring disease progression and treatment efficacy, posing a challenge to HIV/AIDS management. It can be conducted evaluations of viral load and CD4 classification in adults receiving ART care, employing machine learning algorithms [47]. Table 1 represents a comprehensive study focusing on infectious diseases through the lens of artificial intelligence.

4 Methodology

The section encompasses a diverse set of components, encompassing various types of data, techniques for data pre-processing, methods for feature extraction, and the specific focus on the detection or classification of infectious diseases.

(a) *Data and Data Types*

AI algorithms can analyze vast amounts of data from various sources, such as social media, healthcare records, and environmental data. This reduces the chances of misdiagnosis and ensures that infected individuals receive appropriate treatment promptly. By continuously monitoring this data, AI can detect patterns and anomalies that may indicate the emergence of a new infectious disease or the spread of an existing one much faster than traditional methods [69].

For medical images data such as X-rays, computed tomography (CT) scans, and magnetic resonance imaging (MRI) provide visual insights into disease progression, localization of infections, and organ damage [17]. Using social media and internet data, digital surveillance can provide early signals of disease

Table 1 A comprehensive study of the infectious disease based on AI

Reference	Problem area	Data type	Data size	Techniques	Results
Ahishali et al. [3]	COVID-19 diagnosis	X-ray images	1065 samples (pneumonia with COVID-19 and 12,544 samples (normal)	DenseNet-121	Accuracy of 99.2%, sensitivity 95% and specificity 99.74%
Yamac et al. [81]	COVID-19 recognition	X-ray images	2760 samples (bacterial pneumonia), 1485 samples (viral pneumonia), 462 samples (COVID-19) and 1579 normal samples	Convolution support estimation network (CSEN2)	Accuracy of 95.9%, sensitivity 98.5% and specificity 95.7%
Qiblawey et al. [59]	COVID-19 detection and severity	CT images	1139 patients with 51,027 CT samples	DenseNet201 FPN	Accuracy of 95.96%, precession of 96.47% sensitivity of 99.64%, specificity of 98.72%, and F1-score of 98.03%
Rahman et al. [61]	COVID-19 detection	Chest X-ray images	18,479 samples including 3616 COVID-19 samples	Pre-trained model (ResNet18, ResNet50, ResNet101, InceptionV3, DenseNet201, and ChexNet)	The highest accuracy is 96.29%, F1-score is 96.28% and sensitivity is 97.28%
Degerli et al. [19]	COVID-19 detection and severity grading	Chest X-ray images	119,316 where 2951 samples of COVID-19	U-Net DenseNet-121	Accuracy is 99.73%, precision 96.40%, F1-score 95.67%, sensitivity 94.96%, and specificity 99.88%.
Degerli et al. [20]	COVID-19 detection	Chest X-ray images	121,378 samples including 9258 COVID-19 samples	OSegNet (DenseNet-121 and inception-v3)	The maximum accuracy of 99:65% with 98:09% precision
Brioschi et al. [14]	COVID-19 detection	Thermal images	2558 cases from 227,261 workers in five countries	CNN	Accuracy of 98.98% and a PPV of 18.18%
Azeem et al. [10]	COVID-19 detection	Chest radiography images	10,192 benign 3616 malignant	ConXNet	Accuracy of 97.8%, precision is 97.93% and F1-measure is 97.92%

Lee et al. [44]	Malaria prediction	Blood smear images	Over 10,000 cases from 1956 to 2019	SVM, RF, MLP, AdaBoost, GB, and CatBoost	Accuracy of SVM: 93.8%, RF: 93%, MLP:91.4%, AdaBoost: 93.2%, GB: 93%, and CatBoost: 94.9%
Kumar et al. [42]	Malaria detection	Blood smear images	27,558 cases from 200 patients	CNN	Accuracy of 95.4%
Gan et al. [25]	Forecast Hepatitis B	Text data	10,486,959 cases	Hybrid model (BP-ANN and GM)	MAE: 3.9704 × 104, RMSE: 4.863 × 103, R: 0.9495
Harabor et al. [28]	Prediction of Hepatitis B and C	Clinical data	1359 patients	SVM, RF, NB, and KNN	The KNN achieves highest accuracy of 98.1%, SVM and RF with equal accuracies (97.6%) and NB (95.7%)
Doyle et al. [22]	Undiagnosed patient detection of Hepatitis C	Clinical data	9,721,923 patients	LR, GB trees, RF, and stacked ensemble	The highest AUCROC of 96%, specificity of 99.9%, and precision of 97%
Saleh and Rabie [66]	Monkeypox diagnose	Image data	MPX 296 samples and others 204 samples	NB, kNN, and DL	Accuracy: 98.48%, precision: 91.1%, and recall:88.91%
Islam and Shin [33]	Monkeypox detection	Image data	MPX 1428 samples and others 1764 samples	ResNet18 and FL	Accuracy of 99.81%
Turbé et al. [78]	Rapid HIV diagnostic	Image data	11,374 images	MobileNetV2, MobileNetV3, ResNet50, SVM	Sensitivity: 97.8%, specificity: 100%
Seboka et al. [68]	HIV/AIDS treatment activities	Demographics and clinical data	2907 adults	kNN, DT, NB, GNB, SVM, LR, GB, XGB, RF	Accuracy of 96%, sensitivity 97%, AUC: 0.99, F1-measure: 96%

outbreaks, public sentiment, and information dissemination [1]. Similarly, the genomic data of pathogens, obtained through techniques like DNA sequencing, help identify the specific microorganism responsible for an infectious disease [26]. Consequently, wearable devices and sensors can collect real-time data on physiological parameters like body temperature, heart rate, and respiratory rate [72]. Thus, AI algorithms can detect anomalies that might indicate the presence of an infectious disease.

In infectious disease detection, a diverse range of data types such as clinical data, imaging data, genomic data, social media and web data, sensor data, drug and treatment data, healthcare system data, etc. are harnessed to gain insights into the presence, spread, and characteristics of diseases. Each type of data offers unique information that enhances our ability to detect and manage infectious diseases effectively when combined and analyzed using advanced AI techniques.

(b) *Data preprocessing*

Data preprocessing involves preparing and cleaning raw data to ensure that it is suitable for analysis by AI algorithms. Also, data preprocessing aims to enhance the quality, reliability, and effectiveness of AI models. There are some key aspects of data preprocessing such as data cleaning (removing or correcting errors, inconsistencies, and missing values), data integration (combining data from different sources as well as ensuring data compatibility and standardization), normalization (bringing different features to a similar scale), data augmentation (increase the diversity of the dataset), handling imbalanced data, dimensionality reduction and so on [32, 56]. The traditional data preparation techniques are illustrated in Fig. 3.

(c) *Feature Extraction and Detection*

The feature extraction techniques involve transforming raw data into a set of relevant and informative features that capture the essential characteristics of the data. Feature extraction helps highlight patterns, anomalies, and relationships that can aid AI models in making accurate predictions. Usually, there are different types of features such as statistical features, text and Natural Language Processing (NLP) features, image and signal processing features, molecular and genetic features, composite features, and so forth [12]. Several methods of feature extraction are utilized in the identification of infectious diseases. In textual data, NLP techniques can be used to extract features like word frequencies, TF-IDF scores, n-grams, and topic modeling [24]. For image data, features might include textures, edges, shapes, color histograms, and moments that describe different aspects of the image [30]. In addition, pre-trained deep learning models, such as convolutional neural networks (CNNs) or transformer-based models, can be used to extract high-level features from data like images, text, or audio [40]. In addition, Cross-validation techniques may also be used to evaluate and tune the model's hyperparameters.

In traditional machine learning, feature extraction involves manually selecting and transforming specific aspects of the data to create meaningful inputs

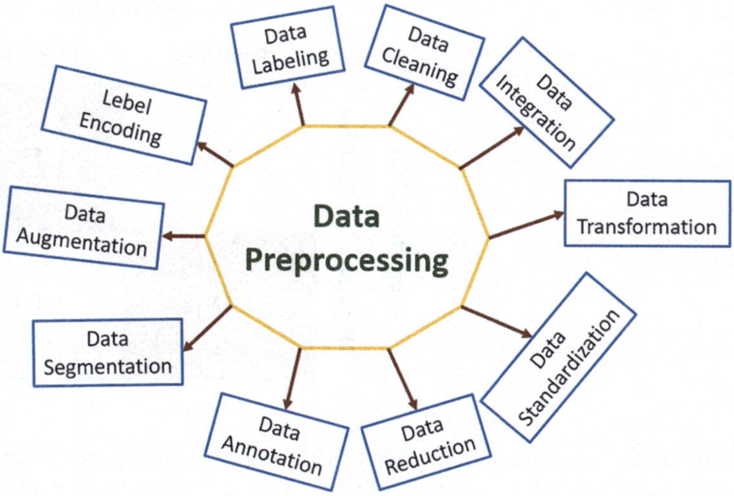

Fig. 3 Conventional data preprocessing techniques in AI

for the model. However, in deep learning, neural networks are designed to automatically learn hierarchical representations of data through layers of interconnected nodes (neurons). Each layer in a neural network learns to recognize increasingly complex patterns or features from the data. This ability to learn features internally is one of the key advantages of deep learning. For example, in an image classification task, traditional machine learning might require manually extracting features like edges, textures, or shapes from the images before feeding them into the model. In contrast, a deep learning model like Fig. 2, a convolutional neural network (CNN) can automatically learn to detect edges, textures, and other relevant features directly from the raw pixel values of the images. Similarly, in natural language processing tasks, deep learning models like recurrent neural networks (RNNs) or transformers can learn to understand the underlying semantic structure of text without requiring explicit manual feature engineering. This internal feature extraction capability of deep learning methods not only simplifies the model-building process but also often leads to improved performance, as the models can adapt and learn relevant features from the data on their own [43].

5 Performance Metrics

The Confusion Matrix is the common performance evaluation tool used in the field of machine learning and statistics to assess the performance of a classification model. The Confusion Matrix is a square matrix that summarizes the predictions

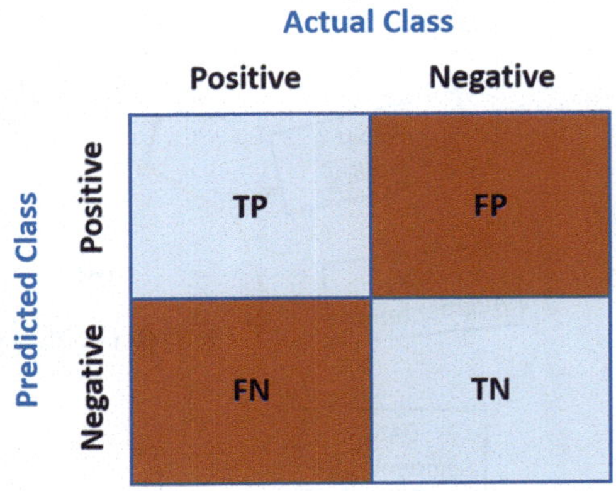

Fig. 4 Binary Confusion Matrix

made by a classification model on a set of data points with known ground truth labels. It provides a breakdown of correct and incorrect predictions made by the model for each class in the dataset. The matrix is of size N × N, where N is the number of classes in the dataset. For a binary classification problem, N will be 2, and for a multi-class problem, N will be greater than 2.

When N = 2, the general structure of a Confusion Matrix is shown in Fig. 4.

- True Positive (TP): The number of positive data points that were successfully categorized as positive (correctly forecasted as positive) outcomes.
- False Positive (FP): The number of negative data points that were incorrectly categorized as positive (or incorrectly forecasted as positive)
- True Negative (TN): The number of negative data points that were successfully categorized as negative (correctly forecasted as negative) outcomes.
- False Negative (FN): The number of positive data points that were incorrectly categorized as negative (incorrectly forecasted as negative) outcomes.

The aforementioned information is used to formulate many performance indicators that describe numerous aspects of how well the model performs [45]. From the Confusion Matrix, the following typical metrics can be derived:

Accuracy is an important performance parameter for assessing an AI model's effectiveness. It estimates the percentage of correctly forecast instances (or data points) among all of the instances (instances belonging to the class) in the dataset.

$$Accuracy = \frac{TP + TN}{TP + TN + FP + FN}$$

Accuracy can be misleading, especially when dealing with unbalanced datasets. An unbalanced dataset is one where the distribution of classes is heavily skewed, meaning that one class has significantly more examples than the other(s). In such cases, accuracy alone may not provide a clear and accurate picture of a model's performance. For example, if we have a dataset with 95% of instances belonging to Class A and only 5% to Class B, a model that predicts Class A for all instances would still achieve an accuracy of 95%, even though it is not actually making any meaningful predictions.

Recall, also known as Sensitivity or True Positive Rate, is a performance metric that focuses on the ability of a classification model to correctly identify all relevant instances of a particular class. When considered in terms of the confusion matrix, recall is calculated by considering the true positives (TP) and false negatives (FN) for a specific class.

$$Recall = \frac{TP}{TP + FN}$$

Recall is particularly important when the consequences of missing positive instances (false negatives) are more severe than misclassifying negative instances (false positives). In other words, recall is useful when we want to minimize the risk of failing to identify instances of a certain class [80]. A high recall indicates that the model is effectively capturing most of the positive instances in the dataset, while a low recall suggests that the model is missing a significant number of positive instances. However, achieving high recall might come at the cost of increased false positives, which in turn reduces the precision.

Specificity or the True Negative Rate is a performance metric used in the evaluation of a classification model's ability to correctly identify the negative instances. It complements the concept of recall, which focuses on the model's ability to correctly identify positive instances. In other words, specificity is the recall rate of the negative class. Regarding the confusion matrix, specificity is calculated by considering the true negatives (TN) and false positives (FP) for the negative class. A high specificity indicates that the model is effective at correctly classifying negative instances, while a low specificity suggests that the model includes a considerable number of false positives in its negative predictions.

$$Specificity = \frac{TN}{TN + FP}$$

Precision Focuses on the accuracy of positive predictions made by a classification model. It provides a measure of how well the model is at avoiding false positive errors (false alarms). In terms of the confusion matrix, precision is calculated by considering the true positives (TP) and false positives (FP) for a specific class. A high precision indicates that the model is making accurate positive predictions, while a low precision suggests that the model is including a substantial number of false positives in its positive predictions [36].

$$Precision = \frac{TP}{TP + FP}$$

The F1 Score is a performance metric used in machine learning applications to provide a combined metric of the precision and recall. It is particularly useful when we want to assess a model's performance in situations where both false positives and false negatives have significant consequences [73]. Thus, the F1 score is calculated as the harmonic mean of precision and recall. From the standpoint of the confusion matrix, the F1 score is derived from the true positives (TP), false positives (FP), and false negatives (FN). The F1 score ranges between 0 and 1, where a higher value indicates better performance.

$$F1\ Score = \frac{2 \times Precision \times Recall}{Precision + Recall}$$

A Receiver Operating Characteristic Curve or An ROC curve plots the true positive rate (sensitivity or recall) on the y-axis and the false positive rate on the x-axis as vary the prediction threshold. The true positive rate is the proportion of actual positive instances that the model correctly identifies, while the false positive rate is the proportion of actual negative instances that the model incorrectly classifies as positive [27].

Let us imagine a medical diagnostic test that is designed to detect a certain disease. The test provides a numerical score for each patient, and based on that score, a decision is made whether the patient is positive or negative for the disease. Assume that, we have data for 100 patients who were tested using this diagnostic test. We also have the true outcomes for each patient: whether they actually had the disease or not (true positive or true negative). Based on the test scores and true outcomes, we can calculate the True Positive Rate (TPR) and False Positive Rate (FPR) for different threshold values.

Plotting the five values on a graph in Fig. 5 where TPR on the y-axis and FPR on the x-axis, will give the ROC curve. The curve typically starts at the bottom left corner (0, 0) and moves towards the top right corner (1, 1). A diagonal line from the bottom left to the top right would represent a random classifier.

Intersection over Union (IoU) Is a performance metric commonly used in the field of computer vision, especially in tasks such as object detection, instance segmentation, and image segmentation. It assesses the accuracy of an algorithm's predictions by evaluating the overlap between the predicted and ground truth regions. Particularly, we can evaluate how well the predicted bounding boxes or segmented sections of a model match the real objects in the image [60]. IoU values range from 0 to 1, with higher values indicating better alignment between predictions and ground truth. The IoU is determined by the following formula:

$$IoU = \frac{Intersection\ Area}{Union\ Area}$$

Mean Average Precision (mAP) Is particularly suited for evaluating the performance of object detection and instance segmentation algorithms when dealing

Fig. 5 A sample ROC curve

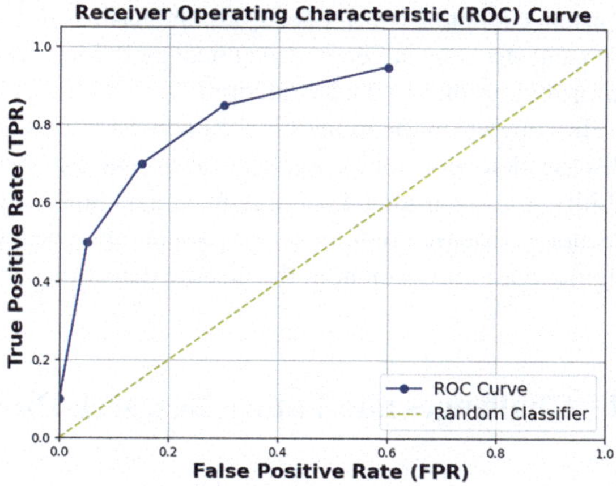

with multiple classes and varying levels of detection confidence. It provides a comprehensive view of how well a model can detect and localize objects of different classes in an image [29]. It takes into account both precision and recall and provides a single value that summarizes the model's performance. In mathematically, the AP values for all classes are averaged to compute the mean average precision. In this term, The AP_k refers to the AP of class k and N is the number of classes.

$$mAP = \frac{1}{n}\sum_{k=1}^{k=n} AP_k$$

6 Results and Discussion

AI offers advanced tools and techniques that can significantly enhance our ability to combat infectious diseases effectively. In the field, ML algorithms are instrumental in predicting disease outbreaks by analyzing epidemiological data and identifying factors contributing to disease spread [4]. Boosting algorithms like XGBoost or LightGBM can process large datasets containing various features (e.g., population density, travel patterns) to predict the likelihood of an outbreak in different regions [39]. By examining time-series data on disease incidence, recurrent neural networks (RNNs) are able to forecast future trends in outbreaks based on historical patterns [79].

In the case of multimodal data integration, the success of the AI models can be attributed to the integration of multimodal data sources. By combining clinical, molecular, and environmental data, AI algorithms could capture complex interactions and subtle signals indicative of infectious diseases [9]. This underscores the importance of data fusion in enhancing detection accuracy. While AI offers promising results, ethical concerns related to patient data privacy and informed consent cannot be overlooked. [65] emphasizes the need for robust data anonymization and stringent adherence to ethical guidelines when utilizing sensitive healthcare information for AI-based detection.

In conclusion, deep learning models have demonstrated significant potential in disease detection and classification across various medical domains [76]. Their ability to learn intricate patterns from data holds promise for improving diagnostic accuracy, disease prediction, and patient outcomes. In Table 1, the results indicate a significant improvement in the disease detection accuracy in AI methods.

7 Challenges and Future Research Directions

Collecting and cleaning diverse data sources for AI model training in the context of infectious disease detection presents several significant challenges. The quality, quantity, and diversity of data play a crucial role in the effectiveness of AI models [51]. Infectious disease datasets may have imbalanced class distributions, where certain diseases or outcomes are rare. Diverse data sources often have varying formats, structures, and levels of granularity. Integrating data from sources such as electronic health records, medical images, and genomic sequences requires careful preprocessing to ensure compatibility. Also, infectious disease data can be vast and rapidly accumulating during outbreaks. Ensuring that AI models can handle large datasets efficiently while maintaining high performance is a technical challenge. Furthermore, incomplete, inaccurate, or inconsistent data can lead to biased or unreliable AI models. Data quality issues may arise from errors in data entry, mislabeling, or variations in recording practices [74].

Data collected from electronic health records, patient records, and other sources may contain sensitive personal information. Concerns about patient data privacy and security arise when using AI systems. Ensuring compliance with privacy regulations and obtaining informed consent adds complexity to data collection. Besides, accessing data from different healthcare systems, institutions, or countries can be challenging due to data ownership, sharing agreements, and interoperability issues [53]. Biases present in the data can be inadvertently learned by AI models, leading to unfair or inaccurate predictions. Biases can stem from demographic, geographic, or socioeconomic factors, reflecting disparities in healthcare access and outcomes [5]. Models trained on data from one population or region might not generalize well to other populations or regions due to variations in disease prevalence, genetic factors, or environmental conditions [55].

Data augmentation is the process of transforming the original data in order to generate newly formed training samples. This technique increases the diversity and quantity of the training dataset, helping the model learn robust and invariant features [58]. In the context of infectious disease detection, data augmentation can be particularly useful when dealing with limited or imbalanced data [71]. For medical image analysis, techniques like rotation, flipping, scaling, cropping, and adding noise can create variations of images without altering their clinical meaning.

In cases of clinical notes or medical text, techniques like synonym replacement, random insertion/deletion of words, and paraphrasing can increase text diversity.

Data Normalization is crucial for preventing certain features from dominating the learning process due to their scale, which can negatively impact model convergence and performance [13]. In infectious disease detection, where features can vary widely, normalization helps stabilize training and improves model convergence [34]. Apart from this, AI systems need to process and analyze data in real-time for fast disease detection and response, a requirement for effective computing infrastructure and algorithms.

8 Conclusion

AI can identify subtle disease markers that might be challenging to detect through traditional methods, enhancing diagnostic precision. These successful applications highlight AI's ability to analyze complex data, identify patterns, and provide insights that contribute to more accurate diagnoses, personalized treatments, and improved patient outcomes. Given these achievements, it's evident that AI holds immense potential for transforming infectious disease detection and management, leveraging similar data-driven approaches to enhance early detection, prediction, and intervention. As a result, AI streamlines healthcare processes, automates routine tasks, and optimizes resource utilization, leading to cost savings and improved healthcare delivery. Ongoing research, collaboration, and responsible deployment are crucial for harnessing AI's full capabilities in this critical domain.

References

1. M. Abisado, A. Trillanes, A. Lacasandile, A. De La Cruz, Using low-resourced language in social media platforms towards disease surveillance for public health monitoring using artificial intelligence. ACM Int. Conf. Proc. Ser., 77–85 (2022). https://doi.org/10.1145/3571513.3571527
2. C. Affonso, A.L.D. Rossi, F.H.A. Vieira, A.C.P.D.L.F. de Carvalho, Deep learning for biological image classification. Expert Syst. Appl. **85**, 114–122 (2017). https://doi.org/10.1016/J.ESWA.2017.05.039
3. M. Ahishali, A. Degerli, M. Yamac, et al., Advance warning methodologies for COVID-19 using chest X-ray images. IEEE Access **9**, 41052–41065 (2021). https://doi.org/10.1109/ACCESS.2021.3064927
4. M.M. Ahsan, S.A. Luna, Z. Siddique, Machine-learning-based disease diagnosis: A comprehensive review. Healthcare **10**, 541 (2022). https://doi.org/10.3390/HEALTHCARE10030541
5. S. Alelyani, Detection and evaluation of machine learning bias. Appl. Sci. (Switzerland), 11 (2021). https://doi.org/10.3390/app11146271
6. B. Alkouz, Z. Al Aghbari, M.A. Al-Garadi, A. Sarker, Deepluenza: Deep learning for influenza detection from Twitter. Expert Syst. Appl. **198**, 116845 (2022). https://doi.org/10.1016/J.ESWA.2022.116845

7. M. Alshamrani, IoT and artificial intelligence implementations for remote healthcare monitoring systems: A survey. J. King Saud Univ. Comput. Inf. Sci. **34**, 4687–4701 (2022). https://doi.org/10.1016/J.JKSUCI.2021.06.005
8. K. Arumugam, M. Naved, P.P. Shinde, et al., Multiple disease prediction using machine learning algorithms. Mater. Today Proc. **80**, 3682–3685 (2023). https://doi.org/10.1016/J.MATPR.2021.07.361
9. M.A. Azam, K.B. Khan, S. Salahuddin, et al., A review on multimodal medical image fusion: Compendious analysis of medical modalities, multimodal databases, fusion techniques and quality metrics. Comput. Biol. Med. **144**, 105253 (2022). https://doi.org/10.1016/J.COMPBIOMED.2022.105253
10. M. Azeem, S. Javaid, R.A. Khalil, et al., Neural networks for the detection of COVID-19 and other diseases: Prospects and challenges. Bioengineering **10**, 850 (2023). https://doi.org/10.3390/bioengineering10070850
11. M. Baharom, N. Ahmad, R. Hod, M.R.A. Manaf, Dengue early warning system as outbreak prediction tool: A systematic review. Risk Manag. Healthc. Policy **15**, 871–886 (2022). https://doi.org/10.2147/RMHP.S361106
12. A.L. Blum, P. Langley, Selection of relevant features and examples in machine learning. Artif. Intell. **97**, 245–271 (1997). https://doi.org/10.1016/S0004-3702(97)00063-5
13. D. Borkin, A. Némethová, G. Michaľčonok, K. Maiorov, Impact of data normalization on classification model accuracy. Res. Pap. Fac. Mater. Sci. Technol. Slovak Univ. Technol. **27**, 79–84 (2019). https://doi.org/10.2478/RPUT-2019-0029
14. M.L. Brioschi, C. Dalmaso Neto, M. de Toledo, et al., Infrared image method for possible COVID-19 detection through febrile and subfebrile people screening. J. Therm. Biol. **112**, 103444 (2023). https://doi.org/10.1016/J.JTHERBIO.2022.103444
15. K. Chadaga, S. Prabhu, N. Sampathila, et al., Application of artificial intelligence techniques for Monkeypox: A systematic review. Diagnostics **13** (2023)
16. V. Chang, V.R. Bhavani, A.Q. Xu, M.A. Hossain, An artificial intelligence model for heart disease detection using machine learning algorithms. Healthc. Anal. **2**, 100016 (2022). https://doi.org/10.1016/J.HEALTH.2022.100016
17. G. Currie, K.E. Hawk, E. Rohren, et al., Machine learning and deep learning in medical imaging: Intelligent imaging. J. Med. Imaging. Radiat. Sci. **50**, 477–487 (2019). https://doi.org/10.1016/J.JMIR.2019.09.005
18. D. Das, S.K. Biswas, S. Bandyopadhyay, A critical review on diagnosis of diabetic retinopathy using machine learning and deep learning. Multimed. Tools Appl. **81**(18), 25613–25655 (2022). https://doi.org/10.1007/S11042-022-12642-4
19. A. Degerli, M. Ahishali, M. Yamac, et al., COVID-19 infection map generation and detection from chest X-ray images. Health Inf. Sci. Syst. **9**, 1–16 (2021). https://doi.org/10.1007/S13755-021-00146-8/TABLES/8
20. A. Degerli, S. Kiranyaz, M.E.H. Chowdhury, M. Gabbouj, OSEGNET: Operational segmentation network for COVID-19 detection using CHEST x-ray images. Proc. Int. Conf. Image Proc. ICIP, 2306–2310 (2022). https://doi.org/10.1109/ICIP46576.2022.9897412
21. R. Dias, A. Torkamani, Artificial intelligence in clinical and genomic diagnostics. Genome Med. **11**, 1–12 (2019). https://doi.org/10.1186/S13073-019-0689-8/FIGURES/1
22. O.M. Doyle, N. Leavitt, J.A. Rigg, Finding undiagnosed patients with hepatitis C infection: An application of artificial intelligence to patient claims data. Sci. Rep. **10** (2020). https://doi.org/10.1038/s41598-020-67013-6
23. W.L. Flowers, Genetic and phenotypic variation in reproductive traits of AI boars. Theriogenology **70**, 1297–1303 (2008). https://doi.org/10.1016/J.THERIOGENOLOGY.2008.06.016
24. S. Fu, D. Chen, H. He, et al., Clinical concept extraction: A methodology review. J. Biomed. Inform. **109**, 103526 (2020). https://doi.org/10.1016/J.JBI.2020.103526
25. R. Gan, X. Chen, Y. Yan, D. Huang, Application of a hybrid method combining grey model and back propagation artificial neural networks to forecast hepatitis b in China. Comput. Math. Methods Med. **2015** (2015). https://doi.org/10.1155/2015/328273

26. S. Goswami, S. Sharma, DNA sequencing using artificial intelligence, in *International Conference on Edge Computing and Applications, ICECAA 2022 – Proceedings*, (2022), pp. 1033–1037. https://doi.org/10.1109/ICECAA55415.2022.9936101
27. D.J. Hand, Measuring classifier performance: A coherent alternative to the area under the ROC curve. Mach. Learn. **77**, 103–123 (2009). https://doi.org/10.1007/S10994-009-5119-5/METRICS
28. V. Harabor, R. Mogos, A. Nechita, et al., Machine learning approaches for the prediction of hepatitis B and C seropositivity. Int. J. Environ. Res. Public Health **20**, 2380 (2023). https://doi.org/10.3390/IJERPH20032380
29. P. Henderson, V. Ferrari, End-to-end training of object class detectors for mean average precision, in *Lecture Notes in Computer Science (Including Subseries Lecture Notes in Artificial Intelligence and Lecture Notes in Bioinformatics) 10115 LNCS*, (2017), pp. 198–213. https://doi.org/10.1007/978-3-319-54193-8_13/COVER
30. A. Hosny, C. Parmar, J. Quackenbush, et al., Artificial intelligence in radiology. Nat. Rev. Cancer **18**(8), 500–510 (2018). https://doi.org/10.1038/s41568-018-0016-5
31. Z. Hu, J. Zhang, Y. Ge, Handling vanishing gradient problem using artificial derivative. IEEE Access **9**, 22371–22377 (2021). https://doi.org/10.1109/ACCESS.2021.3054915
32. T. Iliou, C.N. Anagnostopoulos, M. Nerantzaki, G. Anastassopoulos, A novel machine learning data preprocessing method for enhancing classification algorithms performance, in *ACM International Conference Proceeding Series 2015*, (2015). https://doi.org/10.1145/2797143.2797155
33. A. Islam, S.Y. Shin, A blockchain-based privacy sensitive data acquisition scheme during pandemic through the facilitation of federated learning, in *International Conference on ICT Convergence*, (2022), pp. 83–87. https://doi.org/10.1109/ICTC55196.2022.9952440
34. I. Izonin, B. Ilchyshyn, R. Tkachenko, et al., Towards data normalization task for the efficient mining of medical data, in *2022 12th International Conference on Advanced Computer Information Technologies*, (ACIT, 2022), pp. 480–484. https://doi.org/10.1109/ACIT54803.2022.9913112
35. D. Jiang, M. Hao, F. Ding, et al., Mapping the transmission risk of Zika virus using machine learning models. Acta Trop. **185**, 391–399 (2018). https://doi.org/10.1016/j.actatropica.2018.06.021
36. M. Junker, R. Hoch, A. Dengel, On the evaluation of document analysis components by recall, precision, and accuracy, in *Proceedings of the International Conference on Document Analysis and Recognition*, (ICDAR, 1999), pp. 717–720. https://doi.org/10.1109/ICDAR.1999.791887
37. S.S. Kabir, M.F. Bulbul, F.F. Ahmed, et al., A deep learning approach for Covid-19 detection in chest x-rays, in *Computer Vision and Image Analysis for Industry 4.0*, (CRC Press, 2023), pp. 120–137
38. M.A. Khan, W.U.H. Abidi, M.A. Al Ghamdi, et al., Forecast the influenza pandemic using machine learning. Comput. Mater. Continua **66**, 331–340 (2021). https://doi.org/10.32604/cmc.2020.012148
39. H. Koçak, G. Çetin, The diagnosis of diabetes mellitus with boosting methods. El-Cezeri **10**, 409–419 (2023). https://doi.org/10.31202/ECJSE.1242207
40. P. Kora, C.P. Ooi, O. Faust, et al., Transfer learning techniques for medical image analysis: A review. Biocybern. Biomed. Eng. **42**, 79–107 (2022). https://doi.org/10.1016/J.BBE.2021.11.004
41. Y. Kumar, A. Koul, R. Singla, M.F. Ijaz, Artificial intelligence in disease diagnosis: A systematic literature review, synthesizing framework and future research agenda. J. Ambient Intell. Hum. Comput. **14**(7), 8459–8486 (2022). https://doi.org/10.1007/S12652-021-03612-Z
42. S. Kumar, S. Priya, A. Kumar, *Malaria detection using Deep Convolution Neural Network* (2023)
43. A. Latif, A. Rasheed, U. Sajid, et al., Content-based image retrieval and feature extraction: A comprehensive review. Math. Probl. Eng. **2019** (2019). https://doi.org/10.1155/2019/9658350
44. Y.W. Lee, J.W. Choi, E.H. Shin, Machine learning model for predicting malaria using clinical information. Comput. Biol. Med. **129**, 104151 (2021). https://doi.org/10.1016/J.COMPBIOMED.2020.104151

45. J. Liang, *Confusion Matrix: Machine Learning* (POGIL Activity Clearinghouse, 2022), p. 3
46. R. Manne, S.C. Kantheti, *Application of Artificial Intelligence in Healthcare: Chances and Challenges* (2021)
47. J.L. Marcus, W.C. Sewell, L.B. Balzer, D.S. Krakower, Artificial intelligence and machine learning for HIV prevention: Emerging approaches to ending the epidemic. Curr. HIV/AIDS Rep. **17**, 171–179 (2020). https://doi.org/10.1007/S11904-020-00490-6/METRICS
48. M. Meraj, S.P. Singh, P. Johri, M.T. Quasim, An investigation on infectious disease patterns using Internet of Things (IoT), in *Proceedings of the International Conference on Smart Technologies in Computing, Electrical and Electronics, ICSTCEE*, vol. 2020, (2020), pp. 599–604. https://doi.org/10.1109/ICSTCEE49637.2020.9276922
49. M.A. Mercioni, S. Holban, A brief review of the Most recent activation functions for neural networks, in *2023 17th International Conference on Engineering of Modern Electric Systems, EMES 2023*, (2023). https://doi.org/10.1109/EMES58375.2023.10171705
50. T. Mikolov, S. Kombrink, L. Burget, et al., Extensions of recurrent neural network language model, in *ICASSP, IEEE International Conference on Acoustics, Speech and Signal Processing – Proceedings*, (2011), pp. 5528–5531. https://doi.org/10.1109/ICASSP.2011.5947611
51. Y. Mohamadou, A. Halidou, P.T. Kapen, A review of mathematical modeling, artificial intelligence and datasets used in the study, prediction and management of COVID-19. Appl. Intell. **50**, 3913–3925 (2020). https://doi.org/10.1007/s10489-020-01770-9
52. G. Montavon, W. Samek, K.R. Müller, Methods for interpreting and understanding deep neural networks. Digit. Signal Process. **73**, 1–15 (2018). https://doi.org/10.1016/J.DSP.2017.10.011
53. A. Munappy, J. Bosch, H.H. Olsson, et al., Data management challenges for deep learning, in *Proceedings – 45th Euromicro Conference on Software Engineering and Advanced Applications, SEAA 2019*, (2019), pp. 140–147. https://doi.org/10.1109/SEAA.2019.00030
54. C. Nabet, A. Acherar, A. Huguenin, et al., Artificial intelligence and malaria. Artif. Intell. Med., 1353–1368 (2022). https://doi.org/10.1007/978-3-030-64573-1_273/COVER
55. A. Naeem, M.S. Farooq, A. Khelifi, A. Abid, Malignant melanoma classification using deep learning: Datasets, performance measurements, challenges and opportunities. IEEE Access **8**, 110575–110597 (2020). https://doi.org/10.1109/ACCESS.2020.3001507
56. C.C. Olisah, L. Smith, M. Smith, Diabetes mellitus prediction and diagnosis from a data preprocessing and machine learning perspective. Comput. Methods Prog. Biomed. **220**, 106773 (2022). https://doi.org/10.1016/J.CMPB.2022.106773
57. D. Paul, G. Sanap, S. Shenoy, et al., Artificial intelligence in drug discovery and development. Drug Discov. Today **26**, 80 (2021). https://doi.org/10.1016/J.DRUDIS.2020.10.010
58. L. Perez, J. Wang, *The Effectiveness of Data Augmentation in Image Classification using Deep Learning* (2017)
59. Y. Qiblawey, A. Tahir, M.E.H. Chowdhury, et al., Detection and severity classification of COVID-19 in CT images using deep learning. Diagnostics **11**, 893 (2021). https://doi.org/10.3390/DIAGNOSTICS11050893
60. M.A. Rahman, Y. Wang, Optimizing intersection-over-union in deep neural networks for image segmentation, in *Lecture Notes in Computer Science (Including Subseries Lecture Notes in Artificial Intelligence and Lecture Notes in Bioinformatics) 10072 LNCS*, (2016), pp. 234–244. https://doi.org/10.1007/978-3-319-50835-1_22/COVER
61. T. Rahman, A. Khandakar, Y. Qiblawey, et al., Exploring the effect of image enhancement techniques on COVID-19 detection using chest X-ray images. Comput. Biol. Med. **132**, 104319 (2021). https://doi.org/10.1016/J.COMPBIOMED.2021.104319
62. M.S. Rahman, M.N. Hoque, S.R. Chowdhury, et al., Temporal dynamics and fatality of SARS-CoV-2 variants in Bangladesh. Health Sci. Rep. **6** (2023). https://doi.org/10.1002/hsr2.1209
63. A.M. Rahmani, E. Azhir, M. Naserbakht, et al., Automatic COVID-19 detection mechanisms and approaches from medical images: A systematic review. Multimed. Tools Appl. **81**, 28779–28798 (2022). https://doi.org/10.1007/S11042-022-12952-7/FIGURES/9
64. M. Roodschild, J. Gotay Sardiñas, A. Will, A new approach for the vanishing gradient problem on sigmoid activation. Prog. Artif. Intell. **9**, 351–360 (2020). https://doi.org/10.1007/S13748-020-00218-Y/METRICS

65. L. Rubinger, A. Gazendam, S. Ekhtiari, M. Bhandari, Machine learning and artificial intelligence in research and healthcare. Injury **54**, S69–S73 (2023). https://doi.org/10.1016/J.INJURY.2022.01.046
66. A.I. Saleh, A.H. Rabie, Human monkeypox diagnose (HMD) strategy based on data mining and artificial intelligence techniques. Comput. Biol. Med. **152**, 106383 (2023). https://doi.org/10.1016/J.COMPBIOMED.2022.106383
67. N.A.M. Salim, Y.B. Wah, C. Reeves, et al., Prediction of dengue outbreak in Selangor Malaysia using machine learning techniques. Sci. Rep. **11**, 1–9 (2021). https://doi.org/10.1038/s41598-020-79193-2
68. B.T. Seboka, D.E. Yehualashet, G.A. Tesfa, Artificial intelligence and machine learning based prediction of viral load and CD4 status of people living with HIV (PLWH) on anti-retroviral treatment in Gedeo Zone Public Hospitals. Int. J. Gen. Med. **16**, 435–451 (2023). https://doi.org/10.2147/IJGM.S397031
69. T. Shaik, X. Tao, N. Higgins, et al., Remote patient monitoring using artificial intelligence: Current state, applications, and challenges. Wiley Interdiscip. Rev. Data Min. Knowl. Discov. **13**, e1485 (2023). https://doi.org/10.1002/WIDM.1485
70. T. Sharma, M. Shah, A comprehensive review of machine learning techniques on diabetes detection. Vis. Comput. Ind. Biomed. Art, 4 (2021)
71. C. Shorten, T.M. Khoshgoftaar, A survey on image data augmentation for deep learning. J. Big Data **6** (2019). https://doi.org/10.1186/s40537-019-0197-0
72. A.T. Shumba, T. Montanaro, I. Sergi, et al., Leveraging IoT-aware technologies and AI techniques for real-time critical healthcare applications. Sensors **22**, 7675 (2022). https://doi.org/10.3390/S22197675
73. M. Sokolova, N. Japkowicz, S. Szpakowicz, Beyond accuracy, F-score and ROC: A family of discriminant measures for performance evaluation, in *AAAI Workshop – Technical Report WS-06-06*, (2006), pp. 24–29. https://doi.org/10.1007/11941439_114/COVER
74. W.W. Stead, Clinical implications and challenges of artificial intelligence and deep learning. JAMA **320**, 1107–1108 (2018). https://doi.org/10.1001/JAMA.2018.11029
75. K. Stokes, R. Castaldo, C. Federici, et al., The use of artificial intelligence systems in diagnosis of pneumonia via signs and symptoms: A systematic review. Biomed. Signal Process Control **72**, 103325 (2022). https://doi.org/10.1016/J.BSPC.2021.103325
76. S. Suganyadevi, V. Seethalakshmi, K. Balasamy, A review on deep learning in medical image analysis. Int. J. Multimed. Inf. Retr. **11**, 19–38 (2021). https://doi.org/10.1007/S13735-021-00218-1
77. G. Thergarajan, S.D. Sekaran, Diagnostic approaches for dengue infection. (2023). https://doi.org/10.1080/14737159.2023.2234815
78. V. Turbé, C. Herbst, T. Mngomezulu, et al., Deep learning of HIV field-based rapid tests. Nat. Med. **27**(7), 1165–1170 (2021). https://doi.org/10.1038/s41591-021-01384-9
79. M. Villegas, A. Gonzalez-Agirre, A. Gutiérrez-Fandiño, et al., Predicting the evolution of COVID-19 mortality risk: A recurrent neural network approach. Comput. Methods Progr. Biomed. Update **3**, 100089 (2023). https://doi.org/10.1016/J.CMPBUP.2022.100089
80. J.P. Winkler, J. Grönberg, A. Vogelsang, Optimizing for recall in automatic requirements classification: An empirical study, in *Proceedings of the IEEE International Conference on Requirements Engineering*, (IEEE Computer Society, 2019), pp. 40–50
81. M. Yamac, M. Ahishali, A. Degerli, et al., Convolutional sparse support estimator-based COVID-19 recognition from X-ray images. IEEE Trans. Neural Netw. Learn. Syst. **32**, 1810–1820 (2021). https://doi.org/10.1109/TNNLS.2021.3070467
82. M.S. Yeasir, A. Tusher, H. Kabir, et al., Artificial intelligence for Parkinson's disease diagnosis: A review, in *Artificial Intelligence for Disease Diagnosis and Prognosis in Smart Healthcare*, (CRC Press, 2023), pp. 157–168
83. A.N. Belkacem, S. Ouhbi, A. Lakas, E. Benkhelifa, C Chen, End-to-end AI-based point-of-care diagnosis system for classifying respiratory illnesses and early detection of COVID-19: a theoretical framework. Front. Med. **8**, 585578 (2021). https://doi.org/10.3389/fmed.2021.585578

84. S. Agrebi, A. Larbi, Use of artificial intelligence in infectious diseases, in *Artificial Intelligence in Precision Health*, ed. by D. Barh, (Elsevier, Amsterdam, 2020), pp. 415–438. https://doi.org/10.1016/B978-0-12-817133-2.00018-5
85. J.S. Brownstein, B. Rader, C.M. Astley, H. Tian, Advances in artificial intelligence for infectious-disease surveillance. New Engl. J. Med. **388**(17), 1597–1607 (2023). https://doi.org/10.1056/NEJMra2119215
86. H. Chen, D. Zeng, D.L. Buckeridge, M.I. Izadi, A. Verma, A. Okhmatovskaia, X. Hu, X. Shen, Z. Cao, F.Y. Wang, X. Zheng, AI for global disease surveillance. IEEE Intell. Syst. **24**(6), 66–82 (2009). https://doi.org/10.1109/MIS.2009.126
87. P. Cunningham, M. Cord, S.J. Delany, *Supervised Learning*, (Cognitive Technologies, 2008), pp. 21–49
88. J. Bell, *What is Machine Learning? Machine Learning and the City*, (2022), pp. 207–216. https://doi.org/10.1002/9781119815075.ch18
89. C.J. Kelly, A. Karthikesalingam, M. Suleyman, G. Corrado, D. King, Key challenges for delivering clinical impact with artificial intelligence. BMC Med. **17**, 1–9 (2019). https://doi.org/10.1186/s12916-019-1426-2
90. T. Hastie, R. Tibshirani, J. Friedman, *Unsupervised Learning*, (2009), pp. 485–585. https://doi.org/10.1007/978-0-387-84858-7_14
91. M. Ziegler, The Black Death and the Future of the Plague. Med. Globe **1**(1), 259–283 (2015). https://doi.org/10.17302/TMG.1-1.10

A Comprehensive Review of Algorithms Developed for Rapid Pathogen Detection and Surveillance

Amna Zar, Lubna Zar, Sara Mohsen, Yosra Magdi, and Susu M. Zughaier

1 Introduction

Surveillance and early detection of infectious diseases are critical for prevention. Some communicable diseases pose significant threats to human health with high mortality and morbidity as evidenced by the recent COVID-19 pandemic. Advances in Artificial Intelligence (AI) applications are aiding the early detection and surveillance of emerging infectious diseases which help mitigate the risk. Moreover, Antimicrobial Resistance (AMR) is the current silent pandemic and poses a critical threat to public health as the rate of antimicrobial-resistant pathogens is increasing globally. Advances in AI provide solutions and algorithms that facilitate antimicrobial resistance monitoring and the discovery of novel antimicrobial therapeutics. This chapter provides a comprehensive review of current advances in AI applications for surveillance, rapid pathogen detection methods, antibiotics and vaccine candidate discovery, AMR stewardship, data sharing and collaboration as well as predictive analytics that all help in the prevention and control of infectious diseases.

2 AI in Pathogen Identification and Characterization

Pathogen identification has traditionally been conducted using traditional microbial culture techniques and, more recently, genomic methods such as polymerase chain reaction (PCR). Although these techniques have led to great advancements in the

A. Zar · L. Zar · S. Mohsen · Y. Magdi · S. M. Zughaier (✉)
Department of Basic Medical Sciences, College of Medicine, QU Health, Qatar University, Doha, Qatar
e-mail: szughaier@qu.edu.qa

M. E. H. Chowdhury, S. Kiranyaz (eds.), *Surveillance, Prevention, and Control of Infectious Diseases*, https://doi.org/10.1007/978-3-031-59967-5_2

field of microbiology, they are usually tedious, time-consuming, and demand a lot of resources [1]. In recent years, AI and Machine Learning (ML) algorithms have led to groundbreaking discoveries in microbiology and the persistent battle against AMR. In this section, we will review different methods including the traditional techniques of pathogen identification using AI/ML.

2.1 Bacterial Identification from Microscopic Morphology Using ML Algorithms

The automation of bacteria identification can be useful in situations where there is a shortage of skilled microbiologists and clinicians at a time of great need. One of the earlier methods proposed by researchers in 2014 was the use of morphological images of different bacterial strains to extract features and classify them using the Naïve Bayes classifier [2]. The Naïve Bayes classifier is an ML algorithm used for classification tasks. Since it only required a small training dataset, it was applied in the proposed bacterial identification system to approximate the factors required for the classification process. The proposed system achieved around 80% accuracy in the classification of the three major classes of bacteria. Another study was conducted using the Speeded Up robust features (SURF) algorithm, which detects key points in the gram stain images and produces an input vector for the classifier [3]. The classifier was then trained on key point vectors to predict which of the three classes the specific bacteria belonged to. This method had a lower accuracy of 75% in the test set. Both of these approaches required manual feature extraction methods and therefore were less efficient.

A few years later, Hay et al. [4] used Google's open-source TensorFlow framework as their 3D convolutional neural network (ConvNet) to distinguish bacteria and non-bacterial objects in 3D light sheet fluorescence microscopy images of larval zebrafish intestines. ConvNets are a type of ML algorithm that uses layers consisting of multiple kernels, which are numerical arrays acting as filters. These kernels are convolved across the input, taking advantage of locally correlated information. The kernels are updated as the algorithm is fed labeled data, converging by numerical optimization methods on the weights that best match the training data (Fig. 1). The network also has numerous layers generating different parameters. Furthermore, the accuracy generated by this model was on par with human experts and outcompeted traditional feature-based methods such as random forest and support vector machine classifiers. It also generalized well to different bacterial species through the use of transfer learning.

Inspired by previous work, Ahmad et al. [5] further improved the classification of bacterial images by combining two machine learning techniques: The inception V3 CNN model [6]. The researchers used bacterial images from online repositories. Inception V3 is a pre-trained model that underwent training using a dataset comprising one million images categorized into one thousand distinct categories. The initial

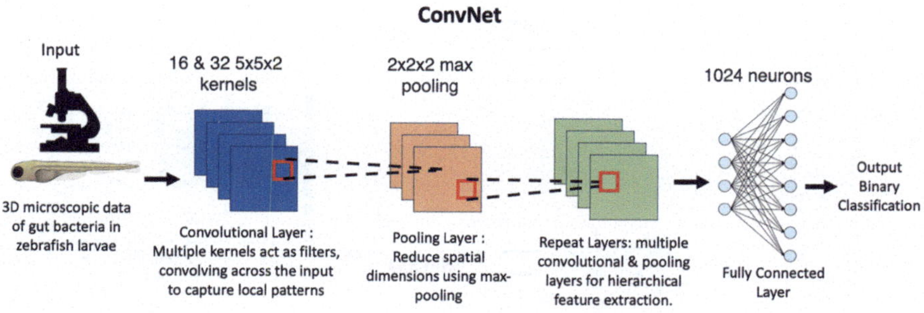

Fig. 1 depicts the Convolutional Neural Network used to distinguish bacterial from non-bacterial objects from 3D light sheet fluorescence microscopy images of larval zebrafish intestines

Inception V3 CNN model was altered and subsequently retrained using a training dataset that encompassed over 800 microscopic images featuring seven different bacterial species, employing the transfer-learning approach. After this retraining, the CNN model captured one-dimensional characteristics from the images, which were then utilized to train the SVM classifier. The combination of CNN and SVM have led to the accurate classification of microscopic bacteria images. Finally, they achieved a predictive accuracy of 96.07% using a test dataset of 200 samples. This method overcame the challenges the previous studies faced; this updated model developed an automatic method of feature extraction without the need for manual classification of bacterial images.

2.2 *Raman Spectroscopy and Deep Learning*

Raman spectroscopy is a technique that uses laser light to measure the vibrational modes of molecules, providing a unique spectral fingerprint that can be used to identify the molecules. In recent years, Raman spectroscopy has been used to identify bacteria, predict antibiotic susceptibility, and recommend suitable treatments for different cases.

In 2019, Ho et al. [7] published an extensive dataset of bacterial Raman spectra. The study aimed to develop a rapid system to identify bacterial isolates and determine their antibiotic resistance by combining Raman spectroscopy and deep learning. To achieve this, the researchers trained a CNN to classify noisy bacterial spectra by isolate, empiric treatment, and antibiotic resistance. The CNN architecture used in this study is based on ResNet and consists of an initial convolution layer, 6 residual layers, and a final fully connected classification layer, totaling 26 layers. Skip connections within the residual layers enhance gradient propagation and training stability. The initial convolution layer has 64 filters, and hidden layers have 100 filters, chosen through a grid search. The network was trained on the largest known dataset of bacterial Raman spectra, which included

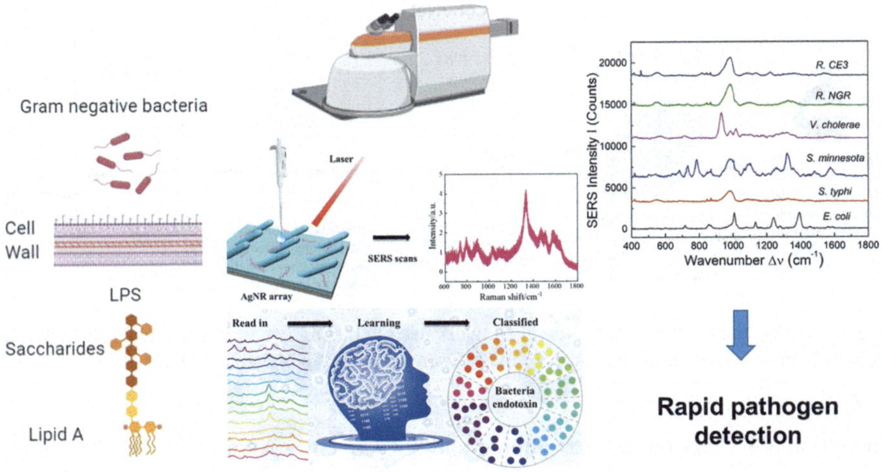

Fig. 2 Raman spectroscopy surface enhanced fingerprints (SERS) can be used for the rapid detection of bacterial biomarkers using an algorithm trained to identify molecular biomarkers and predict pathogens

30 of the most common bacterial pathogens. The CNN was able to distinguish between methicillin-resistant and -susceptible isolates of *Staphylococcus aureus* (MRSA and MSSA) with 89 ± 0.1% accuracy. Furthermore, the results from initial clinical validation (data from 50 patients) showed that the network has achieved 99.0 ± 1.9% species identification accuracy using just 10 bacterial spectra from each of 25 isolates. The study represented an important proof-of-concept for the rapid identification of bacterial isolates and antibiotic resistance using Raman spectroscopy and deep learning.

Various studies have made efforts to develop culture-free diagnostic methods for infectious diseases using Surface Enhanced Ramen Spectrum (SERS). In 2014, Wu et al. [8] used SERS to detect pyocyanin, a crucial biomarker of *Pseudomonas aeruginosa*, in sputum samples. This technique was tested on 15 sputum samples and achieved a sensitivity of 95.6% and a specificity of 93.3%. Then, in 2021, the team used SERS to differentiate between endotoxins from various pathogenic bacteria, including *E. coli*, *Vibrio cholerae*, *Salmonella typhimurium*, and *Salmonella Minnesota* [9] (Fig. 2).

To combat the rise in Antimicrobial Resistance (AMR) many research groups have developed fast and accurate methods of detection of antibiotic susceptibility. The research paper published by Thomsen et al. [10] discussed the development of a ML technique that uses Raman spectroscopy for the identification of bacteria and the distinction between methicillin-resistant and methicillin-susceptible bacteria. The paper introduces a novel spectral transformer (ST) ML model that is efficient in training on both small and large Raman spectroscopy bacteria datasets. The researchers used a home-built Raman microscope to acquire training and validation datasets of minimally prepared bacteria samples. They used a home-built system as it allowed them to optimize the Raman microscope's signal-to-noise ratio (SNR). The SNR is a measure of the strength of the signal compared to the background noise. Optimizing it can improve the accuracy and reliability of the measurements. By tailoring the system to the task of detecting bacteria, the researchers were able to acquire Raman spectra using very short measurement times down to 0.1 s. This was important because it allowed for faster and more efficient analysis of large numbers of samples, which is crucial for clinical applications. Additionally, using a home-built system is relatively cheap compared to commercial Raman microscopes. The authors aimed to simplify and reduce sample preparation time and complexity by transferring bacteria samples from a bacterial monoculture directly to a calcium fluoride (CaF2) objective slide followed by Raman raster-scan measurements. The researchers in this study used ML techniques to improve the accuracy and speed of Raman spectroscopy for identifying different types of bacteria. They tested their system on a dataset containing 15 different classes of bacteria and achieved an overall classification accuracy of more than 96%. The paper concluded that the developed ML technique using Raman spectroscopy has the potential to be a fast and reliable diagnostic tool for the identification of bacteria and the distinction between methicillin-resistant and methicillin-susceptible bacteria.

Furthermore, Han et al. [11] published a proof-of-principle study in which they proposed a protocol for rapid antibiotic susceptibility testing of bacteria from patients' blood using SERS. The results of the study showed that the protocol based on SERS could obtain consistent antibiotic susceptibility test results from clinical blood-culture samples within 4 h. The characteristic spectral signatures of *Staphylococcus aureus* and *Escherichia coli* became prominent after an effective pretreatment procedure removed strong interferences from blood constituents. Using these spectral signatures as the biomarkers of bacterial metabolic responses to antibiotics, the protocol reported the susceptibility profiles of tested drugs against these two bacteria with high specificity, sensitivity, and speed. The protocol demonstrated the potential to overcome the limitations of the standard microbiological diagnosis of infection, which usually lasts days using conventional methods compared to a few hours. Due to the reduced time of antibiotic susceptibility detection, empirical broad-spectrum antibiotics will be administered for a shorter time period.

Problems arise in the interpretation and analysis of Raman spectra data due to its highly dimensional nature. Raman spectra are usually long, and the energy distribution plots may not be suitable for the use of CNNs. Furthermore, CNNs are known for their ability to handle spatial invariance, which means that they can recognize patterns regardless of their location in an image. However, this property may not be suitable for analyzing Raman spectra data, which has unique properties and patterns. Despite this limitation, CNNs are still more capable than traditional ML techniques due to their sparse connection and weight-sharing properties. To overcome the limitations of CNNs and leverage their strengths, a recent article published by Ibtehaz et al. [12] proposed a novel deep learning model called RamanNet. The model uses shifted densely connected layers, which are similar to multi-layer perceptrons (MLP) but with shifted connections. This allows the model to extract significant features across the entire spectrum without being limited by spatial or temporal invariance. Furthermore, RamanNet employs triplet loss in the hidden layers to make the embeddings more separable and informative in lower-dimensional space. This helps to reduce the dimensionality of the data and improve the efficiency of the model. The authors used publicly available bacterial Raman spectroscopy data [7] to evaluate the performance of RamanNet (only three hidden layers) to a deep CNN with 25 hidden layers. RamanNet outperformed the CNN model by 85.5% compared to 82.2%. Overall, RamanNet can greatly help in identifying and classifying different types of bacteria more accurately and with fewer hidden layers compared to the far more complex state-of-the-art models. However, further research is needed to evaluate the model's performance on large-scale datasets and investigate its denoising capabilities.

Raman spectroscopy has also been used for viral detection. Yang et al. [13] used SERS to detect SARS-CoV-2 RNA in nasopharyngeal swab specimens. Most previously used indirect detection, which involved identifying the SERS spectrum of a chemical tag that is chemically linked to the analyte, such as RNA. However, the use of additional chemical tags increased the complexity and cost of the detection process. Yang et al. used direct detection, where the SERS spectrum is measured directly from the analyte itself. This was deemed to be a more straightforward approach since it did not require the use of any additional chemical tags or labels. The challenge arises when differentiating between DNA and RNA using this method because RNA and DNA have similar nucleic acid bases. To overcome the problem, the researchers used a Recurrent Neural Network (RNN) model to analyze the SERS spectra and identify the specific peaks that correspond to the RNA of SARS-CoV-2. The algorithm was trained on a dataset of positive and negative specimens to learn the patterns in the SERS spectra that correspond to the presence or absence of the RNA of SARS-CoV-2. Positive and negative specimens were accurately predicted by the RNN model at 97.7% and 100%, respectively. The study demonstrated that Raman spectroscopy working with deep learning could serve as a rapid diagnostic method for detecting COVID-19.

Another study developed a SERS aptasensor to rapidly detect SARS-CoV-2 viral particles. A crucial component of the aptasensor was a locking amplifier, which only activated when it recognized the aptamer of SARS-CoV-2. By amplifying the signal generated by the aptamer-virus interaction, viral detection was made easier with more accurate results. Thus, the SERS aptasensor can be used for rapid detection of SARS-CoV-2 and aid in controlling the spread of infectious diseases [14].

2.3 Innovative Methods of Pathogen Detection

There are many innovative ways in which artificial intelligence has been utilized to identify pathogens in recent years. In 2023, researchers were able to develop a rapid method to identify potential pathogen contamination in food products [15] and thus prevent foodborne illnesses and outbreaks. The study combined artificial intelligence (AI) and optical imaging to detect bacteria at the micro-colony stage within 3 h of inoculation. The approach developed in this study was used to distinguish between a diverse bacterial species including *Salmonella enterica (serotypes Enteritidis and Typhimurium) and Listeria monocytogenes, Pseudomonas fluorescens, Bacillus spp. (Bacillus coagulans and Bacillus subtilis), and Listeria innocua.* The study also aimed to evaluate the feasibility of using the trained You Only Look Once version 4 (YOLOv4) [16] detector for the detection of *E. coli* in romaine lettuce, where diverse microbiota and food debris are present. The method used in this study involved: first, the microcolonies were incubated and imaged using white light, then, the real-time detection was performed using the object detection and classification algorithm YOLOv4. YOLOv4 incorporates advanced techniques, including data augmentation methods like CutMix and Mosaic, regularization with DropBlock, and label smoothing for the backbone. It also utilizes special features like Mish activation, Cross-Stage Partial Connections (CSP), and Multi-Input Weighted Residual Connections (MiWRC). For the detector, it employs CIoU-loss, Cross-Stage Batch Normalization (CmBN), Mosaic data augmentation, Self-Adversarial Training, and other enhancements. Additionally, it utilizes Mish activation, SPP-block, SAM-block, PAN path-aggregation block, and DIoU-NMS (Distance-IoU) Non-Maximum Suppression to improve object detection performance. The main strength of the algorithm was its high speed (30 frames per second) as it could detect objects in real-time at a rate faster than the human eye can. The study was able to successfully distinguish *E. coli* from other bacterial species with a precision of 93.3%. Using YOLOv4, the six *E. coli* strains were classified with a precision range of 87.3–97.2%, indicating that strain-level classification was possible with this method.

Another recent study conducted by Kim et al. used three-dimensional quantitative phase imaging (3DQPI) and a 4 layered CNN model to identify pathogens from single to few cells images or tomograms [17]. The 3DQPI consists of a label-free imaging technique used to obtain the 3D refractive index tomogram of a live cell. The training process of the ANN involved a gradient-based optimization of the network parameters using a dataset of known species. The network model mainly consisted of 3D convolution operations, which could effectively recognize the 3D structure in 3D RI tomograms. It utilized dense blocks, each consisting of two 3D convolution operations followed by concatenation. Then the feature-maps were rescaled between dense blocks by a transition unit. The first convolution had 64 feature maps, and each following convolution operation had feature maps increased by 32. The dense connections between the convolution operations in the ANN induced it to revisit the feature maps of the shallower layers even at the deep layers. This helped in improving the accuracy of the classification process. Training involves minimizing cross-entropy loss between ground truth and predictions. Data is split into training, validation, and blind test datasets. Stochastic gradient descent is used with a mini-batch size of 48 and cosine annealing for learning rate scheduling. Data augmentation techniques, including cropping, rotation, and noise, are applied to prevent overfitting. The time required for training was approximately 290 h. In the final phase of the blind test, a classifier is established by aggregating predictions from several top-performing ANN models. The process involved exploring four key parameters for model integration: the number of models, the balance between considering training and validation accuracies, output normalization, and the specific method employed for integration (including averaging, exponential averaging, voting, or maximum projection). The ultimate choice of parameters, guided by the pursuit of the highest validation accuracy, formed the basis for the blind test algorithm, ensuring its effectiveness in making accurate predictions. This study was important because it allowed for rapid and accurate identification of bacterial species from a small sample size, which is crucial in the early treatment of infections. The use of a single 3D QPI and ANN achieved an accuracy of 82.5% in identifying 19 bacterial species that caused bloodstream infections from an individual bacterial cell or cluster (minute quantity), which is comparable to the gold standard mass spectroscopy. The accuracy of the classification process increased with multiple measurements, reaching 99.9% with seven different measurements of cells or clusters. The proposed framework could serve as a beneficial advisory tool for clinicians during the initial treatment of infections, as it provides rapid and accurate identification of the pathogen from single to few cells.

Weis et al. [18] developed a new ML approach to predict AMR directly from matrix-assisted laser desorption/ionization–time of flight (MALDI-TOF) mass spectra profiles of clinical isolates. The authors created a publicly available database of mass spectra profiles from clinically relevant isolates with linked antimicrobial susceptibility phenotypes, called the Database of Resistance Information on Antimicrobials and MALDI-TOF Mass Spectra (DRIAMS). They trained calibrated classifiers on this dataset and validated their approach on a panel of clinically important pathogens. Thus, they demonstrated the potential of using ML to substantially accelerate AMR determination and enhance clinical management. Three different ML models were used for classification: logistic regression, gradient-boosted decision trees (LightGBM), and a deep multilayer perceptron (MLP). The performance of each model was evaluated using two metrics: the area under the receiver operating characteristic curve (AUROC) and the area under the precision-recall curve (AUPRC). These metrics quantified the ability of the model to correctly classify samples as resistant or susceptible while minimizing false positives and false negative rates. Overall, the study found that LightGBM and MLP were the best-performing models in terms of AUROC, indicating that they were able to accurately predict antimicrobial resistance from clinical mass spectra. The authors suggested that future research can build upon their findings and use unlabeled MALDI-TOF mass spectra in DRAIMS (Database of Resistance-Associated Isolates and Microbial Species) for pre-training a classifier. The purpose of this pre-training is to potentially improve the prediction performance of the classifier. This pre-training would be done in a semi-supervised fashion, meaning that the classifier would learn from both labeled and unlabeled data.

A recent study developed a HarDNet algorithm, which could distinguish between bacterial, fungal, and viral pneumonia using computed tomography (CT) images. Each HarD block had the same L-layer structure, then the channel weight ($m = 1.6$), the convolutional channel (k), and the greatest integer when one is divided by

2n(n) were used to calculate the channel number of layer 1. Wang et al. [19] trained the algorithm, called Pneumonia-Plus, using 2763 chest CT images. Then, the algorithm was tested on 173 images. Viral, fungal, and bacterial pneumonia had AUCs of 0.816, 0.715, and 0.934, respectively. Meanwhile, a radiologist with 12 years of experience achieved sensitivities of 0.694 and 0.580 for bacterial and fungal pneumonia respectively. The study demonstrated that the Pneumonia-Plus algorithm can accurately classify different types of pneumonia based on CT images, improving the diagnosis and treatment of patients.

3 Early Detection and Diagnosis of Infectious Diseases

AI offers rapid and precise preliminary screening for COVID-19 using chest X-rays. In a recent study, COVID-19 screening has been accomplished by applying Machine Learning algorithms to chest X-ray (CXR) images using the Operational Segmentation Network (OSegNet), an artificial intelligence model specifically created to improve the reliability of COVID-19 pneumonia detection by segmenting affected regions within CXR images [20]. The study utilized the QaTa-COV19 dataset, which is the largest available collection of COVID-19 CXR images, encompassing more than 121,000 images. Remarkably, OSegNet has achieved an accuracy rate of 99.65%, which is the highest compared to state-of-the-art deep learning models.

Similarly, another AI model effectively classified chest X-ray images into different categories: COVID-19, non-COVID-19, pneumonia, tuberculosis (TB), and normal [21]. The model demonstrated a testing accuracy of 100% for non-COVID-19, pneumonia, and tuberculosis. However, it exhibited a lower accuracy in other categories: 14.29% for normal, 20% for COVID-19, and 14.67% for new COVID-19 cases. In addition to chest X-rays, alternative radiological images can be utilized for diagnostic purposes. For example, a study developed and validated an automated AI framework called COVIA for COVID-19 detection using chest CT scans [22]. COVIA achieved an AUC of 0.882 in discriminating between COVID-19 positive and negative cases. The model utilized 45 radiomics features, including measures of texture complexity, correlation, distance, and image intensity, extracted from lung segmentations using a CNN. This fully automated framework could provide rapid and accurate diagnosis, aiding in timely intervention and isolation procedures for suspected COVID-19 cases.

In addition, clinical notes have been analyzed using AI to diagnose COVID-19. An AI model was trained on a dataset consisting of sentences related to cardiovascular, pulmonary, metabolic diseases, and COVID-19 symptoms [23]. To apply the model to COVID-19 diagnosis, it was used to analyze clinical notes from COVID-19 positive and negative patients. The notes from 7 days prior to the SARS-CoV-2 diagnostic test were considered, and the model identified the set of symptoms present for each patient at that time. The presence of a symptom was determined based on the model's classification of "Yes" or "Maybe" for that symptom. To validate the accuracy of the model for COVID-19 symptoms, a manual verification step was performed on a subset of sentences. The model achieved a true positive rate ranging from 93% to 100% for Fever/Chills, Cough, Respiratory Difficulty, Headache, Fatigue, Myalgia/Arthralgia, Dysuria, Change in appetite/intake, and Diaphoresis. However, the true positive rate was slightly lower (82.2%) for Altered or diminished sense of taste and smell. Overall, the model achieved an accuracy of 94.0% and a precision and recall of 96% for both positive and negative sentiment classification. This knowledge can potentially assist healthcare providers in identifying and monitoring patients who exhibit specific symptoms, allowing for earlier intervention and appropriate testing to mitigate the spread of the virus.

Likewise, laboratory notes can be employed for the detection of COVID-19 infection. In Iran, seven data mining algorithms were used to create models based on a dataset from 19 hospitals [24]. The dataset consisted of individuals who were hospitalized between February and May 2020 and had tested positive for COVID-19 using polymerase chain reaction (PCR) tests, including their demographic details and the results of 16 laboratory tests. The results showed that the Random Forest (RF) and Gradient Boosted Trees models had the highest accuracy percentages of 86.45% and 84.80%, respectively. By identifying specific laboratory tests that are strongly associated with patient outcomes, the model can aid in risk stratification, treatment planning, and resource allocation for COVID-19 patients.

A novel serological test platform has been developed to quantify neutralizing antibodies in serum as an alternative to the complex and time-consuming neutralization test (NT) method [25]. Serum samples were collected from two groups: patients with confirmed COVID-19 and healthy individuals. An enzyme-linked immunosorbent assay (ELISA) system was used to measure antibody responses, focusing on the S1 protein and receptor-binding domain (RBD). By utilizing a two-variable generalized additive model (GAM) regression model, the researchers accurately predicted the neutralization titer (NT) of the antibodies based on the optical density (OD) readings of S1 and RBD.

Pulmonary tuberculosis is another infectious disease that has been an important target for AI-powered diagnosis. A systematic review and meta-analysis assessed the performance of AI-based software for diagnosing pulmonary tuberculosis (PTB) [26]. The analysis included 13 development studies and 23 clinical studies. The results indicated that the AI software exhibited high accuracy in diagnosing PTB, with pooled sensitivities greater than 0.9 in both clinical and development studies. To exemplify, three recent studies focused on the application of computer-aided detection (CAD) technologies in the diagnosis and screening of tuberculosis TB and related lung diseases. One study examines the detection of active pulmonary TB using deep learning algorithms, outperforming human radiologists with an AUC of 0.89 [27]. A second study discusses the high accuracy of CAD in detecting occupational lung diseases, specifically silicosis, and pulmonary TB, among ex-miners from South African gold mines [28]. A third study evaluates the diagnostic accuracy of three CAD systems for TB detection on chest radiographs during screening, targeting a multinational population of migrants. While all studies employ CAD technologies for TB detection, they differ in terms of their target populations, research objectives, and specific focus within the context of TB screening and diagnosis [29].

Another example of infectious diseases that have been targeted by AI-powered detection is sexually transmitted diseases, particularly HIV. In recent years, the application of machine learning algorithms and predictive models has emerged as a promising strategy to address missed opportunities in early HIV diagnosis and assess HIV risk using electronic health records and clinical notes. Researchers in South Carolina employed two machine learning models to retrospectively analyze individuals diagnosed with HIV, utilizing the Least Absolute Shrinkage and Selection Operator (LASSO) for feature selection and Poisson regression to develop prediction models [30]. These models identified several predictors, including facility type, physician specialty, age, gender, and substance use, demonstrating acceptable discrimination with the area under the receiver operating characteristic curve (AUC) values of 0.82 and 0.78. Similarly, Feller et al. utilized natural language processing (NLP) and machine learning techniques to develop predictive models for HIV risk assessment using electronic health records and clinical notes [31]. These models outperformed the baseline model, exhibiting good precision and recall in identifying individuals at elevated risk of HIV. Additionally, Xiang et al. investigated the impact of network context on detecting unknown HIV infections among young men who have sex with men (MSM) by collecting social network data [32]. Their ensemble approach, combining Graph Convolutional Networks (GCN) with logistic regression and random forest, significantly improved the prediction of HIV status within the social network, achieving high accuracy (96.6%) and F1 measure (94.6%), surpassing baseline methods. By utilizing this GCN, the study demonstrates the potential of incorporating social network information into HIV detection approaches, leading to more effective targeting of interventions and prevention strategies among at-risk populations.

4 AI in Drug and Vaccine Development

Drug and vaccine development has significantly been accelerated by the use of AI techniques. By analyzing genomic sequences of pathogens, AI can also aid in the discovery of new vaccines by designing antigens that can stimulate a protective immune response [33]. In the field of drug discovery, AI has revolutionized the process by speeding up the identification of lead molecules with desired pharmacodynamics and pharmacokinetic properties [34]. Traditional drug discovery strategies are time-consuming and costly, with a high failure rate. However, ML approaches have been successful in accelerating the identification of potential drug candidates. Various machine learning algorithms, such as random forest, deep learning, support vector machine, and Lasso, have been used to assess protein-ligand interactions and generate models for drug discovery [35]. The application of AI in drug discovery and vaccine development is not without challenges. One of the main limitations is the lack of technologies to identify potential candidates from the vast chemical space. Additionally, there is a dilemma between performance and interpretability within machine intelligence, which has limited its application in drug discovery [34]. Despite these challenges, AI has shown great promise in expediting the process of drug and vaccine development. By leveraging machine learning algorithms and analyzing large datasets, AI can identify potential drug targets, simulate drug interactions, predict treatment efficacy, and design antigens for vaccine development. These advancements have the potential to significantly improve public health outcomes by accelerating the availability of effective drugs and vaccines.

4.1 Drug Discovery and Repurposing

The implementation of AI techniques in drug discovery, repurposing, and vaccine development has vastly increased due to the COVID-19 outbreak. AI-driven drug development has resulted in faster and more efficient drug discovery processes. Not only have AI-based drug discovery tools been used to develop treatments for COVID-19, but these tools have also led to several promising new antimicrobial treatments. Moreover, AI is being used to analyze existing drugs, to see if they can be repurposed to treat COVID-19. Finally, AI is used to speed up the development of vaccines.

Many studies have focused on identifying small molecule therapeutic drugs with inhibitory effects on the main protease (Mpro), also known as 3CL protease, of SARS-CoV-2. Mpro is vital for virus replication and infection, which makes it the perfect target for antiviral treatment [36]. AI-guided INTerprotein's Engine for New Drug Design (INTENDD) was developed by Komatsu et al. [37] to detect 20 potential Mpro ligands, 13 of which demonstrated Mpro-binding signals through surface plasmon resonance (SPR). SPR is a method used to detect and measure molecules' binding to surfaces. It is used to study interactions between proteins and small molecules, such as drugs." Six of these drugs were newly discovered in this study (Fig. 3).

A similar study aimed to discover novel compounds targeting Mpro. Two SMILES-based Long Short-Term Memory (LSTM) autoencoders were employed in this study. The embeddings model was unsupervised while the energy model was semi-supervised. In the embeddings model, there was an encoder, a Gaussian noise entry into the latent layer, and a decoder. It received vectorized SMILES as input that passed through the LSTM layer. Next, the energy model utilized another parameter (free energy binding value) to learn compounds from the training set based on molecular docking results. The binding free energy of each compound was estimated using scoring functions calculated by three methods: AutoDock Vina, RF-Score-4, and NNScore 2.0. The values of each scoring function were then employed to calculate the ranks of compounds, and the value of the exponential consensus ranking (ECR) function. Compounds were ranked by ECR, and the most promising

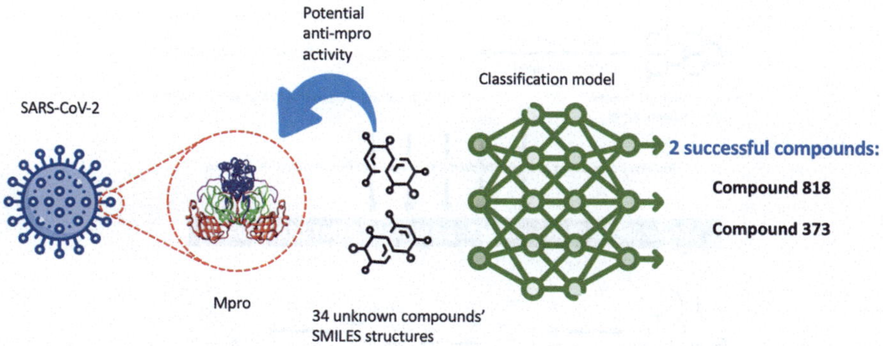

Fig. 3 SMILES structures of 34 unknown compounds with potential anti-mpro activity. Compound 818 is a reversible 8-methyl-γ-carboline analogue and compound 737 is an N-pyridyl-isatin with irreversible activity against Mpro

ones were selected for further study. Overall, the seven compounds with the best scores demonstrated low binding free energy values compared to those of potent inhibitors of Mpro, suggesting that they could be potential targets for anti-SARS-CoV-2 therapeutics [38].

Another study aimed to detect potential inhibitors of Mpro using an AI-driven approach followed by in vitro validation. The model was trained on SMILES representations of compounds with known biological activity against Mpro activity. The model was developed to generate compounds with potential anti-Mpro activity. Then, a trained classifier was employed to predict the compounds' bioactivity against Mpro. The three most promising molecules were tested in vitro against SARS-CoV-2 in Vero E6 and Calu-3 cells. One compound outshone the others as it was active in both cell models and demonstrated low cytotoxicity [39].

Drug repurposing is an attractive alternative to novel drug discovery, especially in emergency epidemics. Repurposing is a fast and cost-effective approach that involves repurposing existing drugs and re-testing them for new indications. This approach has proven successful in the past, and it can be used to develop treatments for new diseases quickly and efficiently. Beck et al. [40] identified commercially available drugs that could inhibit SARS-CoV-2 viral proteins including proteinase, RNA-dependent RNA polymerase (RdRp), and helicase. The study used a drug-target interaction model called the Molecule Transformer-Drug Target Interaction (MT-DTI) model. After being trained using manually curated databases, the model utilized two 1D string inputs: SMILES strings and amino acid sequences (Fig. 4). This allowed the model to visualize 3D crystal structures of proteins with unconfirmed 3D structures. Atazanavir, an antiretroviral medication administered for HIV infection prevention and treatment, proved to be the strongest competitor in the study, with an inhibitory potency of 94.94 nM against Mpro. Other drugs that demonstrated inhibitory effects were Remdesivir, Efavirenz, Ritonavir, and Dolutegravir.

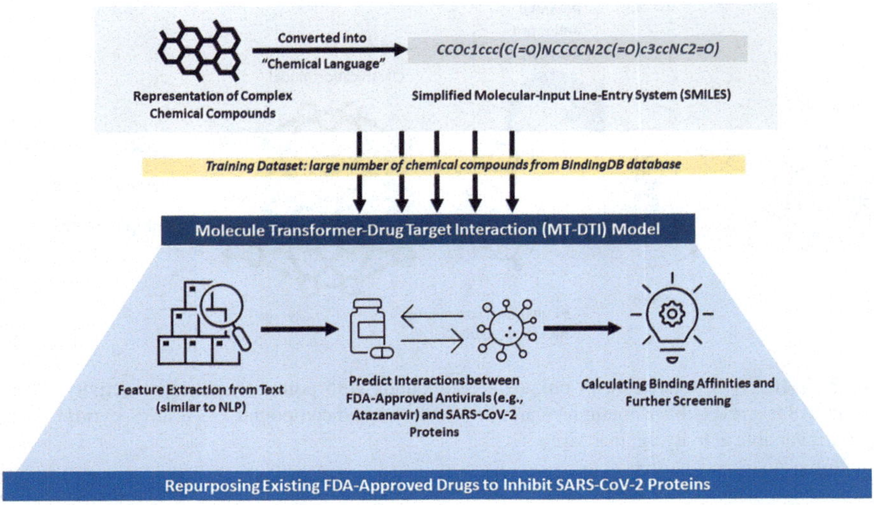

Fig. 4 Drug repurposing using Molecule Transformer-Drug Target Interaction (MT-DTI) Model

Another study aimed to repurpose drugs using a network-based knowledge mining algorithm called CoV-DTI. The algorithm screened a list of potential drugs targeting SARS-CoV-2. By learning a network topology-preserving embedding for each node, the algorithm extracted information about virus-related features and correctly predicted drug candidates. The study found that CVL218, a poly-ADP-ribose polymerase 1 (PARP1) inhibitor in a phase I trial, demonstrated inhibitory effects on inflammatory cytokine production and interaction with the nucleocapsid (N) protein. This study proved that an integrative drug repurposing framework could reveal new indications for existing drugs, accelerating the drug development process [41].

AI has revived the interest in antibiotic discovery. Stokes et al. [42] utilized a directed message-passing neural network to predict the antibacterial effects of 107 million molecules extracted from the ZINC15 database. The model identified a molecule called Halicin, a drug under investigation for treating diabetes patients, which demonstrated bactericidal activity against a large number of pathogens, including carbapenem-resistant *Enterobacteriaceae* and *Mycobacterium tuberculosis* among others. This study proves that deep learning approaches can increase antibacterial drug options and greatly aid the fight against antibiotic-resistant bacteria.

4.2 Vaccine Development

"Reverse vaccinology" is a process by which protective antigens and epitopes are identified through microbial genome analysis and monoclonal antibodies. Recent studies have shown that this method can be used to develop vaccines for a variety of infectious diseases, including COVID-19 and malaria [43]. In May 2020, Ong et al. [44] developed a supervised machine learning classification model, which they named Vaxign-ML, could most accurately predict bacterial protective antigens (BPAgs) when trained using the eXtreme Gradient Boosting (XGB) algorithm. XGBoost enables nonlinear relationships between features and outcomes to be captured through a tree ensemble model. A regularized learning objective also prevents overfitting and optimizes the model's data generalization ability [45]. A year later, Ong et al. [46] used Vaxign2 to demonstrate that the Spike protein of SARS-COV-2 was an effective vaccine candidate. Dalsass et al. [47] aimed to identify suitable antigens for bacterial vaccines using reverse vaccinology programs. They compared six different RV programs (NERVE, Vaxign, VaxiJen, Jenner-predict, Bowman-Heinson, and VacSol) and focused on 11 pathogens with known bacterial protective antigens (BPAs). However, all of the programs could not recall 100% of the BPAs, and the protein output lists were not consistent. The machine-learning approach proposed by Bowman and enhanced by Heinson showed the most effective balance between predicting suitable candidates and recalling BPAs.

One of the direct applications of AI in vaccine development is the identification of antigenic peptides presented by major histocompatibility complex class II (MHC-II) molecules. Machine learning has been used to develop programs that predict antigen presentation, allowing for the design of vaccines that can elicit an immune response [48, 49]. AI-related tools have also been used to analyze viral peptide presentation on MHC molecules from patients infected with SARS-CoV-2, providing insights into natural immunity [50].

5 Artificial Intelligence in Antimicrobial Stewardship

Antimicrobial stewardship refers to coordinated efforts to promote the appropriate use of antimicrobials to preserve their effectiveness [51]. Explainable AI can predict the likelihood of antibiotic drug resistance based on patient data [52]. AI can identify the efficacy of empiric treatment for various infections, such as recurrent urinary tract infections (rUTIs) in women [53]. ML-based clinical decision support systems (ML-CDSS) can be used in critical situations, such as sepsis, as the protection of the most effective antibiotics can be lifesaving [54]. These efforts reduce risks of adverse effects, minimize unnecessary costs, and slow antimicrobial resistance.

According to Cavallaro et al. [52], explainable AI can predict the likelihood of antimicrobial drug resistance by analyzing a patient's characteristics, past medical history, and past drug treatments and culture results. Predictions were made using a gradient-boosted decision tree algorithm and a Shapley explanation model. The gradient-boosted decision tree (GBDT) algorithm combines many weak decision tree models into a single prediction. The Shapley explanation model compares the full model's predictions to those of a model without a specific feature. This was averaged over all combinations of features to calculate the Shapley value. These values are plotted, and the features are ranked based on Shapley values. The Shapley value of a feature represents its contribution to the final prediction. Thus, this model successfully justified the predictions that it made. The results of the study showed that the AI-based system substantially reduced the risk of mismatched treatment compared with observed prescriptions. Explainable AI offers transparency and interpretability to models' predictions. This is crucial in healthcare where incorrect predictions can have severe consequences. By understanding the model's prediction, healthcare professionals can better understand the rationale behind it and make informed decisions about patient care. It also contributes to building trust in AI models and promoting their use in healthcare. The paper shows how explainable AI can predict antimicrobial resistance, allowing healthcare professionals to make informed decisions about antibiotic prescriptions, and slowing antimicrobial resistance.

A recent study developed an ANN using Neural Networks Predict ® and ROC analysis that could predict the clinical efficacy of empiric antimicrobial treatment in females with rUTI. The model was trained on clinical and microbiological data from 725 patients and validated on 318 patients to predict the probability of Fosfomycin therapy-based failure. The model achieved a sensitivity of 87.8% and specificity of 97.3%. Furthermore, the study identified certain variables that were crucial in determining the failure of specific types of antimicrobial therapy. For example, patients with *Escherichia coli* infections who had previously used fluoroquinolones and cephalosporins were less likely to be treated successfully with cotrimoxazole. Thus, the study concluded that ANNs could be useful tools in recommending the most suitable antibiotic when treating rUTI patients, enhancing antimicrobial stewardship [53].

Another study applied a backward step-wise AIC model to predict antibiotic susceptibilities based on patient data. The model was used to perform a logistic regression and additional algorithms such as random forest and recursive partitioning were used. All models were five-fold cross-validated. The error estimation was estimated three times and the average was used for parameter fitting. The ratio of training to testing data was 80:20. This can guide appropriate empiric antibiotic therapy, especially in resource-limited settings. Data from 243 patients with bloodstream infections in a Columbian hospital were analyzed. The aim was to determine whether the infections could be treated with ampicillin and gentamicin, ceftriaxone, or neither option. On average, the random forest classifier gave the most accurate predictions among the algorithms tested. Time from admission to blood culture, patient age, hospital versus community-acquired infection, and age-adjusted weight score were the most critical determinants of susceptibility to treatment. This study proved that ML could save patients in critical conditions, in addition to slowing down AMR [54].

Antimicrobial stewardship program includes multiple elements such as education, research, environmental factors, and of course the misuse of antibiotics. The One Health Initiative covers the AMR problem and environmental interface [55]. AI has significantly aided the fight against infectious diseases in many ways. However, it is important to avoid exaggerating its capabilities or downplaying uncertainties.

For example, after the COVID-19 outbreak, zoonotic risk technology was developed to predict future emerging zoonotic diseases. Despite being undeniably valuable in the emerging disease toolkit, these models are essentially reliant on virology research and experimental work for providing data and validation. Therefore, it is advised not to focus investments on machine learning endeavors while compromising more important components of outbreak prevention and control, like health system preparation. Investing in scientific research is fundamental for data collection, which allows development in zoonotic risk technology as well as aids in outbreak control.

6 Artificial Intelligence in Data Sharing and Collaboration

6.1 Methods of Privacy Preservation

Data sharing has many challenges, the most significant being privacy concerns. Federated learning is an emerging approach that addresses these concerns by allowing multiple institutions to collaborate and collectively train the model. This is done without sharing the patients' data. The model is trained locally on each institution's data, and the resulting weights are averaged across participants. This approach enables privacy-preserving collaboration between multiple institutions. This approach also prevents overfitting as it allows the use of larger datasets. This results in improved accuracy and better generalization of the model. This shared model can then be used to make predictions on data from any of the participating institutions without compromising the privacy of the data. Furthermore, this approach allows for the development of models that are more powerful and accurate than any one institution could create on its own [56].

Dayan et al. [57] used a federated learning model named the Electronic medical record chest X-ray AI Model, abbreviated as EXAM, which could predict the future oxygen requirements of symptomatic COVID-19 patients uses inputs of vital signs, laboratory data, and chest X-rays. The model was trained on 16,148 cases, with 70% of the cases used for training, 10% for alidation and the rest for testing. The average area under the curve (AUC) of locally trained models without federated learning was 0.795. Federated learning improved the average AUC by 16% across all participating institution sites. The EXAM model achieved an AUC of 0.92 for predicting outcomes 24 and 72 h after the initial emergency room presentation. Generalizability increased by 38% when using federated learning compared to models trained at a single site. The study demonstrated the effectiveness of federated learning in facilitating rapid data science collaboration without data exchange. It also generated a model that could be generalized across heterogeneous, unharmonized datasets for clinical outcomes prediction for COVID-19 patients. Another study designed a framework that used decentralized privacy-preserving predictive modeling to allow multiple institutions to adopt a more generalizable model for healthcare or genomic data by sharing partially trained models rather than individual-level data while avoiding risks such as a single point of control [58].

Ghavamipour et al. [59] presented two protocols that perform logistic regression using the Newton-Raphson method. The protocols were based on secure Multi-Party Computation (MPC) and tailored to the honest majority and dishonest majority security settings. The MPC cryptographic technique allows multiple parties to compute a function together based on their private inputs without revealing information about those inputs. It works in two settings: the honest majority and the dishonest majority. In the honest majority setting, most parties are truthful and follow the protocol correctly, except for a malicious minority. In the dishonest majority setting, the majority is pernicious and colludes to learn more about the other parties' inputs, with only a few being honest. The aim was to enable logistic regression between multiple data holders while preserving privacy. Assuming the data were horizontally partitioned, the data holders had the same variables with different values for each variable. The efficiency and accuracy of the protocols were assessed against synthetic and real-world datasets. The scores were then compared to ordinary logistic regression. The experimental results demonstrated that the proposed protocols were highly efficient and accurate. A multi-class logistic regression that keeps private information secure would enable doctors to use this model for various data classification tasks without worrying about leaking patient data.

6.2 Genome Sequencing

A crucial step in developing machine learning models is by nourishing them with data, which are supplied through data collected from scientific research. Data sharing became much easier during the outbreak of the COVID-19 pandemic due to changes in data sharing protocols. In March 2020, the Bulletin of the World Health Organization issued a protocol for immediate online posting of research manuscripts relevant to the coronavirus emergency. This allowed ML developers to avoid conventional privacy and data ownership hurdles when retrieving training data [60]. Dugan et al. [61] developed a standardized metadata format for human pathogen/vector genomic sequences to enable effective analysis of genomic sequences for genotype-phenotype association studies and phylogenetic studies. The authors aimed to develop a metadata standard that can be extended to support additional project-specific data fields and integrated with other data represented with comparable standards.

Another study used a CNN classifier to develop a specific primer set for accurate SARS-CoV-2 detection. First, they classified the 583 sequences into 5 classes using one-hot label encoding based on their seasonality and the number of sequences available. The CNN was ten-fold stratified cross-validated, demonstrating a 98.7% accuracy. Over 90% of the sequences were correctly classified even in the underrepresented classes. The data, which was retrieved from the National

Genomics Data Center repository, was split into training (80%), validating (10%) and testing data (10%). The technique allowed the researchers to analyze the network's behavior and pinpoint sequences the model identified as specific to SARS-CoV-2 [62].

7 Predictive Analytics

AI has been used to analyze large amounts of data to identify trends, relationships, and patterns that can be used to forecast future behavior. This has been especially useful in the prediction of the prognosis and spread of the COVID-19 pandemic. An AI model used demographic and clinical data from COVID-19 patients admitted to Wuhan Infectious Diseases Hospital [63]. Predictors of mortality were identified using Least Absolute Shrinkage and Selection Operator (LASSO) regression and LASSO-based ANN models. The study found that severity of illness, age, platelet count, leukocyte count, pre-albumin, C-reactive protein (CRP), total bilirubin, Acute Physiology and Chronic Health Evaluation (APACHE) II score, and Sequential Organ Failure Assessment (SOFA) score were independent prognostic factors for mortality. The LASSO regression and LASSO-based ANN models showed high accuracy and predictive performance, with correct classification rates ranging from 0.98 to 0.990 and AUC values of 0.980 to 0.990 in both training and testing cohorts. Another study was conducted in Spain aimed to predict the severity of COVID-19 cases based on early biochemical analysis [64]. The data included the first blood analysis after COVID-19 diagnosis and demographic information. Statistical analyses were conducted, comparing variables between severe and non-severe cases. A software called AutoDiscovery was used for feature selection and model creation, using multi-class classifiers such as Random Forest. The top-performing model achieved an accuracy of 67.33% and demonstrated that specific variables could be potential predictors of disease severity, aiding in early-stage assessment. Another research protocol uses geotagged Twitter data and other sources to analyze human movement and population flows for monitoring COVID-19 spread and predicting infectious risk [65]. A database is created to store the collected data, and an Origin-Destination-Time (ODT) data cube is constructed to quantify movement between locations over time. The ODT cube is used to develop population-level infectious risk maps and a fused neural network is developed to predict future risk. Privacy protection and ethical considerations are given significant importance in the research protocol. The project's findings will be shared through various channels, including interactive web portals and research articles.

In addition to COVID-19, AI was used to predict the transmission of HIV among special populations. A paper by Bao et al. compared multiple AI models that were developed to predict HIV and sexually transmitted infections (STIs) among men who have sex with men (MSM) [66]. Data from clinic records, including demographic, clinical, behavioral, and laboratory information, were used to compare AUCs of various models, such as gradient boosting machine (GBM), random forest (RF), deep learning (DL), and extreme gradient boosting (XGBoost). The GBM model performed the best, achieving an AUC of 0.763. Key predictors of diagnosis included past infection history, symptoms, sexual behavior, and demographic factors. Another AI model, MySTIRisk, was trained with clinic consultation data from the Melbourne Sexual Health Centre [67]. The model assessed the risk of acquiring HIV, syphilis, gonorrhea, and chlamydia based on predictors such as gender, age, sexual behavior, number of casual partners, and condom use. The model achieved AUC values ranging from 0.70 to 0.84 for different STIs on testing data sets. The model's performance was also stable and reliable when validated with external datasets.

8 Contact Tracing and Social Distancing

During disease outbreaks, AI plays a crucial role in contact tracing efforts and enforcing social distancing measures. By analyzing data from multiple sources, such as mobile phone records, GPS data, and public transportation logs, AI can identify individuals who may have come into contact with an infected person, allowing public health agencies to promptly notify and isolate potentially exposed individuals [68]. This helps in containing the spread of the disease and preventing further transmission.

AI-powered contact tracing systems utilize technologies such as Bluetooth and BLE to track and record interactions between individuals [69]. These systems can provide real-time information on potential exposure, allowing for timely intervention and reducing the risk of further transmission [70]. Additionally, AI can be used to analyze the data collected from contact tracing efforts to identify patterns and trends, which can inform public health strategies and interventions [71]. In the context of social distancing, AI can be utilized to monitor compliance with social distancing measures and provide recommendations for crowd management. For example, AI algorithms can analyze real-time data from surveillance cameras to detect overcrowding in public spaces and provide alerts to authorities [72]. This enables proactive measures to be taken to disperse crowds and ensure compliance with social distancing guidelines [73].

Furthermore, AI can assist in the development of smart IoT-driven solutions for social distancing enforcement. These solutions utilize computer vision and biometric sensing machines to identify symptomatic individuals and prevent them from entering crowded public places, thereby limiting the spread of infections [74]. By leveraging AI algorithms, these systems can accurately detect and track individuals, ensuring effective enforcement of social distancing measures. However, the implementation of AI in contact tracing and social distancing efforts is not without challenges. Privacy preservation is a significant concern, as the collection and analysis of personal data raise ethical and legal considerations. It is crucial to develop robust privacy-preserving mechanisms to protect individuals' sensitive information while still enabling effective contact tracing and social distancing enforcement [75].

There are studies that explore the use of robotics integrated with AI in the context of the COVID-19 pandemic for social distancing and patient monitoring/serving. One such study discusses the contribution of robotics integrated with AI in the COVID-19 pandemic. The study highlights the use of robots to protect frontline workers from the virus and addresses the shortage of healthcare workers. The paper evaluates the existing robotics models employed during the pandemic and proposes the Simultaneous Fast Filtering Localization and Mapping (SFFLAM) model for the hospital environment. The SFFLAM model utilizes extended Kalman filtering integrated with sectorial error probability for robot localization. The study emphasizes the improved performance of the proposed model in terms of localization and processing [76].

AI plays a vital role in contact tracing and social distancing efforts during disease outbreaks. By analyzing data from various sources, AI can identify potential contacts, facilitate timely notifications and isolation, and provide insights for public health strategies. Additionally, AI can help to monitor compliance with social distancing measures and assist in crowd management. However, privacy preservation remains a critical challenge that needs to be addressed to ensure the ethical and effective implementation of AI in these efforts.

9 Public Awareness and Communication

Public awareness and communication are crucial in managing disease outbreaks, and AI-powered chatbots and virtual assistants have emerged as valuable tools in this regard. These AI systems can provide accurate and timely information about infectious diseases to the public, answering frequently asked questions, offering guidance on preventive measures, and dispelling misinformation [77]. By analyzing social media conversations, AI can also identify rumors or misinformation spreading rapidly and help authorities respond effectively with accurate information [78].

During the onset of the COVID-19 pandemic, social media platforms were flooded with misinformation, including rumors about the virus and its transmission. The spread of such misinformation can lead to confusion and hinder effective public health responses [79]. To address this issue, researchers have utilized AI techniques to detect and analyze rumors on social media platforms. For example, they developed a novel feature space that includes psycholinguistic features to detect rumor instances with high accuracy [77]. By incorporating psycholinguistic features, the study aimed to improve the detection accuracy of rumors on social media. In addition to detecting rumors, AI can also play a role in quantifying the amount of COVID-19 content among online opponents of established health guidance. Sear et al. used machine learning to quantify COVID-19 content among the anti-vaccination community on social media platforms [78]. The study found that the anti-vax community exhibited a broader range of COVID-19 topics, potentially appealing to a broader cross-section of individuals seeking COVID-19 guidance online. This highlights the importance of countering misinformation and promoting accurate information to ensure widespread adoption of COVID-19 vaccines and achieve herd immunity.

Furthermore, AI can contribute to public awareness and communication by ensuring the privacy and security of individuals' data. For instance, proposed an epidemiological approach to control the dissemination of fake information in online social networks [80]. By analyzing the spread of misinformation, AI can help identify and mitigate the negative impact of fake news on public health and societal harmony. The use of AI in public awareness and communication is not without challenges. One of the main challenges is the rapid dissemination of misinformation through social media platforms. Researchers have developed AI-based models for the detection of fake news and misinformation, but there is a need for continuous improvement and the development of scalable solutions [81]. Additionally, ensuring the interpretability of AI models is crucial to build trust and transparency in the information provided to the public [82].

In the field of healthcare and infectious diseases, large language models like ChatGPT have shown promise in various applications. AI-powered chatbots, including ChatGPT, have been used to combat the COVID-19 pandemic by increasing public awareness, optimizing the use of health resources, and reducing unnecessary encounters. These chatbots simulate human conversation and utilize artificial intelligence techniques such as natural language processing (NLP) to interact with users. By leveraging NLP platforms like Google Dialogflow, Rasa framework, and IBM Watson, AI chatbots can understand natural language input and act on user requests [83]. One of the key advantages of AI chatbots in public health communication is their ability to provide accurate information and dispel misinformation. These chatbots can analyze social media conversations and identify rumors or misinformation, helping authorities respond effectively [84]. However, it is important to address challenges such as the spread of fake information and the need for explainable AI models to ensure the effectiveness and trustworthiness of AI in public health communication. Explainable AI is a rapidly growing research discipline that aims to address concerns about the safety and ethical usage of AI [85]. AI-powered chatbots and virtual assistants have become valuable tools in public awareness and communication during disease outbreaks. These AI systems can provide accurate information, guidance, and dispel misinformation. By analyzing social media conversations, AI can identify rumors or misinformation and help authorities respond effectively. However, challenges such as the spread of fake information and the need for explainable AI models need to be addressed to ensure the effectiveness and trustworthiness of AI in public health communication.

References

1. C. Institute of Medicine Committee on Emerging Microbial Threats to Health in the 21st, in *Microbial Threats to Health: Emergence, Detection, and Response*, ed. by M.S. Smolinski, M.A. Hamburg, J. Lederberg, (National Academies Press (US). Copyright 2003 by the National Academy of Sciences. All rights reserved, Washington, DC, 2003)
2. N.A. Mohamad, N.A. Jusoh, Z.Z. Htike, S.L. Win, Bacteria identification from microscopic morphology using naïve bayes. Int. J. Comput. Eng. Inf. Technol. **4**(2), 1–9 (2014)
3. V.R. Vijaykumar, Classifying bacterial species using computer vision and machine learning. Int. J. Comput. Appl. **151**, 23–26 (2016)
4. E.A. Hay, R. Parthasarathy, Performance of convolutional neural networks for identification of bacteria in 3D microscopy datasets. PLoS Comput. Biol. **14**(12), e1006628 (2018). https://doi.org/10.1371/journal.pcbi.1006628
5. T. Ahmed, M.F. Wahid, M.J. Hasan, Combining deep convolutional neural network with support vector machine to classify microscopic bacteria images, in *2019 International Conference on Electrical, Computer and Communication Engineering (ECCE)*, (7–9 Feb 2019, 2019), pp. 1–5. https://doi.org/10.1109/ECACE.2019.8679397
6. C. Szegedy, V. Vanhoucke, S. Ioffe, J. Shlens, Z. Wojna, Rethinking the inception architecture for computer vision, in *2016 IEEE Conference on Computer Vision and Pattern Recognition (CVPR)*, (27–30 June 2016, 2016), pp. 2818–2826. https://doi.org/10.1109/CVPR.2016.308
7. C.S. Ho et al., Rapid identification of pathogenic bacteria using Raman spectroscopy and deep learning (in eng). Nat. Commun. **10**(1), 4927 (2019). https://doi.org/10.1038/s41467-019-12898-9
8. X. Wu, J. Chen, X. Li, Y. Zhao, S.M. Zughaier, Culture-free diagnostics of Pseudomonas aeruginosa infection by silver nanorod array based SERS from clinical sputum samples. Nanomedicine **10**(8), 1863–1870 (2014). https://doi.org/10.1016/j.nano.2014.04.010
9. X. Wu, Y. Zhao, S.M. Zughaier, Highly sensitive detection and differentiation of endotoxins derived from bacterial pathogens by surface-enhanced Raman scattering. Biosensors (Basel) **11**(7) (2021). https://doi.org/10.3390/bios11070234
10. B.L. Thomsen et al., Accurate and fast identification of minimally prepared bacteria phenotypes using Raman spectroscopy assisted by machine learning. Sci. Rep. **12**(1) (2022). https://doi.org/10.1038/s41598-022-20850-z
11. Y.-Y. Han et al., Rapid antibiotic susceptibility testing of bacteria from patients' blood via assaying bacterial metabolic response with surface-enhanced Raman spectroscopy. Sci. Rep. **10**(1), 12538 (2020). https://doi.org/10.1038/s41598-020-68855-w
12. N. Ibtehaz, M.E.H. Chowdhury, A. Khandakar, S. Kiranyaz, M.S. Rahman, S.M. Zughaier, RamanNet: A generalized neural network architecture for Raman spectrum analysis. Neural Comput. & Applic. (2023). https://doi.org/10.1007/s00521-023-08700-z
13. Y. Yang et al., Rapid detection of SARS-CoV-2 RNA in human nasopharyngeal specimens using surface-enhanced Raman spectroscopy and deep learning algorithms. ACS Sens. **8**(1), 297–307 (2023). https://doi.org/10.1021/acssensors.2c02194
14. C. Tian, L. Zhao, G. Qi, J. Zhu, S. Zhang, One-pot and rapid detection of SARS-CoV-2 viral particles in environment using SERS aptasensor based on a locking amplifier. Sensors Actuators B Chem. **371**, 132445 (2022). https://doi.org/10.1016/j.snb.2022.132445
15. L. Ma, J. Yi, N. Wisuthiphaet, M. Earles, N. Nitin, Accelerating the detection of bacteria in food using artificial intelligence and optical imaging (in eng). Appl. Environ. Microbiol. **89**(1), e0182822 (2023). https://doi.org/10.1128/aem.01828-22
16. A. Bochkovskiy, C.-Y. Wang, Y. Hong, YOLOv4: Optimal speed and accuracy of object detection. arXiv pre-print server. arxiv:2004.10934 (2020)
17. G. Kim et al., Rapid species identification of pathogenic bacteria from a minute quantity exploiting three-dimensional quantitative phase imaging and artificial neural network. Light Sci. Appl. **11**(1), 190 (2022). https://doi.org/10.1038/s41377-022-00881-x

18. C. Weis et al., Direct antimicrobial resistance prediction from clinical MALDI-TOF mass spectra using machine learning. Nat. Med. **28**(1), 164–174 (2022). https://doi.org/10.1038/s41591-021-01619-9
19. F. Wang et al., Pneumonia-plus: A deep learning model for the classification of bacterial, fungal, and viral pneumonia based on CT tomography. Eur. Radiol. (2023). https://doi.org/10.1007/s00330-023-09833-4
20. S.K.A. Degerli, M.E.H. Chowdhury, M. Gabbouj, Osegnet: Operational segmentation network for Covid-19 detection using chest X-ray images, in *2022 IEEE International Conference on Image Processing (ICIP)*, (2022), pp. 2306–2310. https://doi.org/10.1109/ICIP46576.2022.9897412
21. A. Sharma, S. Rani, D. Gupta, Artificial intelligence-based classification of chest X-ray images into COVID-19 and other infectious diseases. Int. J. Biomed. Imaging **2020**, 8889023 (2020). https://doi.org/10.1155/2020/8889023
22. J. Guiot et al., Development and validation of an automated radiomic CT signature for detecting COVID-19. Diagnostics (Basel) **11**(1) (2020). https://doi.org/10.3390/diagnostics11010041
23. T. Wagner et al., Augmented curation of clinical notes from a massive EHR system reveals symptoms of impending COVID-19 diagnosis. elife **9** (2020). https://doi.org/10.7554/eLife.58227
24. F. Khounraz et al., Prognosis of COVID-19 patients using lab tests: A data mining approach. Health Sci. Rep. **6**(1), e1049 (2023). https://doi.org/10.1002/hsr2.1049
25. K.T. Liu et al., Quantifying neutralizing antibodies in patients with COVID-19 by a two-variable generalized additive model. mSphere **7**(1), e0088321 (2022). https://doi.org/10.1128/msphere.00883-21
26. Y. Zhan, Y. Wang, W. Zhang, B. Ying, C. Wang, Diagnostic accuracy of the artificial intelligence methods in medical imaging for pulmonary tuberculosis: A systematic review and meta-analysis. J. Clin. Med. **12**(1) (2022). https://doi.org/10.3390/jcm12010303
27. S. Kazemzadeh et al., Deep learning detection of active pulmonary tuberculosis at chest radiography matched the clinical performance of radiologists. Radiology **306**(1), 124–137 (2023). https://doi.org/10.1148/radiol.212213
28. R. Ehrlich et al., Accuracy of computer-aided detection of occupational lung disease: Silicosis and pulmonary tuberculosis in ex-miners from the South African gold mines. Int. J. Environ. Res. Public Health **19**(19) (2022). https://doi.org/10.3390/ijerph191912402
29. S.M. Gelaw, S.V. Kik, M. Ruhwald, S. Ongarello, T.S. Egzertegegne, O. Gorbacheva, et al., Diagnostic accuracy of three computer-aided detection systems for detecting pulmonary tuberculosis on chest radiography when used for screening: Analysis of an international, multicenter migrants screening study. PLOS Glob. Public Health **3**(7), e0000402 (2023). https://doi.org/10.1371/journal.pgph.0000402
30. S. Weissman, X. Yang, J. Zhang, S. Chen, B. Olatosi, X. Li, Using a machine learning approach to explore predictors of healthcare visits as missed opportunities for HIV diagnosis. AIDS **35**(Suppl 1), S7–S18 (2021). https://doi.org/10.1097/QAD.0000000000002735
31. D.J. Feller, J. Zucker, M.T. Yin, P. Gordon, N. Elhadad, Using clinical notes and natural language processing for automated HIV risk assessment. J. Acquir. Immune Defic. Syndr. **77**(2), 160–166 (2018). https://doi.org/10.1097/QAI.0000000000001580
32. Y. Xiang, K. Fujimoto, J. Schneider, Y. Jia, D. Zhi, C. Tao, Network context matters: Graph convolutional network model over social networks improves the detection of unknown HIV infections among young men who have sex with men. J. Am. Med. Inform. Assoc. **26**(11), 1263–1271 (2019). https://doi.org/10.1093/jamia/ocz070
33. L.A. Jackson et al., An mRNA vaccine against SARS-CoV-2—Preliminary report. N. Engl. J. Med. (2020). https://doi.org/10.1056/nejmoa2022483
34. A. Sadybekov, V. Katritch, Computational approaches streamlining drug discovery. Nature (2023). https://doi.org/10.1038/s41586-023-05905-z
35. M.Y. Ansari, V. Chandrasekar, A.K. Singh, S.P. Dakua, Re-routing drugs to blood brain barrier: A comprehensive analysis of machine learning approaches with fingerprint amalgamation and data balancing. IEEE Access (2023). https://doi.org/10.1109/access.2022.3233110

36. T. Pillaiyar, M. Manickam, V. Namasivayam, Y. Hayashi, S.H. Jung, An overview of severe acute respiratory syndrome-coronavirus (SARS-CoV) 3CL protease inhibitors: Peptidomimetics and small molecule chemotherapy. J. Med. Chem. **59**(14), 6595–6628 (2016). https://doi.org/10.1021/acs.jmedchem.5b01461
37. H. Komatsu et al., Identification of SARS-CoV-2 main protease inhibitors from FDA-approved drugs by artificial intelligence-supported activity prediction system. J. Biomol. Struct. Dyn. **41**(5), 1767–1775 (2023). https://doi.org/10.1080/07391102.2021.2024260
38. A.M. Andrianov, M.A. Shuldau, K.V. Furs, A.M. Yushkevich, A.V. Tuzikov, AI-driven de novo design and molecular modeling for discovery of small-molecule compounds as potential drug candidates targeting SARS-CoV-2 main protease. Int. J. Mol. Sci. **24**(9) (2023). https://doi.org/10.3390/ijms24098083
39. L.C. Saramago et al., AI-driven discovery of SARS-CoV-2 Main protease fragment-like inhibitors with antiviral activity in vitro. J. Chem. Inf. Model. **63**(9), 2866–2880 (2023). https://doi.org/10.1021/acs.jcim.3c00409
40. B.R. Beck, B. Shin, Y. Choi, S. Park, K. Kang, Predicting commercially available antiviral drugs that may act on the novel coronavirus (SARS-CoV-2) through a drug-target interaction deep learning model. Comput. Struct. Biotechnol. J. **18**, 784–790 (2020). https://doi.org/10.1016/j.csbj.2020.03.025
41. Y. Ge et al., An integrative drug repositioning framework discovered a potential therapeutic agent targeting COVID-19. Signal Transduct. Target. Ther. **6**(1), 165 (2021). https://doi.org/10.1038/s41392-021-00568-6
42. J.M. Stokes et al., A deep learning approach to antibiotic discovery. Cell **181**(2), 475–483 (2020). https://doi.org/10.1016/j.cell.2020.04.001
43. S. Black, D.E. Bloom, D.C. Kaslow, S. Pecetta, R. Rappuoli, Transforming vaccine development. Semin. Immunol. **50**, 101413 (2020). https://doi.org/10.1016/j.smim.2020.101413
44. E. Ong, H. Wang, M.U. Wong, M. Seetharaman, N. Valdez, Y. He, Vaxign-ML: Supervised machine learning reverse vaccinology model for improved prediction of bacterial protective antigens. Bioinformatics **36**(10), 3185–3191 (2020). https://doi.org/10.1093/bioinformatics/btaa119
45. T. Chen, C. Guestrin, XGBoost. ACM (2016). [Online]. Available https://doi.org/10.1145/2939672.2939785
46. E. Ong et al., Vaxign2: The second generation of the first web-based vaccine design program using reverse vaccinology and machine learning. Nucleic Acids Res. **49**(W1), W671–W678 (2021). https://doi.org/10.1093/nar/gkab279
47. M. Dalsass, A. Brozzi, D. Medini, R. Rappuoli, Comparison of open-source reverse vaccinology programs for bacterial vaccine antigen discovery. Front. Immunol. **10**, 113 (2019). https://doi.org/10.3389/fimmu.2019.00113
48. A.P. Hederman, M.E. Ackerman, Leveraging deep learning to improve vaccine design. Trends Immunol. **44**(5), 333–344 (2023). https://doi.org/10.1016/j.it.2023.03.002
49. S. Xu, X. Wang, C. Fei, A highly effective system for predicting MHC-II epitopes with immunogenicity. Front. Oncol. **12**, 888556 (2022). https://doi.org/10.3389/fonc.2022.888556
50. M.S. Sohail, S.F. Ahmed, A.A. Quadeer, M.R. McKay, In silico T cell epitope identification for SARS-CoV-2: Progress and perspectives. Adv. Drug Deliv. Rev. **171**, 29–47 (2021). https://doi.org/10.1016/j.addr.2021.01.007
51. O.J. Dyar, B. Huttner, J. Schouten, C. Pulcini, Esgap, What is antimicrobial stewardship? Clin. Microbiol. Infect. **23**(11), 793–798 (2017). https://doi.org/10.1016/j.cmi.2017.08.026
52. M. Cavallaro, E. Moran, B. Collyer, N.D. McCarthy, C. Green, M.J. Keeling, Informing antimicrobial stewardship with explainable AI. PLOS Digit Health **2**(1), e0000162 (2023). https://doi.org/10.1371/journal.pdig.0000162
53. T. Cai et al., Artificial intelligence can guide antibiotic choice in recurrent UTIs and become an important aid to improve antimicrobial stewardship. Antibiotics (Basel) **12**(2) (2023). https://doi.org/10.3390/antibiotics12020375
54. M. Oonsivilai et al., Using machine learning to guide targeted and locally-tailored empiric antibiotic prescribing in a children's hospital in Cambodia. Wellcome Open Res. **3**, 131 (2018). https://doi.org/10.12688/wellcomeopenres.14847.1

55. WHO, One health initiative. https://www.who.int/teams/one-health-initiative. Accessed 1 Sept 2023
56. C.J. Carlson et al., The future of zoonotic risk prediction. Philos. Trans. R. Soc. Lond. Ser. B Biol. Sci. **376**(1837), 20200358 (2021). https://doi.org/10.1098/rstb.2020.0358
57. I. Dayan et al., Federated learning for predicting clinical outcomes in patients with COVID-19. Nat. Med. **27**(10), 1735–1743 (2021). https://doi.org/10.1038/s41591-021-01506-3
58. T.T. Kuo, R.A. Gabriel, L. Ohno-Machado, Fair compute loads enabled by blockchain: Sharing models by alternating client and server roles. J. Am. Med. Inform. Assoc. **26**(5), 392–403 (2019). https://doi.org/10.1093/jamia/ocy180
59. A.R. Ghavamipour, F. Turkmen, X. Jiang, Privacy-preserving logistic regression with secret sharing. BMC Med. Inform. Decis. Mak. **22**(1), 89 (2022). https://doi.org/10.1186/s12911-022-01811-y
60. V. Moorthy, A.M. Henao Restrepo, M.P. Preziosi, S. Swaminathan, Data sharing for novel coronavirus (COVID-19). Bull. World Health Organ. **98**(3), 150 (2020). https://doi.org/10.2471/BLT.20.251561
61. V.G. Dugan et al., Standardized metadata for human pathogen/vector genomic sequences. PLoS One **9**(6), e99979 (2014). https://doi.org/10.1371/journal.pone.0099979
62. A. Lopez-Rincon et al., Classification and specific primer design for accurate detection of SARS-CoV-2 using deep learning. Sci. Rep. **11**(1), 947 (2021). https://doi.org/10.1038/s41598-020-80363-5
63. S. Zhang et al., Identification and validation of prognostic factors in patients with COVID-19: A retrospective study based on artificial intelligence algorithms. J. Intensive Med. **1**(2), 103–109 (2021). https://doi.org/10.1016/j.jointm.2021.04.001
64. A. Roncancio-Clavijo et al., Early biochemical analysis of COVID-19 patients helps severity prediction. PLoS One **18**(5), e0283469 (2023). https://doi.org/10.1371/journal.pone.0283469
65. Z. Li et al., Monitoring the spatial spread of COVID-19 and effectiveness of control measures through human movement data: Proposal for a predictive model using big data analytics. JMIR Res. Protoc. **9**(12), e24432 (2020). https://doi.org/10.2196/24432
66. Y. Bao et al., Predicting the diagnosis of HIV and sexually transmitted infections among men who have sex with men using machine learning approaches. J. Inf. Secur. **82**(1), 48–59 (2021). https://doi.org/10.1016/j.jinf.2020.11.007
67. X. Xu et al., Web-based risk prediction tool for an individual's risk of HIV and sexually transmitted infections using machine learning algorithms: Development and external validation study. J. Med. Internet Res. **24**(8), e37850 (2022). https://doi.org/10.2196/37850
68. S.K. Brooks et al., The psychological impact of quarantine and how to reduce it: Rapid review of the evidence. Lancet (2020). https://doi.org/10.1016/s0140-6736(20)30460-8
69. S. Shiraki, S. Shioda, Contact information-based indoor pedestrian localization using bluetooth low energy beacons. IEEE Access (2022). https://doi.org/10.1109/access.2022.3222301
70. E. Hernández-Orallo, P. Manzoni, C.T. Calafate, J.-C. Cano, Evaluating how smartphone contact tracing technology can reduce the spread of infectious diseases: The case of COVID-19. IEEE Access (2020). https://doi.org/10.1109/access.2020.2998042
71. H. Ryu, A. Abulali, S.-M. Lee, Assessing the effectiveness of isolation and contact-tracing interventions for early transmission dynamics of COVID-19 in South Korea. IEEE Access (2021). https://doi.org/10.1109/access.2021.3064371
72. L. Valcarenghi et al., Managing physical distancing through 5G and accelerated edge cloud. IEEE Access (2022). https://doi.org/10.1109/access.2022.3210262
73. A.H. Mutlag, S.Q. Mahdi, S.K. Gharghan, O.N.M. Salim, A. Al-Naji, J. Chahl, Improved control system based on PSO and ANN for social distancing for patients with COVID-19. IEEE Access (2022). https://doi.org/10.1109/access.2022.3183124
74. H. Friji, A. Khanfor, H. Ghazzai, Y. Massoud, An end-to-end smart IoT-driven navigation for social distancing enforcement. IEEE Access (2022). https://doi.org/10.1109/access.2022.3192860
75. M.A. Alsahli, A. Alsanad, M.M. Hassan, A. Gumaei, Privacy preservation of user identity in contact tracing for COVID-19-like pandemics using edge computing. IEEE Access (2021). https://doi.org/10.1109/access.2021.3110762

76. M.M. Haque, C. Sheikder, R. Djembong, M.T.W. Piash, Retroactive about robotics application with artificial intelligence toward the global pandemic scenario. Eur. J. Elect. Eng. Comput. Sci. (2023). https://doi.org/10.24018/ejece.2023.7.2.494
77. S. Mahbub, E. Pardede, A.S.M. Kayes, COVID-19 rumor detection using psycho-linguistic features. IEEE Access (2022). https://doi.org/10.1109/access.2022.3220369
78. R.P. Sear et al., Quantifying COVID-19 content in the online health opinion war using machine learning. IEEE Access (2020). https://doi.org/10.1109/access.2020.2993967
79. N. Kandel, S. Chungong, A. Omaar, J. Xing, Health security capacities in the context of COVID-19 outbreak: An analysis of international health regulations annual report data from 182 countries. Lancet (2020). https://doi.org/10.1016/s0140-6736(20)30553-5
80. R. Singh, A. Galletta, Controlling of fake information dissemination in online social networks: An epidemiological approach. IEEE Access (2023). https://doi.org/10.1109/access.2023.3262737
81. A. Altheneyan, A. Alhadlaq, Big data ML-based fake news detection using distributed learning. IEEE Access (2023). https://doi.org/10.1109/access.2023.3260763
82. K. Gaiger, O. Barkan, S. Tsipory-Samuel, N. Koenigstein, Not all memories created equal: Dynamic user representations for collaborative filtering. IEEE Access (2023). https://doi.org/10.1109/access.2023.3263931
83. A. Mahdavi, M. Amanzadeh, M. Hamedan, R. Naemi, Artificial intelligence based chatbots to combat COVID-19 pandemic: A scoping review. Syst. Rev. (2023). https://doi.org/10.21203/rs.3.rs-2565141/v1
84. M.O. Lwin et al., Global sentiments surrounding the COVID-19 pandemic on Twitter: Analysis of Twitter trends. JMIR Public Health Surveill. (2020). https://doi.org/10.2196/19447
85. Y. Zhang, Q.V. Liao, R.K.E. Bellamy, Effect of confidence and explanation on accuracy and trust calibration in AI-assisted decision making, in *FAT '20: Proceedings of the 2020 Conference on Fairness, Accountability, and Transparency*, (2020). https://doi.org/10.1145/3351095.3372852

Application of Big Data in Infectious Disease Surveillance: Contemporary Challenges and Solutions

Adiba Tabassum Chowdhury, Mehrin Newaz, Purnata Saha, Molla E. Majid, Adam Mushtak, and Muhammad Ashad Kabir

1 Introduction

Because of the confluence of technical developments and the ongoing dangers posed by new diseases, the area of infectious disease monitoring has experienced a significant transition recently. In a world that is becoming more interconnected, data-driven decision-making has become the cornerstone of public health efforts, and this transition is taking place against this backdrop. The novel term "Big Data," which has acquired popularity because of the exponential increase of enormous and varied datasets, is at the center of this movement [11]. Big Data defies the conventional limitations of data management and analysis due to its sheer volume, velocity, diversity, and accuracy. It offers a wide-ranging lens through which we can acquire insights into the complex web of global health dynamics [14].

The purpose of this work is to conduct a thorough investigation of the wide range of big data applications in infectious disease surveillance. Our goal is to explore deeply into this dynamic confluence, where modern problems are met with creative analytical model solutions. By doing this, we hope to highlight how Big Data has the power to fundamentally alter how infectious diseases are monitored

A. T. Chowdhury (✉) · M. Newaz · P. Saha
Department of Electrical and Electronic Engineering, University of Dhaka, Dhaka, Bangladesh

M. E. Majid
Computer Applications Department, Academic Bridge Program, Qatar Foundation, Doha, Qatar

A. Mushtak
Department of Radiology, Hamad Medical Corporation, Doha, Qatar

M. A. Kabir
School of Computing, Mathematics and Engineering, Charles Sturt University, Bathurst, NSW, Australia
e-mail: akabir@csu.edu.au

M. E. H. Chowdhury, S. Kiranyaz (eds.), *Surveillance, Prevention, and Control of Infectious Diseases*, https://doi.org/10.1007/978-3-031-59967-5_3

and managed. Our capacity to identify, follow, and address disease outbreaks has undergone a fundamental shift because of the widespread use of big data in the field of infectious disease surveillance. As we work our way through the complexities of this rapidly developing sector, we discover that big Data is not just a catchphrase, it has profound consequences for public health [32]. It permits the real-time gathering and analysis of data from numerous sources, including social media, wearable technology, electronic health records, and remote sensing techniques. These sources offer a plethora of data that, when appropriately tapped into, can provide early warnings of disease outbreaks, help with the quick assessment of their spread, and make it easier to establish targeted intervention plans [8].

As we seek to close the gap between research and actual application, the review's relevance goes beyond the theoretical sphere. To demonstrate how Big Data is substantively transforming the landscape of infectious disease surveillance, we will critically examine the state of current research, new trends, and case studies. [1] provides one such example, showing the value of integrating mobile apps and dashboards into infectious disease surveillance systems, streamlining data collection, reporting, and analysis procedures, and ultimately improving our capacity to respond to outbreaks.

This chapter aims to give a thorough overview of the crucial part Big Data plays in infectious disease surveillance. In addition to highlighting the current issues the industry is facing, it also provides creative fixes with analytical models that make use of Big Data. We want to encourage a greater knowledge of how Big Data might result in more efficient and successful tactics for disease monitoring, prevention, and control on a worldwide scale. Through this investigation, we hope to inform and inspire new developments in the field of infectious disease surveillance.

2 Challenges of Traditional Surveillance Method

In the context of infectious diseases, the term "traditional surveillance methods" refers to tried-and-true techniques for keeping an eye on disease occurrence and spread within a population by manual data collecting and human observation. Healthcare professionals, laboratories, and public health organizations collect and report data manually via traditional surveillance approaches. Important elements of conventional surveillance include [27]:

Case Reporting: When diagnosed, certain infectious diseases must be reported to local health authorities by healthcare providers. Since so much of this reporting depends on human interaction, data gathering is frequently delayed and inconsistent.

Diagnostic laboratories are crucial in establishing the existence of infectious illness cases. The procedure of reporting results to public health organizations can be time-consuming and error prone.

Contact Tracing: To find potential sources of transmission, epidemiologists manually track the contacts of affected people. This time-consuming method can miss certain connections and impede quick epidemic containment.

Data analysis: After data has been gathered, it is manually examined to find trends and patterns, enabling decision-making by health experts. This study could be sluggish and might miss any immediate dangers that emerge.

Traditional surveillance techniques have been the cornerstone of infectious disease monitoring, although they have some drawbacks. There are various ways in which these restrictions can compromise the safety and efficiency of public health interventions:

Lack of Timeliness: Manual data collection and reporting can cause delays in outbreak detection and response, like the COVID-19 pandemic, while simultaneously protecting patients' privacy and preventing data abuse, possibly allowing infectious diseases to proliferate unchecked [9].

Underreporting: Not every case is reported, and the data that is reported can be inaccurate in some cases. It can result in an underestimation of the disease burden, which makes it difficult to deploy resources efficiently [30].

Limited Data Integration: Data gathered using conventional methods sometimes exist in silos, making it challenging to combine and evaluate data thoroughly. This makes it more difficult to spot larger trends and anticipate new epidemics [30].

Resource Intensity: Traditional surveillance demands significant financial and human resources, which may not be scalable or sustainable in the event of widespread pandemics or in environments with limited resources. Also, ensuring healthcare data security and patient privacy remains a concern of paramount importance ([6]).

Given these difficulties, there is a growing understanding of the necessity for increasingly sophisticated surveillance techniques that make use of technology and data analytics. In order to overcome these shortcomings and improve the security of public health systems in the face of infectious disease risks, big data analytics surveillance technologies present a possible alternative required [21].

3 Research Methodology

3.1 Search Strategy

To find pertinent studies in electronic databases, a thorough search technique was used.

1. Searching through relevant databases, such as PubMed, Google Scholar, Scopus, IEEE Xplore, and Web of Science
2. Starting by conducting a general search using keywords:

"Big Data" or "Data Analytics" or "Data Mining", and "Communicable Disease" or "Infectious Disease" and "disease surveillance"

3. Including terms that specific to infectious diseases and information sources to broaden the search:

"COVID-19" or "Ebola" or "Dengue" or "Influenza" or "Malaria" or "Tuberculosis" and "Social Media" or "Electronic Health Records" or "Wearable devices" or "remote sensing" or "geospatial data"

4. Setting a time limit of the last 10 years (2013–2023) for the publication date
5. Finding relevant references by backward and forward search

3.2 Inclusion and Exclusion Criteria

In the process of selection, this study adhered to a set of defined inclusion and exclusion criteria to ensure rigor and relevance.

Inclusion Criteria:

1. Research focusing on the utilization of big data to surveil infectious diseases, employing substantial datasets and data-centric methodologies
2. Consideration of peer-reviewed journal articles, conference proceedings, reports, white papers, and relevant gray literature
3. Emphasis on research conducted within the timeframe of the last decade (2013–2023), ensuring contemporary and pertinent findings
4. Incorporation of a diverse range of big data sources, such as social media, mobile phones, satellite imagery, electronic health records, internet searches, etc.
5. Incorporation of studies spanning varied geographical regions, thereby capturing a global outlook on infectious disease surveillance

Exclusion Criteria:

1. Exclusion of studies lacking explicit focus on the use of big data for infectious disease surveillance and sufficient depth regarding methodologies and implications
2. Non-English publications, as the review's scope is limited to English language sources
3. Exclusion of non-peer-reviewed materials unless they present substantial and pertinent data not covered in peer-reviewed literature
4. Exclusion of studies primarily centered on infectious disease surveillance in animals
5. Avoidance of duplicate publications or reports stemming from the same study to minimize redundancy
6. Disregarding studies with extremely small sample sizes that may not contribute meaningful insights

7. Exclusion of studies primarily focused on outdated techniques or tools no longer relevant in modern practices
8. Exclusion of studies lacking full-text availability to ensure an exhaustive and transparent review process

3.3 *Study Selection*

The first phase involved the methodical removal of duplicate papers from the 81 primarily selected papers based on our search criteria to ensure a simplified dataset once the aforementioned search approach is implemented throughout the targeted databases. Then, a thorough screening procedure was carried out, which involved carefully going over titles and abstracts to make sure they matched the study question and predefined inclusion criteria. At this point, 24 articles that categorically lacked relevancy were immediately excluded. The retrieval of full-text versions of the retained studies that had passed the initial screening comprised the next phase. These 40 full-text papers were each thoroughly examined in comparison to the predetermined inclusion and exclusion criteria. Due to the complexity of the assessment process, it was necessary to carefully evaluate the articles to determine whether they met the requirements for the systematic review. Any articles that did not fit the requirements were methodically removed from the final list that contained 24 pieces (4 original works and 20 review works). After backward and forward search, 3 more review articles were added to the database making it a list of 27. Throughout this screening process, a thorough log of the justifications for excluding articles was maintained, as shown in Fig. 1.

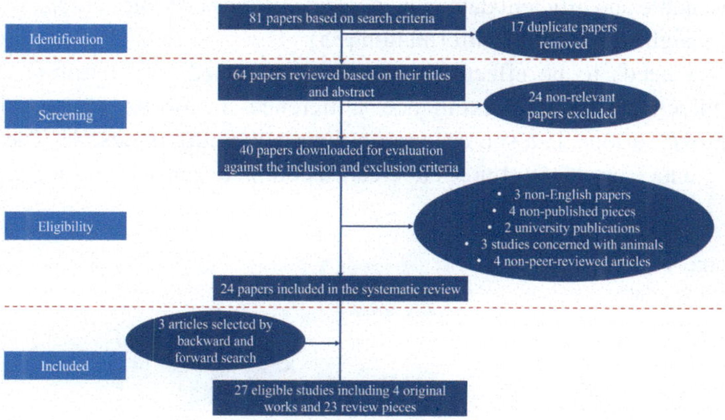

Fig. 1 Search and selection process using PRISMA flowchart

4 Data Collection and Data Management

In the age of Big Data, there is enormous promise for understanding disease dynamics and tackling new health challenges due to the synergy between modern data analytics and infectious disease surveillance. This potential is supported by the complexity of data management, the enormous volume of information, and various gathering techniques [3]. This section explores these fundamental concepts, which are essential for using big data to unravel the complexities of infectious diseases.

Strong data-gathering procedures that capture the complex dynamics of disease transmission are essential for the effective application of big data in infectious disease surveillance and modeling. Data gathering in this context involves a wide range of sources, from conventional health records to modern digital platforms. Electronic health records (EHRs) provide a thorough database of patient data, allowing for the extraction of insightful data on illness patterns and population health [33]. A new era of unprecedented data accessibility has also been ushered in by the growth of digital devices, social media, and wearable technology. These developments have made it possible to access real-time data streams that provide insightful hints about people's activities, mobility patterns, and environmental factors [8]. A summary of the data sources used in this study is illustrated in Fig. 2.

Massive informational quantities, or "big data," are essential for modeling and monitoring infectious illness. A detailed understanding of disease dynamics is made possible by a variety of data sources. An unparalleled amount of information is possible thanks to the data collection from sensors, medical records, and social media [8]. However, this abundance creates problems for data processing, storage, and analysis. To handle the complex task of organizing and processing this flood of data, new computational frameworks, cloud-based architectures, and distributed computing paradigms have evolved [5]. As the amount of data keeps increasing, utilizing scalable and efficient data management systems becomes crucial to provide insightful insights and helpful information [35].

Big Data needs to be effectively integrated, cleaned, and harmonized to be used for infectious disease surveillance. Differences in format, organization, and quality among various data sources present interoperability issues [4]. The process of merging data from many sources to create a complete dataset for comprehending

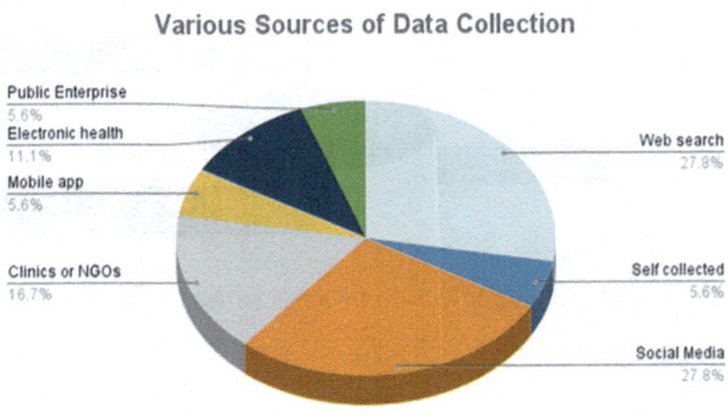

Fig. 2 Sources of data collection for big data analysis

sickness patterns is known as data integration. More data cleansing and validation is needed to correct errors, eliminate duplicates, and enhance analytical accuracy [5]. Data harmonization guarantees consistency among many sources, supporting well-rounded analyses. Strong data management not only makes analysis simpler but also improves the accuracy of the results, allowing academics and public health experts to draw reliable conclusions.

5 Descriptive Summary of the Extracted Bibliographies

The production of research in the field "Application of Big Data in Infectious Diseases" grew remarkably in the last decade, as found in PubMed. But it started becoming significant after 2018. In the remaining months of 2023, it is expected to reach a higher number. Figure 3 depicts that the annual publication production increased steadily over the course of 10 years, from 2013 to 2023, at a pace of 3.46% per year on average.

From these publications, a bibliographic dataset was chosen that included 1653 references, 162 authors, and 27 documents from 26 sources. Four documents (14.8%) are original research pieces, leaving 23 (85.2%) of the 27 documents as review papers. There were 6 articles where we found similar authors or co-authors. Those were represented as author collaborations. Table 1 gives a statistical overview of the key traits of these 38 articles, including their chronological range, authors, and other pertinent details.

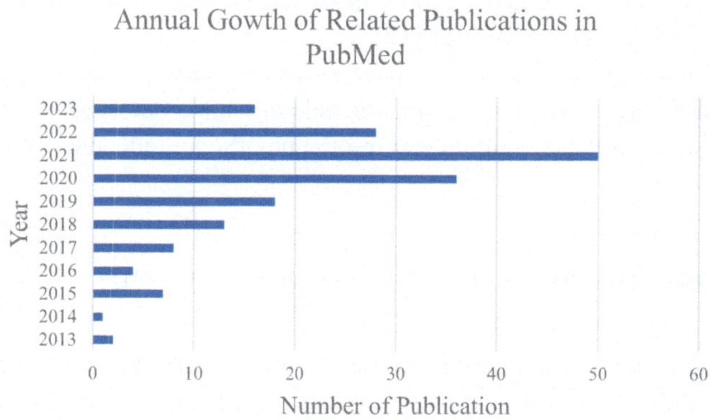

Fig. 3 Annual growth of publications related to big data in infectious diseases in PubMed

Table 1 Main descriptive summary of the extracted bibliographic records from 2013 to 2023

Description	Result
Time Span (Years)	2013–2023
Number of Sources	26
Number of Documents	27
Number of Documents Per Year (Average)	2.7
Number of Average Citations Per Document	92.26
Number of References	1653
Number of Total Authors	162
Number of Single-authored Documents	4
Number of Coauthors Per Document	6
Number of Author Collaborations	6
Percentage of International Co-authorship	40.7

6 Enterprise Solutions for Analyzing Healthcare Data

Numerous businesses have incorporated artificial intelligence (AI) into their operations to improve the effectiveness of analytical processes and meet the issues presented by huge volumes of data. This integration enables the examination of textual material, image-based data, and published findings to produce insightful findings. The leading AI platform for the exchange and analysis of health-related data across hospitals, healthcare providers, and researchers is IBM's Watson Health [12]. Similarly, Flatiron Health is an industry leader in technology-driven healthcare analytics, focusing on advances in cancer research. Beyond these, big industry players like Google Inc. and Oracle Corporation are actively working to develop distributed computing platforms and cloud-based storage solutions in an effort to improve their analytical capabilities [12].

An overwhelming number of new businesses and startups devoted to providing analytics and solutions for the healthcare industry have emerged in recent years. Table 2 lists some of these vendors serving the healthcare industry.

7 Infectious Disease Active Surveillance Systems

An essential element of managing public health is an active surveillance system for infectious diseases. Such systems enable health authorities to quickly spot new hazards and trends by utilizing cutting-edge data collection approaches, such as digital reporting and real-time information sharing. The system's capacity to forecast possible epidemics and distribute resources efficiently is improved by the incorporation of cutting-edge technologies like machine learning and predictive modeling. An optimal surveillance system combines resilience, adaptability, cost-efficiency, and population representation [15]. It demands fast reporting and result confirmation.

Table 2 Large organizations that offer big data analysis solutions in the medical field

Company	Description
IBM Watson Health https://www.ibm.com/watson-health/merative-divestiture	Provides services to assist hospitals, researchers, and providers in exchanging clinical and health-related data
MadeAnalytics https://medeanalytics.com/	Delivers strong health analytics, strategies, and systems, and has a proven track record of success in managing patient data
Health Fidelity https://healthfidelity.com/	Outlines techniques for improving and modifying healthcare organizational procedures and risk management programs
Roam Analytics https://roamanalytics.com/	Offers resources for exploring large amounts of unstructured healthcare data and getting insightful knowledge
Flatiron Health https://flatiron.com/	Applications to enhance oncology data for more effective cancer treatment methods
Enlitic https://www.enlitic.com/	Applying deep learning to massive clinical test datasets for healthcare diagnosis
Digital Reasoning Systems https://digitalreasoning.com/	Offers data analytics tools and services to turn unstructured data into insightful knowledge.
Ayasdi https://www.ayasdi.com/	Provides an upgraded AI platform with clinical variability, population health, risk management, and other healthcare analytics
Linguamatics https://www.linguamatics.com/	Enables the vital insight extraction from unstructured healthcare data using a text mining platform
Apixio https://www.apixio.com/	Offers a framework for cognitive computing that allows for the in-depth analysis of clinical data and PDF health records
Roam Analytics https://roamanalytics.com/	Natural language processing infrastructure in contemporary healthcare systems
Lumiata https://www.lumiata.com	Provides risk management and analytics services to increase the effectiveness of healthcare outcomes
OptumHealth https://www.optum.com/	Presents comprehensive and ground-breaking industry solutions, improves contemporary healthcare infrastructure, and offers healthcare analytics

Additionally, thorough situational awareness depends on several different surveillance data streams, such as death certificates, hospitalization records, ER visits, and outpatient appointments, as well as laboratory-derived data, such as verified cases, genetic sequences, and serological discoveries [29]. This allows health officials to execute focused treatments and lessen the impact on populations. In wealthy countries, systems for monitoring disease incidence and death have existed for centuries, and as shown by the data in Table 3, they have become more intricate and detailed over time [15, 29].

Table 3 Historical overview of disease surveillance and the initial stages of the big data era

Year	Disease	Primary intellectual/Surveillance system	Institution/Country	Area of service	Language	Data source	Data access	User interface	Format
1662	Plague	John Graunt	Bills of Mortality, UK	UK	English	Query	Public	None	Handmade Calculations and Tables
1817	Smallpox	J. C. Moore	London School of Hygiene and Tropical Medicine	UK	English	Query	Public	None	Handmade Calculations and Tables
1847	Influenza	William Farr	General Registrar Office, UK	UK	English	Query	Public	None	Handmade Calculations and Tables
1854	Cholera	John Snow	General Registrar Office, UK	UK	English	Query	Public	None	Handmade Calculations and Tables
1900	All	International Classification of Diseases	WHO	WHO Member States	English	News/Reports	Restricted	Conceptual Framework	Comparable Statistics and Semantic Interoperability
1918	Influenza	121 Cities Mortality Reporting System	CDC	Europe	Spanish	News/Reports	Restricted	Conceptual Framework	Comparable Statistics and Semantic Interoperability
1976	Influenza	Weekly Viral Surveillance	CDC	Europe	Spanish	News/Media Reports	Restricted	Conceptual Framework	Comparable Statistics and Semantic Interoperability
1984	Viral Hepatitis, Mumps, Measles, Influenza	First Computerized Disease Surveillance Network	French Sentinelles Network	France	French	News/Media Reports	Restricted	Conceptual Framework	Comparable Statistics and Semantic Interoperability

1994	SARS	ProMED-Mail	USA	Worldwide	7 Languages	News/ Media Reports	Public	None	Email alert
1997	All	GPHIN	Canada	Worldwide	8 Languages	News/ Media Reports	Subscription	Boolean and Metadata Query System	Website/ Email alert
2000	All	First Medical Claim Forms	Private Companies and Governments	Worldwide	Multiple Languages	News/ Media Reports	Subscription	None	Website/ Email alert
2000	Crohn's disease	GROAN	WHO and UN	Worldwide	English	News/ Media Reports	Restricted	None	Network-based
2004	TB, Cholera	MediSys	EU	EU Member States	43 Languages	Europe Media Monitor	Limited to EU member States	Text Extraction	RSS Feed/ Email/ SMS Alert
2005	Influenza	EpiSimS	USA	USA	English	US Census Data	Restricted	Graphical User Interface and Simulation	XML-based Format
2006	All	BioCaster	Japan	Priority to Asia Pacific region	8 Languages	Query Text Mining	Public	Mapping Interface	RSS Feed
2006	All	EpiSPIDER	USA	North America, Europe, Australia, Asia	English	News/ Media Report, Social Media	Public	Timeline Visualization Mapping, Word Cloud	RSS, Jason, KM Feed
2006	All	Health Map	USA	Worldwide	5 Languages	News/ Media Report, Query, ProMED, WHO	Public	Mapping, Faceted Browsing	Rss Feed
2008	Influenza	Google Flu Trends	Google	28 Countries	39 Languages	Query	Public	Matching Features	Rss Feed

(continued)

Table 3 (continued)

Year	Disease	Primary intellectual/Surveillance system	Institution/Country	Area of service	Language	Data source	Data access	User interface	Format
2008	Influenza	Influenzanet	Europe	11 Countries	10 Languages	Online Questionnaire Response	Public	None	Rss Feed
2010	All	GET WELL	Sweden	Sweden	Swedish	Query	Restricted	Time-series Graphs	HTML Page
2015	Influenza	Birth of Hybrid Systems	Public-Private Partnership	Worldwide	Multiple Languages	Online Questionnaire Response, News, Media Reports	Public	Timeline Visualization Mapping, Word Cloud	HTML Page
2020	COVID-19	COVID Data Tracker	CDC	Worldwide	English, Spanish	Online Questionnaire Response, News, Media Reports, ED information	Public	Timeline Visualization Mapping, Word Cloud	HTML Page

Apart from Table 3, other infectious disease surveillance (IDS) systems have emerged to rapidly gather, analyze, and address outbreaks. Entities like the American Centers for Disease Control and Prevention, Australia's Health Victoria, and Germany's SurvNet have implemented digital and web-based disease notification platforms. These systems prove advantageous for promptly notifying disease outbreaks across decentralized sites like hospitals or community facilities (such as nursing homes and child care centers) to local public health units (PHUs), even when these sites are geographically dispersed [1].

All these techniques, however, take advantage of changes in how information is sought after, gathered, saved, and shared. These changes have coincided with the development and increased accessibility of the Internet and related technologies [27]. Numerous surveillance systems employ unstructured, event-based digital data, which will be addressed in the following sections.

7.1 NDS-Based Surveillance System

Users can activate information flows called NDS (National Data Streams) that include data from a variety of sources, including school attendance, vital statistics, lab results, health records, and sales of various medications [2]. For tracking and making decisions about public health, it is essential to consider how changing public health concerns, such as shifts in sickness rates, interact with the dynamic NDS. Like traditional data sources, for instance, doctor's appointments or test results, developing NDS-based surveillance systems has its share of difficulties [2].

NDS enhances monitoring through faster access, detail, and investigation of unusual illness characteristics. Google Flu Trends is a good example of this because it converts search queries into flu estimates, helping public health, but criticism is raised because user behavior changes when there are anomalies and when it is compared to other systems [18]. Figure 4 illustrates the interplay between user actions (search choices, demographics), external factors (disease changes), and public health measures impacting the connection between public health matters and NDS. Feedback loops emerge from interventions targeting the core issues, influencing the NDS relationship [18]. Data transparency, source code accessibility, and validation techniques are all part of the evaluation of NDS studies. NDS helps with medical and lab-based surveillance but is not a complete replacement; recurrent training on various data subsets is advised for the building of stable models.

An outline of a three-step process for efficiently integrating NDS into surveillance systems is provided: (1) Clearly describe quantitatively the surveillance objectives; (2) construct surveillance models/systems by gradually adding data until no more improvement in fulfilling the objectives is seen; and (3) extensively validate and test the systems. This strategy is consistent with accepted methods for system evaluation [24].

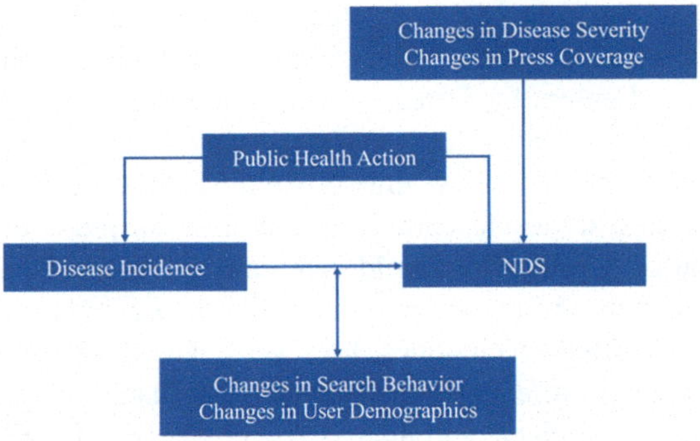

Fig. 4 Interactions and feedback loops between public health issues and NDS

7.2 Smartphone App-Based Surveillance System

Smartphone apps leverage widespread cell phone usage for an Infectious Disease Surveillance (IDS) system, ensuring swift and efficient disease tracking. These software allow medical personnel, public health authorities, and the public to promptly report disease details, symptoms, and outbreaks using their smartphones [13].

Key characteristics of IDS systems based on smartphone apps include [1]:

Real-time Data Collection: Apps allow users to quickly report diseases and symptoms for swift data collection, aiding faster outbreak response.

Maps and geotagging: Geotagging in apps helps map disease spread, aiding authorities in tracking outbreaks' geographic patterns.

Early Warning System: App-based IDS serves as an early warning system by notifying officials about surges in cases or symptoms, enabling quicker responses.

User Engagement: Apps engage the public in disease surveillance, boosting awareness and participation in monitoring efforts.

Data Aggregation and Analysis: App-gathered data is analyzed for trends and clusters, guiding resource allocation and control decisions.

Remote Accessibility: Smartphone apps enable remote disease monitoring, aiding professionals and authorities.

Privacy and Security: Apps prioritize data security with encryption and safeguards.

Support for many languages: Inclusivity is promoted through language options, enhancing diverse user accessibility.

Figure 5 depicts an example guide to an IDS system based on a smartphone app. However, for these systems to be effective on a larger scale, issues pertaining to data accuracy, user engagement, and app uptake must be solved [1].

The presented system consists of a dashboard, cloud server, and mobile app. Staff members utilize the app to input patient data, which is then uploaded to a cloud server for analysis in real time during a disease epidemic. PHU nurses see data on the web dashboard and receive email notifications. The Laravel framework was used to iteratively refine the app depending on PHU feedback, and it is secure

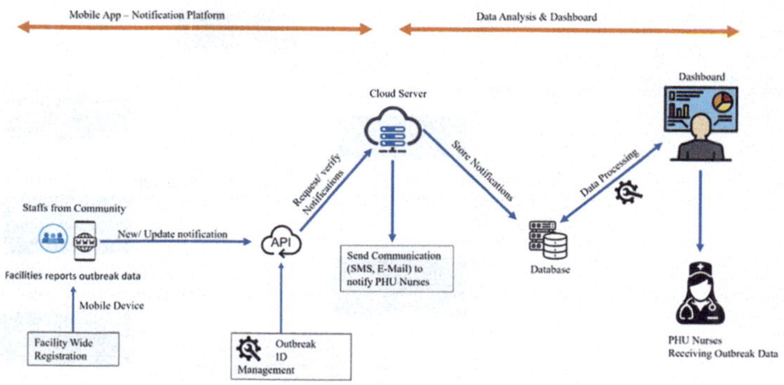

Fig. 5 Overview of a Smartphone app-based IDS System

and encrypted. Data from the app about outbreaks is shown in real time on the dashboard.

7.3 Webpage and Search Engine-Based Surveillance System

For the surveillance of infectious diseases, various technologies provide useful spatial data. Posts on social media are geotagged, GPS signals are sent by mobile devices, and call logs show mobility. Users' locations are revealed by their IP addresses and web searches, and treatment facilities are noted in medical claims. Even cancelled bookings on restaurant reservation websites like OpenTable may provide information about the frequency of sickness in a certain city [25].

Web 2.0's explosion, the information revolution, and rising Internet usage have sparked the development of sophisticated monitoring techniques for early warnings. As observed in the US and Sweden, some Internet-based monitoring technologies are integrated into national security frameworks and are governed at the federal level, reflecting this trend in industrialized countries [10]. Internet search data and disease surveillance data are visualized spatially and temporally to allow for the detection of disease transmission pathways. One famous example is HealthMap that shows current infectious diseases on a map along with connections to online resources for the most recent information [30].

With the development of big data, it is now possible to collect a variety of geographic data, including postings on social media that have been geotagged at different granularities. However, managing geographical misalignment and evaluating this data against conventional public health data present difficulties. Surveillance outcomes are affected by decisions; for instance, research examining microcephaly linked to Zika in Brazilian states reveals regional scale differences between demographic surveys and more detailed data on microcephalic births [25].

Fig. 6 Diagram depicting the process of collecting and processing internet search data

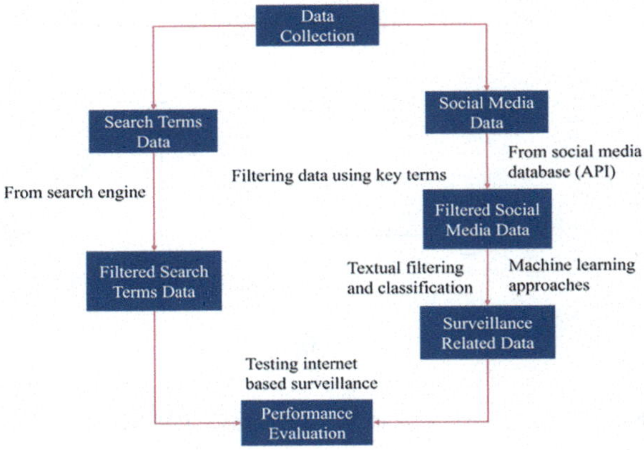

The use of social media as a platform for monitoring individual health data has grown [16]. A growing number of people are interested in using social media to monitor infectious diseases because of the quick data that users on the network produce [20]. Due to their timeliness, social media data are essential for early-stage illness detection, allowing health authorities to involve the public during the early stages of outbreak identification [34]. Infectious illness surveillance has acknowledged Twitter and other blogging platforms as valuable sources of social media data [26, 28].

Following the standardized methods depicted in Fig. 6, the first step entails acquiring pertinent information on infectious diseases from the internet. Studies employed "social media data" via APIs and "internet search data" by examining search traffic from search engines. Most studies gathered information using particular terms, periods of time, and geographical areas [36]. Not all social media data, though, was directly linked to the illnesses indicated. Effective social media data filtering and classification came next in the process. To determine the applicability of gathered social media data to disease episodes, several reviewed studies used machine learning [23]. The final phase compared the accuracy and temporal effectiveness of internet-based surveillance to more traditional surveillance techniques.

It is important to investigate the potential for creating worldwide surveillance systems for newly developing infectious illnesses using internet-based data. Future research should not only focus on inventing new detection methods but also on integrating them into existing systems to augment capabilities, with potential uses extending beyond monitoring to resource management. Although they are impacted by a variety of variables, emerging infectious illnesses are global in scope, demanding international efforts for discovery, monitoring, and control [27].

8 Cautions and Consents for Application of Big Data in Infectious Diseases

A convergence of transformational potential and ethical challenges develops as the incorporation of Big Data into the field of infectious disease surveillance and modeling gains speed. While using large and diverse datasets can lead to groundbreaking discoveries, it also calls for careful consideration of the moral ramifications of handling, processing, and sharing private health data [17]. It is vital to make sure that people are fully informed about how their data will be used and that they have the authority to control that usage, especially when data is passively acquired, such as through social media or mobile apps.

Furthermore, since it affects the rights of people, researchers, and data aggregators, defining who owns and controls the data gathered from different sources is a crucial ethical matter [15]. By ignoring impoverished and marginalized communities while analyzing data primarily from populations with better access, health inequities may unintentionally be perpetuated [17]. To guarantee that Big Data applications in infectious disease research are inclusive, representative, and sensitive to the particular issues faced by varied communities, efforts must be made to resolve these inconsistencies [15].

9 Key Findings

In this section, a compilation of pivotal findings derived from the studies examined in this paper is presented. These findings are integral to the realm of infectious disease surveillance. The accompanying Table 4 succinctly encapsulates these discoveries, offering a consolidated view of the multifaceted strategies, methodologies, and outcomes explored within the context of infectious disease surveillance and modeling.

10 Future Direction and Limitations

The conversations resulting from these recent studies highlight how Big Data has the potential to change disease surveillance by increasing early detection capabilities and offering real-time insights. The ability to take in a range of data sources, such as social media feeds and cell phone data, opens up the possibility for more immediate and accurate sickness monitoring [7, 22]. Collectively, the studies under review show the inherent value of Big Data-driven surveillance in strengthening preparedness and response initiatives, hence lowering the adverse consequences of infectious disease outbreaks on public health [19, 31]. Epidemiologists, data scientists, and public health professionals must work together to overcome obstacles

Table 4 Various big data in infectious disease surveillance discussed in recent works

S.I.	References	Data availability	Mobile/Web deployment	Data ethics	Scalability	Surveillance
1	Ahn et al. [1]	✓	✓	✓	×	✓
2	Althouse et al. [2]	✓	×	×	✓	✓
3	Amusa et al. [3]	✓	×	×	×	✓
4	Bansal et al. [4]	✓	×	✓	×	✓
5	Brownstein et al. [5]	✓	✓	×	×	✓
6	Buckee [6]	✓	×	×	×	✓
7	Buckee et al. [7]	✓	×	✓	×	✓
8	Chae et al. [8]	✓	×	×	×	✓
9	Chen et al. [9]	✓	×	×	×	✓
10	Corsi et al. [11]	✓	×	✓	✓	✓
11	Choi et al. [10]	✓	✓	✓	×	✓
12	Dolley [13]	✓	×	✓	✓	✓
13	Dash et al. [12]	✓	×	×	✓	✓
14	Garattini et al. [15]	✓	×	✓	✓	✓
15	Gilbert et al. [17]	✓	×	✓	✓	✓
16	Hay et al. [19]	×	×	×	✓	✓
17	Jiao et al. [21]	✓	×	×	×	✓
18	Jing et al. [22]	✓	×	×	×	✓
19	Lee et al. [25]	✓	×	✓	✓	✓
20	Milinovich et al. [27]	✓	×	✓	×	✓
21	Simonsen et al. [29]	✓	×	×	×	✓
22	Sun et al. [30]	✓	×	×	×	✓
23	Sylvestre et al. [31]	✓	×	×	×	✓
24	Walsh [32]	✓	×	✓	×	✓
25	Willis et al. [33]	✓	×	×	×	✓
26	Zeng et al. [35]	✓	×	×	×	✓
27	Zhang [36]	✓	×	×	×	✓

including data privacy, data quality, and the ethical issues involved in handling enormous amounts of sensitive data [30]. Surveillance systems, while crucial for monitoring and responding to various issues, possess inherent limitations that can impact their effectiveness. Some of the common limitations of surveillance systems include:

1. Underreporting and Incomplete Data: Surveillance systems often rely on voluntary reporting, which can result in underreporting of cases. Additionally, not all cases may be identified or reported due to lack of awareness, leading to incomplete and inaccurate data.
2. Biases: Surveillance data might be influenced by various biases, such as selection bias (certain groups being overrepresented or underrepresented), reporting bias (cases being selectively reported), and observer bias (data collectors' subjectivity affecting data collection).

3. Data Quality and Accuracy: Inaccuracies in data collection, entry, and coding can lead to erroneous conclusions and decision-making. Poor data quality may arise from errors in recording, transcription, or data entry.
4. Privacy Concerns: Collecting and sharing health-related data can raise privacy and ethical concerns. Balancing the need for data collection with protecting individuals' privacy is a challenge.
5. Resource Constraints: Limited resources, including funding, personnel, and technology, can restrict the scope and effectiveness of surveillance systems.

11 Conclusion

The synergy between advanced data analytics and the intricacies of disease dynamics offers unparalleled insights by revolutionizing traditional surveillance methods. Through harnessing diverse data streams from sources such as social media, electronic health records, and mobile devices, real-time tracking, early detection and predictive modeling have become attainable objectives. However, this paradigm shift is not without challenges. Privacy concerns, data quality issues, and the need for robust analytical frameworks underscore the complexity of integrating big data into surveillance systems. Looking ahead, collaboration between experts in public health, data science, and policy making will play a pivotal role in unlocking the full potential of this approach. As big data continues to reshape infectious disease surveillance, the vision of a safer and healthier global community becomes increasingly attainable.

References

1. E. Ahn, N. Liu, T. Parekh, R. Patel, T. Baldacchino, T. Mullavey, A. Robinson, J. Kim, A mobile app and dashboard for early detection of infectious disease outbreaks: Development study. JMIR Public Health Surveill. **7**(3), e14837 (2021). https://doi.org/10.2196/14837
2. B.M. Althouse, S.V. Scarpino, L.A. Meyers, J.W. Ayers, M. Bargsten, J. Baumbach, J.S. Brownstein, L. Castro, H. Clapham, D.A. Cummings, S. Del Valle, S. Eubank, G. Fairchild, L. Finelli, N. Generous, D. George, D.R. Harper, L. Hébert-Dufresne, M.A. Johansson, et al., Enhancing disease surveillance with novel data streams: Challenges and opportunities. EPJ Data Sci. **4**(1), 17 (2015). https://doi.org/10.1140/epjds/s13688-015-0054-0
3. L. Amusa, H. Twinomurinzi, E. Phalane, N. Phaswana-Mafuya, Big data and infectious disease epidemiology: Bibliometric analysis and research agenda. **12**, e42292 (2023). https://doi.org/10.2196/42292
4. S. Bansal, G. Chowell, L. Simonsen, A. Vespignani, C. Viboud, Big data for infectious disease surveillance and modeling. J. Infect. Dis. **214**(suppl_4), S375–S379 (2016). https://doi.org/10.1093/infdis/jiw400
5. J.S. Brownstein, B. Rader, C.M. Astley, H. Tian, Advances in artificial intelligence for infectious-disease surveillance. N. Engl. J. Med. **388**(17), 1597–1607 (2023). https://doi.org/10.1056/NEJMra2119215

6. C. Buckee, Improving epidemic surveillance and response: Big data is dead, long live big data. Lancet Digit. Health **2**(5), e218–e220 (2020). https://doi.org/10.1016/S2589-7500(20)30059-5
7. C.O. Buckee, M.I.E. Cardenas, J. Corpuz, A. Ghosh, F. Haque, J. Karim, A.S. Mahmud, R.J. Maude, K. Mensah, N.V. Motaze, M. Nabaggala, C.J.E. Metcalf, S.A. Mioramalala, F. Mubiru, C.M. Peak, S. Pramanik, J.M. Rakotondramanga, E. Remera, I. Sinha, et al., Productive disruption: Opportunities and challenges for innovation in infectious disease surveillance. BMJ Glob. Health **3**(1), e000538 (2018). https://doi.org/10.1136/bmjgh-2017-000538
8. S. Chae, S. Kwon, D. Lee, Predicting infectious disease using deep learning and big data. Int. J. Environ. Res. Public Health **15**(8), 1596 (2018). https://doi.org/10.3390/ijerph15081596
9. W. Chen, M. Yao, L. Dong, P. Shao, Y. Zhang, B. Fu, The application framework of big data technology during the COVID-19 pandemic in China. Epidemiol. Infect. **150**, 1–11 (2022). https://doi.org/10.1017/S0950268822000577
10. J. Choi, Y. Cho, E. Shim, H. Woo, Web-based infectious disease surveillance systems and public health perspectives: A systematic review. BMC Public Health **16**(1), 1–10 (2016). https://doi.org/10.1186/s12889-016-3893-0
11. A. Corsi, F.F. de Souza, R.N. Pagani, J.L. Kovaleski, Big data analytics as a tool for fighting pandemics: A systematic review of literature. J. Ambient. Intell. Humaniz. Comput. **12**(10), 9163–9180 (2021). https://doi.org/10.1007/s12652-020-02617-4
12. S. Dash, S. Shakyawar, M. Sharma, S. Kaushik, Big data in healthcare: Management, analysis and future prospects. J. Big Data **6** (2019). https://doi.org/10.1186/s40537-019-0217-0
13. S. Dolley, Big data's role in precision public health. Front. Public Health **6**, 68 (2018). https://doi.org/10.3389/fpubh.2018.00068
14. F. Dorea, C. Revie, Data-driven surveillance: Effective collection, integration, and interpretation of data to support decision making. Front. Vet. Sci. **8**, 633977 (2021). https://doi.org/10.3389/fvets.2021.633977
15. C. Garattini, J. Raffle, D. Aisyah, F. Sartain, Z. Kozlakidis, Big data analytics, infectious diseases and associated ethical impacts. Philos. Technol. **32**, 1–17 (2019). https://doi.org/10.1007/s13347-017-0278-y
16. V. Gianfredi, S. Provenzano, O.E. Santangelo, What can internet users' behaviours reveal about the mental health impacts of the COVID-19 pandemic? A systematic review. Public Health **198**, 44–52 (2021). https://doi.org/10.1016/j.puhe.2021.06.024
17. G.L. Gilbert, C. Degeling, J. Johnson, Communicable disease surveillance ethics in the age of big data and new technology. Asian Bioeth. Rev. **11**(2), 173–187 (2019). https://doi.org/10.1007/s41649-019-00087-1
18. J. Ginsberg, M.H. Mohebbi, R.S. Patel, L. Brammer, M.S. Smolinski, L. Brilliant, Detecting influenza epidemics using search engine query data. Nature **457**(7232), 1012–1014 (2009). https://doi.org/10.1038/nature07634
19. S. Hay, D. George, C. Moyes, J. Brownstein, Big data opportunities for global infectious disease surveillance. PLoS Med. **10**, e1001413 (2013). https://doi.org/10.1371/journal.pmed.1001413
20. N. Huang, M. Slaney, M. Elhilali, Connecting deep neural networks to physical, perceptual, and electrophysiological auditory signals. Front. Neurosci. **12**, 532 (2018). https://doi.org/10.3389/fnins.2018.00532
21. Z. Jiao, H. Ji, J. Yan, X. Qi, Application of big data and artificial intelligence in epidemic surveillance and containment. Intell. Med. **3**(1), 36–43 (2023). https://doi.org/10.1016/j.imed.2022.10.003
22. F. Jing, Z. Li, S. Qiao, J. Zhang, B. Olatosi, X. Li, Using geospatial social media data for infectious disease studies: A systematic review. Int. J. Digit. Earth (2023). https://doi.org/10.1080/17538947.2022.2161652
23. R. Kinoshita, S.-M. Jung, T. Kobayashi, A.R. Akhmetzhanov, H. Nishiura, Epidemiology of coronavirus disease 2019 (COVID-19) in Japan during the first and second waves. Math. Biosci. Eng.: MBE **19**(6), 6088–6101 (2022). https://doi.org/10.3934/mbe.2022284

24. D. Klaucke, J. Buehler, S. Thacker, R. Parrish, F. Trowbridge, Guidelines for evaluating surveillance systems. MMWR Suppl. **37**(5), 1–18 (1988)
25. E. Lee, J. Asher, S. Goldlust, J. Kraemer, A. Lawson, S. Bansal, Mind the scales: Harnessing spatial big data for infectious disease surveillance and inference. J. Infect. Dis. **214**, S409–S413 (2016). https://doi.org/10.1093/infdis/jiw344
26. S. Maxwell, Virtual care technologies, wearable health monitoring sensors, and internet of medical things-based smart disease surveillance systems in the diagnosis and treatment of COVID-19 patients. Am. J. Med. Res. **8**(2), 118 (2021). https://doi.org/10.22381/ajmr8220219
27. G. Milinovich, G. Williams, A. Clements, W. Hu, Internet-based surveillance systems for monitoring emerging infectious diseases. The Lancet infectious diseases **14**(2), 160–168 (2014). https://doi.org/10.1016/S1473-3099(13)70244-5
28. A. Riley, Internet of things-based smart healthcare systems and wireless biomedical sensing devices in monitoring, detection, and prevention of COVID-19. Am. J. Med. Res. **8**(2), 51 (2021). https://doi.org/10.22381/ajmr8220214
29. L. Simonsen, J. Gog, D. Olson, C. Viboud, Infectious disease surveillance in the big data era: Towards faster and locally relevant systems. J. Infect. Dis. **214**, S380–S385 (2016). https://doi.org/10.1093/infdis/jiw376
30. H. Sun, Y. Zhang, G. Gao, D. Wu, Internet search data with spatiotemporal analysis in infectious disease surveillance: Challenges and perspectives. Front. Public Health **10**, 958835 (2022). https://doi.org/10.3389/fpubh.2022.958835
31. E. Sylvestre, C. Joachim, E. Cécilia-Joseph, G. Bouzillé, B. Campillo-Gimenez, M. Cuggia, A. Cabié, Data-driven methods for dengue prediction and surveillance using real-world and Big Data: A systematic review. PLoS Negl. Trop. Dis. **16**(1), e0010056 (2022). https://doi.org/10.1371/journal.pntd.0010056
32. T. Walsh, Modeling COVID-19 with big mobility data: Surveillance and reaffirming the people in the data. Big Data Soc. **10**(1), 205395172311641 (2023). https://doi.org/10.1177/20539517231164115
33. S. Willis, N. Cocoros, L. Randall, A. Ochoa, G. Haney, K. Hsu, A. DeMaria, M. Klompas, Electronic health record use in public health infectious disease surveillance, USA, 2018–2019. Curr. Infect. Dis. Rep. **21** (2019). https://doi.org/10.1007/s11908-019-0694-5
34. Q. Xu, Z. Su, K. Zhang, S. Yu, Fast containment of infectious diseases with E-healthcare mobile social internet of things. IEEE Internet Things J. **8**(22), 16473–16485 (2021). https://doi.org/10.1109/JIOT.2021.3062288
35. D. Zeng, Z. Cao, D.B. Neill, Artificial intelligence–enabled public health surveillance—From local detection to global epidemic monitoring and control, in *Artificial Intelligence in Medicine*, ed. by L. Xing, M.L. Giger, J.K. Min, (Academic, 2021), pp. 437–453. https://doi.org/10.1016/B978-0-12-821259-2.00022-3
36. Q. Zhang, Data science approaches to infectious disease surveillance. Philos. Transact. A Math. Phys. Eng. Sci. **380**(2214), 20210115 (2022). https://doi.org/10.1098/rsta.2021.0115

Development of Low Cost, Automated Digital Microscopes Allowing Rapid Whole Slide Imaging for Detecting Malaria

Md. Sakib Bin Islam, Jahidul Islam, Munshi Sajidul Islam, Md. Shaheenur Islam Sumon, Md. Nahiduzzaman, M. Murugappan, Anwarul Hasan, and Muhammad E. H. Chowdhury

1 Introduction

The Plasmodium parasites that cause malaria continue to be a major public health problem across the world, especially in places with little medical supplies. Female mosquitoes of the genus Anopheles are responsible for transmitting the Plasmodium parasite that causes malaria to humans when they bite [1]. Over 241 million cases of malaria were recorded in 2020 [2], with Africa having the highest prevalence. This is according to the World Health Organisation (WHO). This research discusses the successes and shortcomings of utilising digital microscope images with artificial intelligence (AI) techniques to automate the diagnosis of malaria. Several studies and research publications that focused on the use of digital microscopy imaging and AI techniques were used to examine malaria diagnosis. Timely and precise diagnosis is essential for efficient disease treatment and control. Although commonly utilised,

M. S. B. Islam
Department of Biomedical Engineering, Military Institute of Science and Technology, Dhaka, Bangladesh

J. Islam
Department of Computer Science and Engineering, Dhaka International University, Dhaka, Bangladesh

M. S. Islam
Department of Electrical and Electronic Engineering, University of Dhaka, Dhaka, Bangladesh

Department of Electrical Engineering, Qatar University, Doha, Qatar

M. S. I. Sumon
Department of Biomedical Engineering, Military Institute of Science and Technology, Dhaka, Bangladesh

Department of Electrical Engineering, Qatar University, Doha, Qatar

M. E. H. Chowdhury, S. Kiranyaz (eds.), *Surveillance, Prevention, and Control of Infectious Diseases*, https://doi.org/10.1007/978-3-031-59967-5_4

conventional diagnostic techniques like microscopy may be labor-intensive and time-consuming. However, with the development of digital imaging technology, a new and exciting chance to revolutionise malaria detection has emerged [3]. Digital microscopes, which are often referred to as whole slide imaging (WSI) systems, are capable of capturing digital pictures of physical slides, which helps to automate the process of evaluating samples for the purpose of disease diagnosis.

Female Anopheles mosquitoes transmit fatal malaria through plasmodium parasites in the host's blood cells. Machine learning and deep learning advancements offer quicker and more accurate malaria detection, reducing costs and improving accuracy compared to conventional methods [4]. Malaria's severity and limited diagnostic tools call for innovative solutions. A mobile phone-based polarized light microscopy system is introduced, offering affordable, high-resolution malaria detection, rivaling larger, expensive systems [5]. This user-friendly platform holds promise for accurate and accessible malaria diagnosis, the system may be able to detect malaria with high resolution and specificity.The issue of malaria in global healthcare, which continues to be a severe concern with an estimated 228 million infections and 405,000 fatalities per year [6]. Patients who live in rural areas, which might be the most endemic for the illness, limited access to quality microscopy in some settings and symptomatic diagnosis of malaria risk errors. Rapid diagnostic tests (RDTs) lack parasitemia quantification, hindering infection severity evaluation and treatment monitoring [7]. Over the course of the last several decades, the technology that is used in optical microscopes has not changed, and therefore, neither have the procedures or processes that are utilised with these microscopes. On the other hand, as a result of population growth, there are now more samples to analyse, and the diagnostic criteria have become more difficult [8]. Problems arise when trying to diagnose malaria with the inexpensive microscopes and low-magnification lenses that are the norm in places with limited access to healthcare. The authors [9] suggest a new massive dataset, dubbed M5, which includes high-resolution and low-resolution photographs of the same slide areas taken with different microscopes. Both location of malarial cells and categorization of malarial

M. Nahiduzzaman
Department of Electrical and Computer Engineering, Rajshahi University of Engineering and Technology, Rajshahi, Bangladesh
e-mail: nahiduzzaman@ece.ruet.ac.bd

M. Murugappan
Intelligent Signal Processing (ISP) Research Lab, Department of Electronics and Communication Engineering, Kuwait College of Science and Technology, Doha, Kuwait

A. Hasan
Department of Mechanical and Industrial Engineering, Qatar University, Doha, Qatar
e-mail: ahasan@qu.edu.qa

M. E. H. Chowdhury (✉)
Department of Electrical Engineering, Qatar University, Doha, Qatar
e-mail: mchowdhury@qu.edu.qa

life stages are marked in the dataset. This may further provides many object detectors and domain adaption techniques as benchmarks for the dataset.

The importance of optical microscopes in the field of biological sciences is underscored by the authors in study [10], highlighting their role in education and knowledge sharing.The high cost of these microscopes limits their use in low-resource and high-illness prevalence areas. Cheaper alternatives are needed for remote locations and open science. Effective malaria detection in low-resource areas may be achieved by the integration of inexpensive design and automation. While discussing the difficulties of making digital microscopes available to everybody, we also highlight cutting-edge technology and creative solutions that hold great promise for making large-scale malaria diagnosis more inexpensive and accessible.

Table 1 presents a comprehensive review of the literature on automated digital microscopes for malaria detection that are on the low end of the price spectrum. The purpose of this article is to provide readers with a synopsis of the current knowledge on the technologies, methods, and results that have led to the development of these cutting-edge tools.

In addressing the existing research gap, our study presents a pioneering approach by integrating the YOLOv5 model, demonstrating its efficacy in facilitating malaria-infected blood stain detection while reducing human error and accelerating identification processes. This chapter has focused to create an affordable digital microscope that are fully automated to provide rapid entire slide imaging for precise malaria diagnosis. A 3D printed low cost slide preparation modeule with a low-cost zooming miscrope and control assembly, and standalone single-board computer-based YOLO v5 Customized Detector model for non-parasite and parasite blood cell detection and counting. Figure 1 shows the visual guide of the imprementation process of this low-cost automated microscope.

Our innovative method entails the creation of affordable, fully-automated digital microscopes for rapid whole-slide imaging, designed specifically for accurate malaria diagnosis. We employed the YOLOv5 customised detector model to accurately detect and enumerate non-parasite and parasite blood cells using a low-cost 3D-printed device for blood stain preparation and a microscope for blood image collection. The results demonstrated a very good overall accuracy rate of 92% in classifying samples as infected or uninfected, highlighting the potential transformative impact of our approach on healthcare delivery and surveillance efforts in malaria-endemic regions. The proposed system has following novel contributions to the literature:

- Utilizing an open-soruce autohaem smear+ design to prepare the slide automatically for imaging and further analysis
- A cost-effective microscope with 400× zoom capability and XY-scanning mechanism was introduced for precise whole slide scanning and imaging
- YOLOv5 customised detector model was proposed and deployed to accurately detect and enumerate non-parasite and parasite blood cells
- Finally, an automated end-to-end framework for Malaria detection system is proposed.

Table 1 Comprehensive review of the literature on automated digital microscopes for malaria detection

Author	Goals	Methods	Features used	Limitations
Ruicun Liu [11]	"To create AIDMAN, an AI-based object identification system for malaria diagnosis using smartphone thin-blood smear images"	"Malaria diagnosis from smartphone thin-blood smear photos using YOLO v5 and Transformer models for object identification and classification"	"U-Net utilizes upsampling to make images from various feature layers the same dimension"	The Convulational Neural Network (CNN) classifier's features and feature extraction technique are not described in the paper
Golla Madhu [12]	"Development of precise and efficient malaria parasite identification methods, including AI-based models, using microscopic blood images"	"The method of k-means clustering and singular value decomposition (k-SVD) in conjunction with pursuit strategies for overcoming dictionary learning"	"Shannon Entropy was used to quantify feature extraction and compute grayscale image randomness"	Variability in malaria symptoms and manifestations can make it challenging for AI models to detect the disease accurately in all instances
Rohan Sangameswaran [13]	"To create a low-cost, portable microscope with vision AI to automate malaria detection in distant rural areas"	"MAIScope, a low-cost, portable gadget, has an on-device multi-layered deep learning network and a hardware system"	"EfficientDet-lite employs scaling and convolutional neural networks. Object detection models are pre-trained on COCO"	The gadget is waterproof for use in damp and rainy surroundings, making it unsuitable in tropical areas where malaria is common
Feng Yang [14]	"Digital images of thick blood smears for automated malaria parasite identification and counting"	"Deep learning methods can automatically detect and count malaria parasites in thick blood smear digital images"	"Customized Convolutional Neural Network (CNN) and Support Vector Machine (SVM) Classifier"	When negative patches were randomly picked, the CNN model's accuracy dropped below 75%
Paul Gordon [6]	"Multimodal microscopy system to obtain quantitative parasitemia data fromc thin blood smears at a low cost"	"Counting parasites in Plasmodium-infected blood smears quantitatively"	"Modern sample preparation methods, singlet aspheric objective lens, and bimodal imaging"	The research used a non-commercial prototype technology and did not evaluate patient samples
Carles Rubio Maturana [1]	"To analyse automating malaria detection using digital microscope images and AI techniques"	"RDTs, Quantitive buffy coat (QBC) assay, AI Tools"	"For calculating erythrocyte features in thin blood smear pictures, PyRadiomics 2.2.0 is used"	Limitations like picture quality, laboratory facilities, and the need for a uniform final diagnosis

Rai Tathagato [2]	"Automatic focus technology based on cutting-edge AI research"	"WSI combines digital microscopy with deep CNNs to capture high-resolution slide images"	"Computerised evaluation using an AI system,CNN and Whole Slide Imaging System"	The focusing defects obtained by training with RGB-only images are provided in table
Jesus Salido [10]	"Assess affordable open-hardware optical microscopes as alternatives to expensive commercial models"	"Two broad classes: Handheld field microscopes and versatile automated microscopes"	"Modular light sources, Manual slide manipulation, Hand-focused for high clarity"	The research reviews low-cost microscopes for Open Science, it does not examine their limits and their consequences for diverse applications
Jung Yoon [15]	"Design a fully automated malaria detection and parasitemia measuring microscopic system for quick diagnosis and parasite density monitoring"	"Automatic microscopic malaria parasite detection using a microscope, plastic chip, fluorescent dye, and image processing software"	"SYBR Green I fluorescently stained malaria parasites and other nucleic acid-containing structures"	Giemsa-stained peripheral blood smear quality may affect parasite density monitoring
Jaime García-Villena [8]	"Mobile-based slide scanning microscope that can be controlled from a smartphone"	"Telemedicine web platform integration allows for remote viewing and analysis of digitised microscope images"	"The robotic scanner, with a resolution of around 1 m, has been tested in two clinical settings"	The approach separates people into three infection intensity classifications which may not discover low-intensity illnesses
Alexander Kratz [16]	"Evaluation of digital imaging identification and suggestion for further development"	"Digital image analysis of blood smear through AI algorithms, comparing it to manual microscopy"	"Characterization of different morphological abnormalities, screening for detection"	Lack of standardisation of staining procedures, optical magnifications, colour, hardware, software
Debashish Das [17]	"Diagnosis accuracy of a ML based digital malaria microscopy instrument"	"Machine-learning-based digital microscope designed to detect malaria"	"Identify and flag low-quality blood films and can diagnose malaria, determine White Blood Cell count"	The EasyScan Go's sensitivity was decreased at low parasitemia levels, it may not detect low parasite levels
Kevin De Haan [18]	"Sickle cell disease (SCD) that may aid in early detection even in situations with limited access to healthcare"	"This system used a pair of deep neural networks. Both networks use artificial intelligence"	"Sickle cell identification, image enhancement and DL-based methods for smartphone microscopy"	The limited sample size of 96 individuals, including 32 SCD patients, may restrict the generalizability of the results

(continued)

Table 1 (continued)

Author	Goals	Methods	Features used	Limitations
Rong De [19]	"Automatic detecting Malaria from RBC by using DL model"	"Mask Regions with Convolutional Neural Networks Deep Learning Model which can perform object identification, classification"	"Before the training phase, the images were exported as a json file after being manually annotated"	When cells overlap and lack a border, the model may perform poorly, resulting in inaccurate cell counts
P Pattanaik [20]	"MM-ResNet for completely automated categorization of blood smear pictures as infected with malaria or not"	"Multi-scale residual network for deep learning (MM-ResNet)"	"Evaluations of small-scale deep CNNs performed using mobile phone data"	Due to expert shortages and poor photo quality, segmenting erythrocytes in microscopic blood smear phone images is difficult
Rizki Nurfauzi and Hanung Nugroho [21]	"Hybrid automated malaria parasite identification and segmentation approach based on image processing and DL methods"	"Improved double-Otsu technique"	"Automated hybrid approach for detecting and segmenting malaria parasites through image processing and deep learning"	The PlasmoID dataset utilized for assessment has few pictures, which may restrict the scope of the suggested technique
Wan Rasyidah [22]	"Deep learning algorithm based on Convolutional Neural Network (CNN) and YOLOv5 architectures"	"Images of malaria parasites in infected blood are classified according to their developmental stage using the YOLOv5 algorithm"	"CNN model is utilized, whereas YOLOv5 is used to categorize the different life stages of the parasite"	Lack of dataset quantity and variety limits generalizability.CNN and YOLOv5 feature extraction information are lacking
Niranjana Sampathila [23]	"Automatic cell categorization of malaria parasites with deep learning in Pytorch"	"Detecting Malaria in Segmented Red Blood Cell Images using PyTorch Transfer Learning"	"Pre-trained ImageNet models and fine-tuned them for our dataset of interest"	Lack of information about the dataset used to train and test models, as its size and variety might affect model performance and generalizability
Gonçalo Marques [24]	"Suggest an EfficientNet-based automated method for blood-cell malaria detection"	"Efficient Net-based detection"	"Convolutional neural networks which is verified by 10-fold cross-validation"	Malaria diagnostic picture collections are still weak, limiting CNN algorithm training datasets
Aliyu Abubakar [25]	"To suggest using machine learning algorithms to aid in malaria parasite detection in blood smear images"	"Deep learning features with computational analysis"	"Used VGG16, VGG19, ResNet50 etc. models to extract six distinct features from the images"	The research dataset may include parasites other than malaria, limiting generalizability

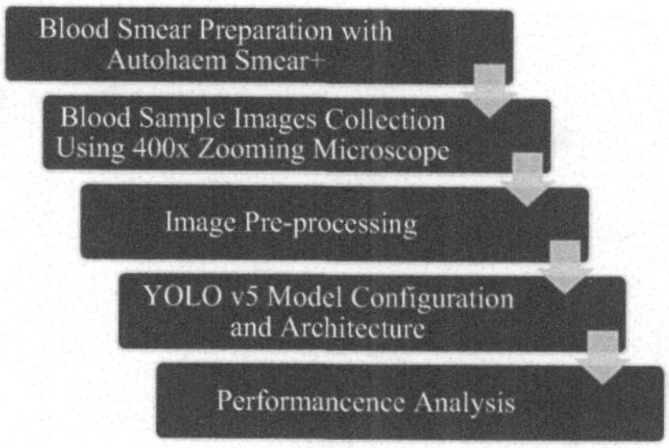

Fig. 1 A visual guide to the comprehensive process

The microscope-based scanning system presented in this chapter represents a significant advancement in low-cost blood sample analysis. By combining a high-resolution microscope, a precision moving frame, and a PC-based controller, the system automates and enhances the imaging process, offering researchers and clinicians a powerful tool for accurate and efficient but low-cost diagnostics. This innovative approach holds the potential to redefine the landscape of biomedical microscopy and contribute to advancements in medical research and patient care.

In this chapter, beginning with a discussion of the intricate design process in the next section, innovative techniques was used to create a cost-effective device with 400× zoom capability microscope are described. The focus then shifts to the development, validation and deployment of the detection algorithm in the experimental phase, casting light on the meticulous approach taken to ensure the accuracy and dependability of our study. Subsequently, we present the results of our exhaustive experimentation, which provide valuable insights into the efficacy and viability of our device and model.

2 Methods and Materials

A cost-effective apparatus and microscope were developed using 3D printing technology, off-the-shelf low-cost devices for the purpose of blood smear preparation and blood image capture, respectively. The subsequent use of the YOLO v5 [26–29] customized detector model included the detection and quantification of both non-parasitic and parasitic blood cells allowed to deploy that solution to a central controller (personal computer). YOLOv5 models are compoundscaled object identification models trained on customised datasets. We've trained our model with a free accessible dataset which contains images with their annotation files in text format. We did not train the model with our collected images because they were not annotated rather we have tested deployed model performance on a small set of image samples to validate the proposed solution. Figure 2 shows the schematic representation of the entire system and the workflow of the methodology. In the following section, different modules of the system will be discussed elaborately:

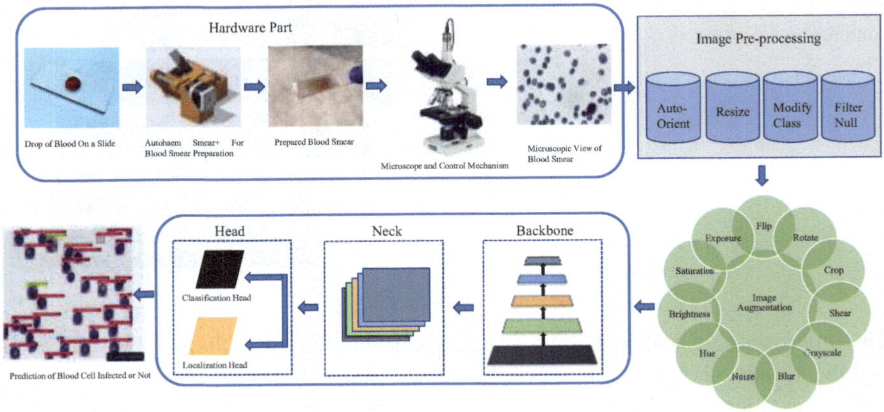

Fig. 2 Schematic representation of the complete system as a workflow diagram

2.1 Low-Cost Mechanical Blood Smear Preparation Device

Haematological illnesses including anaemia and parasitic infections like malaria can be diagnosed using a blood smear. Preparing a smear is a tedious, time-consuming, and physically demanding process. In order to accurately diagnose patients or characterise samples for scientific purposes, it is necessary to analyse blood smears using optical microscopy. To facilitate the creation of blood smears, we have created one electro-mechanical device that is fully described as open-source hardware and can be simply built locally [30]. The gadgets outperform human experts while also being easy to use and potentially improving repeatability and standardisation across facilities. The analysis of blood smears by optical microscopy is now considered the "gold standard" for malaria diagnosis [31]. A microscopic film of the patients' blood is mounted and stained on a microscope slide. The parasites in the smear are counted when the microscopist examines it at different magnifications. The parasite density in the blood may be determined with this method, and it has a good level of sensitivity for application in clinical malaria.

2.1.1 The Autohaem Smear+ Device

The electro-mechanical device Autohaem smear+ is suitable for high-volume blood smear laboratories and hospitals [30]. Alternately, two users could simultaneously use the device, with one user preparing the next blood sample and the other depositing the blood onto the coating mechanism. This apparatus allows the spreader slide to be moved at a predetermined angle and speed while remaining level and in constant contact with the microscope slide. Any smear should be performed at the same speed regardless of the user, and this speed can be programmed (for

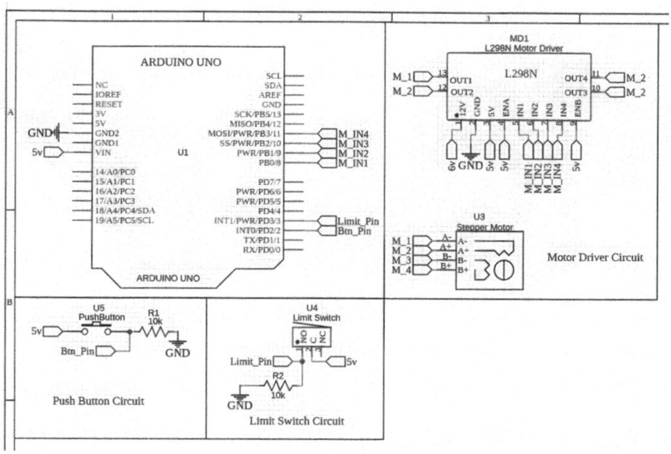

Fig. 3 A schemtatic of autohaem smear+

instance, to optimise for the typical ambient conditions of specific laboratories, which may have an influence on the smear).

2.1.2 Design and Testing of the Hardware

Schematic Design The device shown in Fig. 3 combines electronics components to achieve precise and efficient blood smear preparation. Key components are in this system include the Arduino UNO R3, L298N motor driver, NEMA17 stepper motor, push button, limit switche and 6 V 3A adapter. Through precise integration of these components, the device promises unparalleled accuracy and repeatability, marking a significant advancement in diagnostic technology. In this blood smear device, the Arduino UNO R3 microcontroller takes center stage, orchestrating critical functions. It processes user inputs from push buttons and limit switches, calculates precise stepper motor steps, and regulates motor control via the L298N driver. This centralized control ensures efficient, accurate, and user-friendly blood smear preparation. The push button initiates each blood smear processing cycle, followed by the limit switch establishing the stepper motor's home position. Subsequently, the motor executes pre-calculated steps from the home position, facilitating a seamless single blood smear procedure.

Mechanical Design As can be seen in Fig. 4, the device's primary body is 3D printed. This stores the electronics and includes a slit for the microscope slide. The autohaem smear uses a similar 3D printed slider to keep the slide at a consistent angle. On one end, a lead screw nut is fastened to power its motion. The other end has an inverted hook equipped with a magnet. A metal rod made of ground steel is held above the slide and serves as a guide. The slider can't go in the anti-clockwise

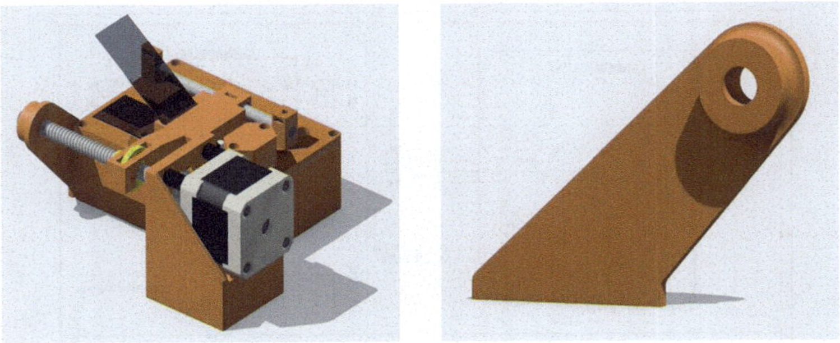

Fig. 4 A modified part for holding threaded rod

direction because of the rod, and it can't go in the correct direction because of the magnet. The Nema 17 motor and limit switch are housed separately.

All of the essential parts of the improved autohaem smear+ design are shown in Fig. 4; the focus is on the new, and supplementary features that reduce vibrations. Recognizing the detrimental impact of vibrations on smear quality, these additional components are seamlessly integrated. Utilizing threaded rods, these elements provide pivotal support, ensuring axis stability and optimal angle maintenance throughout the procedure.

Hardware Setup An Iverntech Nema 17 stepper motor with an integral 100 mm Tr8x8 lead screw moves the slider. This was decided upon because it is widely used in the z-axis drive of 3D printers and is hence easily accessible. Because it is powered by a stepper motor, the slider can be moved to very specific locations and at very controlled rates. The stepper motor is powered by a Polulu DRV8825 driver. This driver was selected because it can provide the large current required by the motor (1.5 A) without requiring any extra cooling. The expansion board for driving stepper motors is used for connecting the driver. The driver of a 3D printer or CNC machine is connected to one of these generic boards, which have solderless pinouts, a motor connection, a decoupling capacitor, and dipswitches for microstepping. Because the motor's lead screw has a pitch of 8 mm and its step-size standard is 1.8, 200 motor steps will move the slider by 8 mm. To improve the smoothness without sacrificing speed as the Arduino Uno can handle 4000 steps per second, this was micro-stepped down to 1/2 step. The consequence is that the motor can move the slider at a maximum speed of 8 cm s1 in 400 discrete increments of 8 mm in length. The motor is powered by a 12 V, 2 A DC power source that is wired into the motor controller expansion board through an external DC connection. Because of its widespread availability and user-friendliness for controlling other electronic components, an Arduino Uno serves as the brain of the Autohaem Smear+. The Arduino's "step," "direction," and "enable" pins are used to connect the motor driver expansion board. In addition to the motor and slider, the Arduino is linked to a limit switch that sets the starting position of the slider and an LED button that lights up when the smear is initiated and stays on as long as the motor is in motion. The "AccelStepper" library17 is used in the Arduino code to provide methods for smoothly accelerating and decelerating the motor, as well as positioning and repositioning the motor.

2.1.3 Operation Priniple of Autohaem Smear+

Plugging the gadget into an electrical outlet initiates its functioning. The slider goes backward until it touches the limit switch, and then forward to the idle position during the device's first calibration phase immediately after power on. The slide for the microscope is inserted into a slot, and the operator turns a slider around the lead screw's axis. The smear maker begins working as soon as the button is pressed. When the gadget is active, an indicator light will turn on, and the slider will begin to advance. The speed of the slider is reduced as it approaches the blood drop. The drop of blood is pulled down the edge of the spreader slide as the slider microscope slide passes through it. The slider advances at a rate set by the user, stopping once it reaches its resting position. To avoid cross-contamination, the user twists the slider and lifts out the spreader slide from underneath. After that, the spreader slide may be sterilised and put back into use as a microscope slide.

Autohaem smear+ allows the user to adjust the angle at which the spreader slide is placed in relation to the microscope slide, as well as the pace at which the slider moves to form the smear. These two settings allow the user to fine-tune the device's optimum angling and velocity. The ability to replicate concepts or work together on future enhancements relies heavily on thorough documentation. A Bill of Materials, detailed instructions with accompanying images for visual aid, electronic diagrams, and a tutorial for uploading the necessary software to the Arduino are all included at.

2.2 Low Cost Microscope and Control Mechanism Design

In the realm of biomedical research and diagnostics, the need for accurate and efficient blood sample analysis has driven the development of advanced microscopy techniques. The system comprises three pivotal components: a powerful microscope with an impressive 400x zooming capability, a precision moving frame enabling controlled movement along both the x and y axes, and a controller unit incorporating a arduino and motor driver for seamless operation. The proposed system not only streamlines blood sample pre-processing but also automates slide positioning, image acquisition, and post-processing, ultimately leading to the generation of a unified, detailed image of the entire slide. OMAX 40X-2500X Digital Lab Trinocular Compound LED Microscope (Fig. 5) with USB Digital Camera and Double Layer Mechanical Stage [32] was used as microscope as this low-cost microscope can acquire high quality image and can be interfaced to computer using USB interface. This work utilized MCL-MANNZ XY micropositioning system for precise image

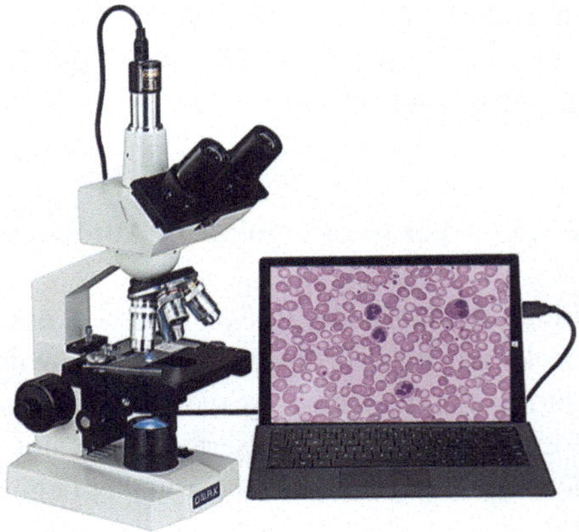

Fig. 5 OMAX 40X-2500X digital lab trinocular compound LED microscope with USB digital camera and double layer mechanical stage

patch acquisition and this allows to introduce a novel but low-cost microscope-based scanning system engineered to deliver high-resolution imaging for blood sample analysis. The acquisiton computer was interfaced to Arduino Uno over USB interface to provide command for XY micropositioning system for precise image patch acquisition and every position of the slide was imaged to capture the patches of the whole slide images.

The proposed system has following features:

Microscope with Enhanced Zooming Capability The cornerstone of the system is a state-of-the-art microscope with an exceptional 400× zooming capacity. This enables the visualization of minute cellular structures, enhancing the accuracy of blood sample analysis. The high zooming capability is achieved through advanced optical components and precision engineering, ensuring minimal aberrations and optimal image quality. Moreover, the microscope should be easily interfacable to single-board computer or personal computer, which is another good feature of the selected off-the-shelf microscope.

Precision Moving Frame for Controlled Motion To facilitate the systematic scanning of entire blood sample slides, a meticulously designed moving frame is employed. This frame offers controlled movement along both the x and y axes, ensuring precise positioning of the slide under the microscope objective. The seamless motion is achieved through a combination of motorized components, MCL-MANNZ and motion control system implemented using two Stepper Motor Driver—TB6600 and an Arduino Uno, which was directly controlled by the personal computer (Fig. 6). The scanning sequence begins with the frame moving the slide under the microscope. The microscope captures a series of high-resolution images, each covering a small segment of the slide.

PC-Based Controller This personal computer is working as the heart of the whole system as it collects patch images, control the scanning system to collect patch images and finally, the trained model was deployed to this computer for stand alone operation. This PC enables the efficient communication between the

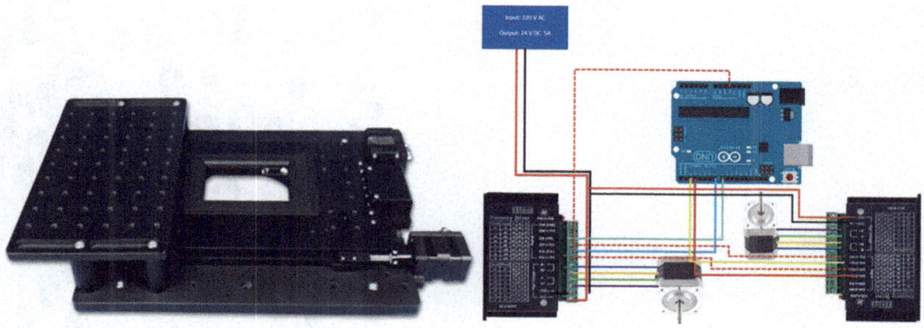

Fig. 6 XY micropositioning system for precise image patch acquisition: slide holder and moving arrangement (left) and interface and control circuitry (right)

different components of the system. This PC serves as the central processing unit, orchestrating the movement of the frame, microscope settings, and image acquisition.

2.3 *Deep Learning-Based Detection and Quantification of Both Non-parasitic and Parasitic Blood Cells*

To develop and deploy the detection and quantification framework, we have utilized publicly accisible and annotated datasets. This development has following five steps:

- Public dataset collection
- Splitting dataset into train, test, and validation,
- YOLOV5 model configuration and architecture,
- Performance evaluation

2.3.1 Public Malaria Dataset Collection

Multiple public datasets were collected with 1364 images (80,000 cells). These datasets are from Stefanie Lopes in Brazil, Benoit Malleret in Southeast Asia, and Gabriel Rangel in the United States. Giemsa reagent was used to stain blood smears. Red blood cells (RBCs), white blood cells (leukocytes), gametocytes, rings, trophozoites, and schizonts are the six types of cells represented in the data. Cells that did not fit neatly into any of the predetermined categories could be flagged as "difficult" by the annotators. There was a significant discrepancy between the percentage of healthy RBCs and the percentage of healthy white blood cells (leukocytes) in the data.

Each cell was assigned a category and its surrounding coordinates were specified. Stefanie Lopes, a malaria researcher at the Dr. Heitor Vieira Dourado Tropical

Fig. 7 An image from Malaria bounding box dataset with annotation

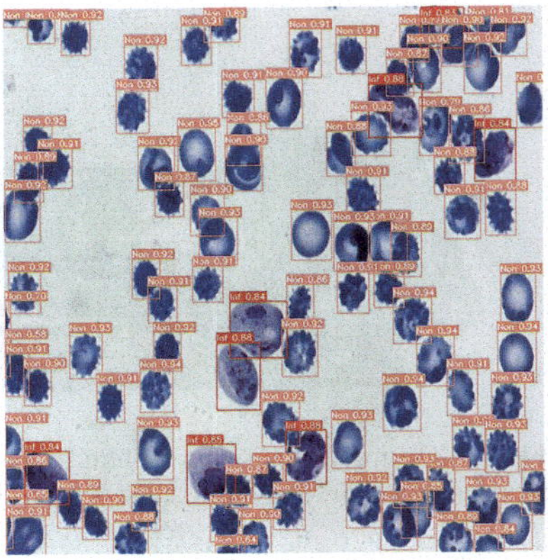

Medicine Foundation hospital, categorised infected cells across all datasets according to their developmental stage or difficulty [33]. The datatset has bounding box to show infected and non-infected cells as shown in Fig. 7.

2.3.2 Splitting Dataset into Train, Test and Validation

It is common practise in deep learning to split data into training, testing, and validation sets so that a model's accuracy may be measured on unseen data. When a model is trained, its parameters are adjusted so that they best fit the training data from the training set. After the model has been trained, its performance is evaluated using the testing set, which consists of new, unexplored data. Depending on the nature of the problem, the testing set may be used to evaluate the model's accuracy, precision, recall, or other metrics. Overfitting occurs when a model is too complex and works well on training data but poorly on new data, therefore the testing set is crucial for preventing this. To ensure the model is not overfit to the training data and can successfully generalise to new data, we split the data into three distinct categories: train, val and test. This technique is crucial in machine learning since it increases the model's precision and robustness. Our images of blood cells based on counting were categorised as follows: 70% for training, 15% for testing, 15% for validation.

Roboflow's augmentation procedure involves using many different types of data augmentation on a dataset's input pictures. In order to improve the variety and amount of the training data without actively gathering additional data, data augmentation is often used in computer vision applications, particularly when training deep learning models. The more augmentations are used, the more the model learns to generalize to new, unknown data [34]. Various transformations are used in image processing and augmentation to improve dataset diversity and model resilience. Horizontal and vertical flips, 90° rotations in clockwise, counter-clockwise, and upside-down directions, cropping with zoom levels ranging from 0% to 20%, rotation within a range of −15° to +15°, horizontal and vertical shearing

Table 2 Displaying a comparative analysis before and after augmentation

Folders	Before augmentation	After augmentation
Train	930	2298
Test	200	281
Validation	197	281
Total	1327	2860

Table 3 Details of training parameters of YOLOv5

Training parameters	YOLOv5
Input dimension	640 × 640 × 3
Batch size	16
Number of epochs	200
Epochs patience	20
Initial learning rate	0.01
Learning rate scheduler	ReduceLR
Learning rate drop factor	0.5
Optimizer	Adam
Weight decay	0.0005
IOU threshold	0.5
Confidence threshold	0.5

up to 15°, grayscale conversion for 25% of images, hue, saturation, brightness, and exposure adjustments within −25% to +25% ranges, blur of up to 2.5 pixels, the introduction of up to 5% pixel-level noise. These changes work together to provide a more diverse and resilient dataset for training machine learning models. The distribution of data samples among distinct folders (Train, Test, Validation) before and after through augmentation is illustrated in the Table 2.

The model's hyperparameters, which are defined before training begins but are not learned in the process, are commonly adjusted using data from the validation set. Some examples of hyperparameters are the neural network's learning rate, the number of hidden layers, and the intensity of regularization (Table 3). The model's performance on test data could be improved by adjusting these hyperparameters. Before splitting we preprocessed the images of dataset with auto-orient, resize to 640 × 640, modify Class, filter null.

2.3.3 YOLOv5 Model Configuration and Architecture

YOLOv5 Model Configuration

A member of the You Only Look Once (YOLO) family of computer vision models is called YOLOv5. For object detection, YOLOv5 is widely utilized. Each of the four sizes of YOLOv5 delivers a higher level of accuracy: small (s), medium (m), large (l), and extra large (x). Also, the training time needed for each kind varies. To get YOLOv5 up and running. The essential Python, PyTorch, NumPy, OpenCV, and Matplotlib packages must first be installed. After everything has been set up, the model need to be trained. Validation data is used to fine-tune the model while test data is used to generate mean average precision (mAP), F1-score, and precision-recall curves, to evaluate the effectiveness of a trained model. To deploy the trained model to test on new images Roboflow platform, an online tool that provides a full suite of operations and services for creating and deploying computer vision models was used [35]. Roboflow has 5 modes: Adding Data, Annotating Images, Train/Test/validation Split, Preprocessing and Augmentations, and Preparing Data for Training [36].

YOLOv5 Model Architecture

YOLOv5 was released in June 2020 and is an improved version of its predecessor, YOLOv4 [24]. YOLOv5 is made up of the following three components: (1) The Cross Stage Partial Network (CSPDarknet) as the backbone, (2) Path Aggregation Network (PANet) as the neck, and (3) Yolo Layer as the head. The data are first supplied into CSPDarknet in order to have features extracted from them, and then they are sent to PANet so that features may be fused together. Yolo Layer is responsible for the final output of detection findings (class, score, location, size). YOLOV5 also has a variety of other features that, together, contribute to the improvement of its performance [37]. The basic configuration of YOLOv5 consists of the following components:

Backbone: A CNN that creates visual characteristics at multiple levels of granularity and then aggregates them.A modified version of the CSPDarknet53 architecture serves as the foundation for YOLOv5, which uses this architecture as its backbone. This is a deep neural network that is made up of many convolutional layers. It also has skip connections, which let information to be transmitted between layers at varying resolutions. The backbone is in charge of retrieving high-level information from the picture that is being fed into it.

Neck: A sequence of layers that will mix and integrate the visual characteristics before passing them on to prediction.YOLOv5's neck is made up of a number of convolutional layers, and these layers are responsible for combining the feature maps that come from the backbone and the detection head. The neck is responsible for producing a cohesive feature representation by merging the low-level and high-level characteristics that are present in the head.

Detection Head: Performs box and class prediction steps while consuming features from the neck. The detection head of YOLOv5 consists of a series of convolutional layers that are used to predict the class and location of objects in the input image. The detection head is responsible for processing the unified feature representation produced by the neck and producing a set of bounding boxes and confidence scores for each detected object.

In general, YOLOv5 is well optimized for speed and precision, and it can do real-time analysis of high-resolution images using a single GPU. This is far superior than

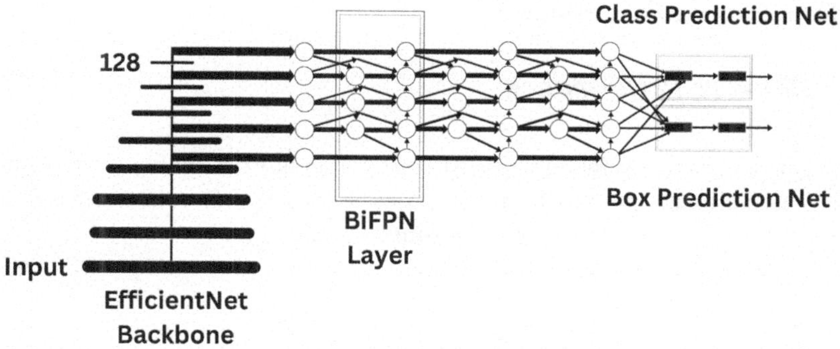

Fig. 8 YoloV5 architecture

its predecessors [38]. Figure 8 explains how an object detector is built and how it operates [39].

2.3.4 Detecting Malaria Infected and Non-infected Blood Cells

The pre-trianed model needs to be loaded to run test on the new test data. In the case of Malaria parasite count and detection, for instance, the test data will consist of a set of images of blood samples, and the goal would be to accurately identify and count the number of blood cells present in each image of WSI. The created model was loaded into memory so that it can be used. To count and detect the cells in a blood sample, the image patches genertaed by the harware system was applied to the model for inference and final decision was taken by counting the cells from all patches from a WSI. The images went through same preprocessing step as we did during the model training so that they are in the correct format and size for the model. Then the inference as done to count the numebr of blood cells present in each test patch and WSI.

2.3.5 Performance Matrics of YoloV5

The effectiveness of an algorithm may be gauged using a variety of assessment measures; model accuracy is among the most frequent. The F1 score is very helpful in finding the sweet spot between a model's accuracy and recall, although it spans a wide range of possible values, from 0 to 1. The F1 score is a common performance metric for classification, and it is generally favoured above other measures such as accuracy when data is imbalanced, like when the number of instances in one class much outnumbers those in the other class. Precision and recall are added together to form the F1 Score. Many applications, such as automated benchmarking and grid search, would benefit greatly from having simply one performance metric rather than multiple [40, 41].

3 Results and Discussion

3.1 *Harware Performance*

The Autohaem Smear+ module, microscope and control assembly were tested to collect sample image patches from the device. Figure 9 shows the sample images collected from the proposed image acquisition system.

3.2 *Performance Evalaution of YoloV5*

Figure 10 and Table 4 provide a high-level perspective of the mdoel. F1 vs confidence, precision vs confidence, precision vs recall, losses over all epochs, confusion matrices, and annotated class counts. In Fig. 10a, it shows that the confidence value maximizes accuracy and recall from the F1 curve is 0.54 (Left) and shows that with a precision of 0.95, this suggests that just 95% of the positive predictions produced by the model were correct (Right).All classes reach at precision value 1 when the confidence value is 0.96. When the confidence threshold is raised, the model becomes more cautious when it comes to generating positive predictions. This results in greater accuracy, but there is a possibility that recall may decrease. The curve may be used to compare the performance of different classification methods. In Fig. 10b, it represents the Precision vs Recall Curve. The graph shows the relationship between the precision and recall scores for the model (Left) and shows all types of Losses (box,object,class) with respect to Epoch during training and validation (Right). According to the examination of the precision-recall curve, the model is 96.2% accurate when classifying a sample as infected, and the precision value for the "infected" class is 0.962. Precision of 0.978 for the "non-infected" class exemplifies a high degree of accuracy (about 97.8%) in determining whether or not a sample is free of infection. As assessed by the mAP at the 0.5 threshold, the model's total performance is 0.968, which indicates a nice middle ground between accuracy and recall for both classes. The precision-recall curve depicts the tradeoff between identifying contaminated samples accurately

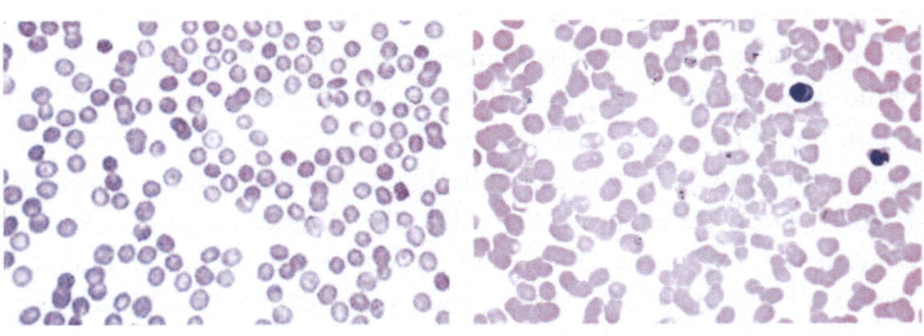

Fig. 9 Sample image patches from the proposed system

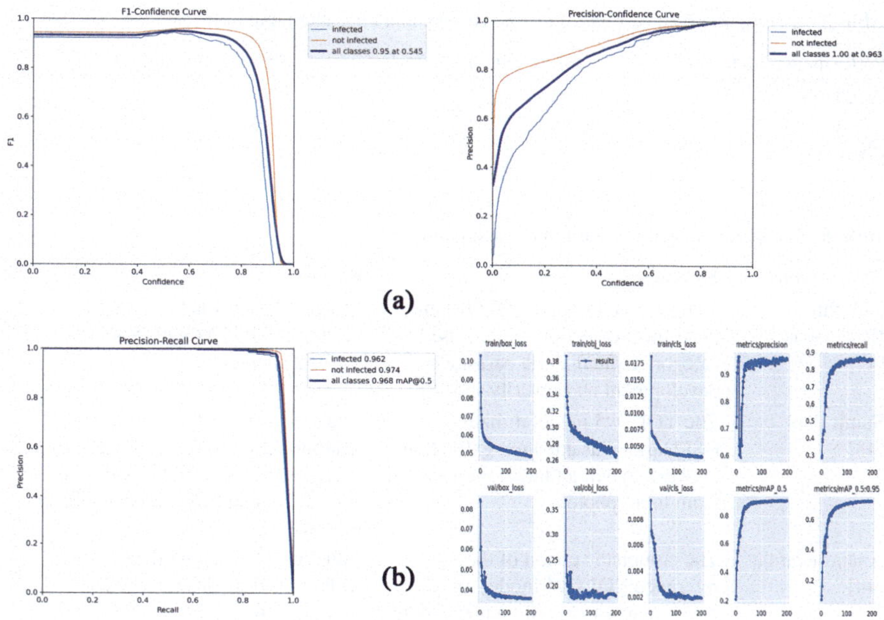

Fig. 10 F1-score vs confidence and precision vs confidence curve (**a**) and precision vs recall and loss vs epoch curve (**b**)

Table 4 The prediction for each classes in confusion matrix

Infected/non-infected	Infected	Not infected (True)	Background
Background	0.05	0.05	0
Not infected (predicted)	0.07	0.95	0.95
Infected	0.89	0	0.05

and incorrectly. These findings point towards the model's promising performance, lending credence to its capacity to effectively discriminate between infected and non-infected instances, a capability essential for efficient Malaria identification and control. As the number of epoch increase, the value of loss decrease.

In Table 4, it displays the number of true positive, false positive, true negative, and false negative predictions made by the model for each class. In assessing a model's performance in detecting infections, we found that it correctly recognized 89% of infected samples, as reflected by a True Positives (TP) score of 0.89. However, it made incorrect predictions for 11% of infected samples, resulting in FN at 0.11. The model, on the other hand, showed a significant capacity to properly categorize non-infected samples, with True Negatives (TN) at 0.95, suggesting a 95% accuracy in detecting samples free of infection. Nonetheless, the model mistakenly identified 5% of infection-free samples as contaminated, resulting in 0.05 False Positives (FP). This thorough evaluation identifies the model's strengths and flaws in discriminating between infected and non-infected samples.

Table 5 A comparison of results for testing (before and after augmentation)

Performance matrics	Before augmentation	After augmentation
Precision	0.95	0.97
Recall	0.83	0.85
mAP_0.5	0.90	0.92

Table 6 Comparative analysis with SOTA techniques

Author name	Methods	Result
Padmini Krishnadas [42]	YOLOv5 and scaled YOLOv4 are two object detection models used to categorize the malaria parasite's development and severity	Scaled YOLOv4 achieved 83% accuracy, while YOLOv5 achieved 78.50% accuracy
Sumit Paul [43]	The YOLOv5 model utilizes CSPDarknet as a feature extraction network to extract target information from input photos	The ensemble YOLOv5 model exhibited accuracy, recall, and mean average precision (mAP) values of 0.76, 0.78, and 0.79, respectively, as reported
Anand Koirala [44]	The complete version of the reference YOLOv4 model for baseline research, with a pixel count of 608 on the input network	Full-YOLOv4 standard and full YOLOv4-41 model achieved mAP@05 IoU value of 90.61 and 91.00 respectively
Ruicun Liu [11]	This malaria parasite identification and classification method used YOLOv5 and transformer models	With a false positive rate of 19.02%, the AAM had an accuracy of 87.10% when diagnosing malaria
Anne de Souza Oliveira [45]	A freshly trained convolutional neural network (CNN)	Precision rates of 76.58% and 71.58% were achieved, respectively, for Image Sets 3 and 4, where the parasite sizes were rather modest
Proposed work	YOLOv5 object detection model	The model has an around 92% accuracy rate overall. This implies that, given the data, the model accurately identifies 92% of samples as either infected or not infected

Table 5 shows comparison unequivocally illustrates the beneficial influence of data augmentation on the performance of the model. The expanded dataset has enhanced the model's predictive capabilities by improving precision, recall, and mAP_0.5 scores, resulting in more precise and comprehensive predictions. The enhancement holds significant importance in practical scenarios where the dependability and precision of object detecting systems are of utmost significance.

Detection and classification of malaria parasites have been crucial research foci, propelling the advancement and improvement of object detection models. This comparative analysis comprises a number of studies, each of which utilizes unique methodologies and frameworks to improve the precision and effectiveness of malaria diagnosis. The Table 6 presents research endeavors that have investigated the effectiveness of well-known models including YOLOv5, YOLOv4, and hybrid architectures that combine convolutional neural networks (CNNs) and transformers. The investigations, carried out by renowned authorities in the discipline, illuminate the diverse degrees of efficacy attained by distinct approaches, thereby providing significant perspectives on the continuous endeavors to address malaria via sophisticated machine learning methodologies.

4 Limitations and Future Work

Although the YOLOv5 model has an impressive 92% accuracy rate, there is still an 8% possibility of misclassification. This could result in false-positive or false-negative results, which could have significant consequences in a healthcare setting. The effectiveness of deep learning models significantly relies on the quantity and quality of the data they are trained on. Inaccurate models may result from insufficient or skewed data. As the original dataset contains only 1327 images before augementation. To improve the accuracy and robustness of the YOLOv5 model, it is essential to collect a large and diverse dataset. The effectiveness of the model is largely dependent on the blood smear quality. Poor preparation of smears may result in inaccurate results. The image quality of the dataset was suboptimal. Although cost-effective, the 3D-printed device and microscope might not offer the same precision and durability as more expensive, professionally manufactured equipment. However, the proposed system should be further validated using a large clinical trial and compared with clinical benhmar device.

Future research should concentrate on improving the model's accuracy and reliability by incorporating advanced deep learning techniques, examining larger and more diverse datasets, and refining the model's training process to accommodate the inherent complexities of malaria-infected blood smear images. There are opportunities to enhance the precision and durability of the 3D-printed device and microscope by refining their design and manufacturing processes. Future research could focus on making the model more robust to variations in blood samples, such as those caused by various types of malaria, patient age, health condition, etc. Finally focus on integrating this technology with existing healthcare systems in order to expedite the process of diagnosis and enhance healthcare delivery in malaria-prone regions.

5 Conclusions

A novel approach for combating malaria that utilises state-of-the-art software and precision hardware. In this work, we proposed innovative approach for Malaria detection and diagnosis using the autohaem smear+ device and a cheap digital microscope with control assesmbly, as well as the incorporation of the YOLOv5 model for quick detection. This all-encompassing method not only improves the rate and precision of whole slide imaging for malaria diagnosis, but also takes on significant obstacles like cost and availability. The fast, whole-slide imaging that a digital microscope makes possible has revolutionised the diagnostic and research processes in the medical and scientific communities, but several low-resource countries and rural parts cannot access these. This study adds to international efforts to control malaria and provides a potentially useful option for early and successful detection in areas with limited access to healthcare resources. This research has the potential to transform malaria diagnosis by expanding availability of good-quality microscopy to such people. To enhance healthcare outcomes and decrease malaria-related mortality, this study offers up promising prospects for expanding the use of automated microscopy and with the help of deep learning in the battle against malaria.

References

1. C.R. Maturana et al., Advances and challenges in automated malaria diagnosis using digital microscopy imaging with artificial intelligence tools: A review. Front. Microbiol. **13**. Frontiers Media S.A. (2022). https://doi.org/10.3389/fmicb.2022.1006659
2. T. Rai Dastidar, R. Ethirajan, Whole slide imaging system using deep learning-based automated focusing. Biomed. Opt. Express **11**(1), 480 (2020). https://doi.org/10.1364/boe.379780
3. R. Varo, N. Balanza, A. Mayor, Q. Bassat, Diagnosis of clinical malaria in endemic settings. Expert Rev. Anti-Infect. Ther. **19**(1), 79–92 (2021)
4. M.R. Islam, M. Nahiduzzaman, M.O.F. Goni, Explainable transformer-based deep learning model for the detection of malaria parasites from blood cell images. MDPI **22**(12), 4358 (2022)
5. C.W. Pirnstill, G.L. Coté, Malaria diagnosis using a mobile phone polarized microscope. Sci. Rep. **5** (2015). https://doi.org/10.1038/srep13368
6. P.D. Gordon, C. De Ville, J.C. Sacchettini, G.L. Coté, A portable brightfield and fluorescence microscope toward automated malarial parasitemia quantification in thin blood smears. PLoS One **17**(4) (2022). https://doi.org/10.1371/journal.pone.0266441
7. E. Rogier et al., Bead-based immunoassay allows sub-picogram detection of histidine-rich protein 2 from Plasmodium falciparum and estimates reliability of malaria rapid diagnostic tests. PLoS One **12**(2), e0172139 (2017)
8. J. García-Villena et al., 3D-printed portable robotic mobile microscope for remote diagnosis of global health diseases. Electronics (Switzerland) **10**(19) (2021). https://doi.org/10.3390/electronics10192408
9. W. Sultani, W. Nawaz, S. Javed, M. S. Danish, A. Saadia, M. Ali, Towards Low-Cost and Efficient Malaria Detection. [Online]. Available: http://im.itu.edu.pk/m5-malaria-dataset/
10. J. Salido, G. Bueno, J. Ruiz-Santaquiteria, G. Cristobal, A review on low-cost microscopes for Open Science. Microsc. Res. Tech. **85**(10), 3270–3283 (2022. Wiley). https://doi.org/10.1002/jemt.24200
11. R. Liu et al., AIDMAN: An AI-based object detection system for malaria diagnosis from smartphone thin-blood-smear images. Patterns **4**(9) (2023). https://doi.org/10.1016/j.patter.2023.100806
12. K.A. Sadiq, A.F. Thompson, O.A. Ayeni, Toward healthcare data availability and security using fog-to-cloud networks, in *Intelligent Interactive Multimedia Systems for e-Healthcare Applications*, (Springer, 2021), pp. 81–103. https://doi.org/10.1007/978-981-16-6542-4_6
13. R. Sangameswaran, *MAIScope: A Low-Cost Portable Microscope with Built-in Vision AI to Automate Microscopic Diagnosis of Diseases in Remote Rural Settings* (2022). [Online]. Available: http://arxiv.org/abs/2208.06114

14. F. Yang et al., Deep learning for smartphone-based malaria parasite detection in thick blood smears. IEEE J. Biomed. Health Inform. **24**(5), 1427–1438 (2020). https://doi.org/10.1109/JBHI.2019.2939121
15. J. Yoon, W.S. Jang, J. Nam, D.C. Mihn, C.S. Lim, An automated microscopic Malaria parasite detection system using digital image analysis. Diagnostics **11**(3) (2021). https://doi.org/10.3390/diagnostics11030527
16. A. Kratz, S.H. Lee, G. Zini, J.A. Riedl, M. Hur, S. Machin, Digital morphology analyzers in hematology: ICSH review and recommendations. Int. J. Lab. Hematol. **41**(4), 437–447 (2019. Blackwell Publishing Ltd). https://doi.org/10.1111/ijlh.13042
17. D. Das et al., Field evaluation of the diagnostic performance of EasyScan GO: A digital malaria microscopy device based on machine-learning. Malar. J. **21**(1) (2022). https://doi.org/10.1186/s12936-022-04146-1
18. K. de Haan et al., Automated screening of sickle cells using a smartphone-based microscope and deep learning. NPJ Digit. Med. **3**(1) (2020). https://doi.org/10.1038/s41746-020-0282-y
19. D.R. Loh, W.X. Yong, J. Yapeter, K. Subburaj, R. Chandramohanadas, A deep learning approach to the screening of malaria infection: Automated and rapid cell counting, object detection and instance segmentation using Mask R-CNN. Comput. Med. Imaging Graph. **88** (2021). https://doi.org/10.1016/j.compmedimag.2020.101845
20. P.A. Pattanaik, M. Mittal, M.Z. Khan, S.N. Panda, Malaria detection using deep residual networks with mobile microscopy. J. King Saud Univ. Comput. Inf. Sci. **34**(5), 1700–1705 (2022). https://doi.org/10.1016/j.jksuci.2020.07.003
21. H.A. Nugroho, R. Nurfauzi, A combination of optimized threshold and deep learning-based approach to improve malaria detection and segmentation on PlasmoID dataset. FACETS **8**, 1–12 (2023). https://doi.org/10.1139/facets-2022-0206
22. W.R.W.M. Razin, T.S. Gunawan, M. Kartiwi, N.M. Yusoff, Malaria parasite detection and classification using CNN and YOLOv5 architectures, in *8th IEEE International Conference on Smart Instrumentation, Measurement and Applications, ICSIMA 2022*, (Institute of Electrical and Electronics Engineers, 2022), pp. 277–281. https://doi.org/10.1109/ICSIMA55652.2022.9928992
23. P. Krishnadas, N. Sampathila, Automated detection of Malaria implemented by deep learning in pytorch, in *Proceedings of CONECCT 2021: 7th IEEE International Conference on Electronics, Computing and Communication Technologies*, (Institute of Electrical and Electronics Engineers, 2021). https://doi.org/10.1109/CONECCT52877.2021.9622608
24. G. Marques, A. Ferreras, I. de la Torre-Diez, An ensemble-based approach for automated medical diagnosis of malaria using EfficientNet. Multimed. Tools Appl. **81**(19), 28061–28078 (2022). https://doi.org/10.1007/s11042-022-12624-6
25. A. Abubakar, M. Ajuji, I.U. Yahya, Deepfmd: Computational analysis for malaria detection in blood-smear images using deep-learning features. Appl. Syst. Innov. **4**(4) (2021). https://doi.org/10.3390/asi4040082
26. S.B. Baray et al., Automated measurement of penile curvature using deep learning-based novel quantification method. Front. Pediatr. **11**, 1149318 (2023)
27. S. Mahmud, T.O. Abbas, A. Mushtak, J. Prithula, M.E.H. Chowdhury, Kidney cancer diagnosis and surgery selection by machine learning from CT scans combined with clinical metadata. Cancers (Basel) **15**(12), 3189 (2023)
28. T.O. Abbas, M. AbdelMoniem, I.A. Khalil, M.S.A. Hossain, M.E.H. Chowdhury, Deep learning based automated quantification of urethral plate characteristics using the plate objective scoring tool (POST). J. Pediatr. Urol. (2023)
29. T.O. Abbas, M. AbdelMoniem, M.E.H. Chowdhury, Automated quantification of penile curvature using artificial intelligence. Front. Artif. Intell. **5**, 954497 (2022)
30. S. McDermott et al., Autohaem: 3D printed devices for automated preparation of blood smears. Rev. Sci. Instrum. **93**(1) (2022)
31. World Health Organization, *Basic Malaria Microscopy* (WHO, 2010)
32. OMAX 40X-2500X LED Digital Trinocular Lab Compound Microscope with USB – Omax. Accessed Oct 17 2023. [Online]. Available: https://omaxmicroscope.com/products/m83ez-c03s

33. V. Ljosa, K.L. Sokolnicki, Corrigendum: Annotated high-throughput microscopy image sets for validation. Carpent. Nat. Methods **9**, 637 (2012)
34. https://app.roboflow.com/thesis-op3m2/malaria-wcux6/4. Malaria Dataset, Roboflow. (2023)
35. S. Ouedraogo, M. Bousso, A. Balde, O. Sall, C. Sall, M. Soumboundou, Automating sickle cell counting using object detection techniques, in *Pan-African Artificial Intelligence and Smart Systems*, ed. by T.M. Ngatched Nkouatchah, I. Woungang, J.-R. Tapamo, S. Viriri, (Springer, Cham, 2023), pp. 224–236
36. F. Mercaldo, F. Martinelli, A. Santone, M. Cesarelli, *Blood Cells Counting and Localisation through Deep Learning Object Detection* (IEEE, 2022), pp. 4400–4409
37. J. Zhao, Y. Cheng, X. Ma, A real time intelligent detection and counting method of cells based on YOLOv5, in *2022 IEEE International Conference on Electrical Engineering, Big Data and Algorithms (EEBDA)*, (2022), pp. 675–679. https://doi.org/10.1109/EEBDA53927.2022.9744842
38. M.A. Rahaman, M.M. Ali, K. Ahmed, F.M. Bui, S.M.H. Mahmud, Performance analysis between YOLOv5s and YOLOv5m model to detect and count blood cells: Deep learning approach, in *Proceedings of the 2nd International Conference on Computing Advancements, in ICCA '22. New York, NY, USA*, (Association for Computing Machinery, 2022), pp. 316–322. https://doi.org/10.1145/3542954.3543000
39. J. Sarkar, S. Ahmadsaidulu, E. Banoth, *Classification and Detection of White Blood Cells using Enhanced YOLOv5 Algorithm* (Optica Publishing Group, 2022), pp. JW48–JW46
40. A. Badithela, T. Wongpiromsarn, R.M. Murray, Evaluation metrics for object detection for autonomous systems. arXiv preprint arXiv, 2210.10298 (2022)
41. H. Mao, X. Yang, W.J. Dally, A delay metric for video object detection: What average precision fails to tell, in *Proceedings of the IEEE/CVF International Conference on Computer Vision*, (2019), pp. 573–582
42. P. Krishnadas, K. Chadaga, N. Sampathila, S. Rao, K.S. Swathi, S. Prabhu, Classification of malaria using object detection models. Informatics **9**(4) (2022). https://doi.org/10.3390/informatics9040076
43. S. Paul, S. Batra, K. Mohiuddin, M.N. Miladi, D. Anand, O.A. Nasr, A novel ensemble weight-assisted Yolov5-based deep learning technique for the localization and detection of malaria parasites. Electronics (Switzerland) **11**(23) (2022). https://doi.org/10.3390/electronics11233999
44. A. Koirala et al., Deep learning for real-time malaria parasite detection and counting using YOLO-mp. IEEE Access **10**, 102157–102172 (2022). https://doi.org/10.1109/ACCESS.2022.3208270
45. A. de Souza Oliveira, M.G.F. Costa, M. das Graças Vale Barbosa, C.F.F.C. Filho, A new approach for malaria diagnosis in thick blood smear images. Biomed. Signal Process Control **78**, 103931 (2022). https://doi.org/10.1016/j.bspc.2022.103931

Innovations in Tuberculosis Disease Screening

Duaa Yousif, Rowan Mesilhy, Roaa Aly, Salma Hegazi, Zahra Yousif, Farhan S. Cyprian, and Abdallah M. Abdallah

1 Introduction

Tuberculosis (TB), an affliction with an enduring legacy has been documented by ancient Egyptians (around 3000 BC), and its existence was identified as early as 9000 years ago, continues to stand as one of the most formidable and persistent contagious diseases, resisting resolution even in the contemporary era [1–3]. It remains the number one cause of death from a single infectious agent and one of the top ten causes of death worldwide despite childhood vaccination. Infections with the bacterium *Mycobacterium tuberculosis* (*Mtb*) are primarily disseminated via airborne droplets. While the lungs are afflicted in more than 75% of cases, virtually any other organ and tissue can be infected. Despite the knowledge acquired since the discovery of *Mtb* as the principal agent of human TB by Robert Koch 140 years ago, TB still remains a major burden to human health globally, with 10 million new cases diagnosed and around 2 million deaths every year [4]. Around 30% of individuals exposed to *Mtb* will develop latent TB infection and, if untreated, around 5% to 10% of these individuals will progress to active TB disease or reactivation of TB [5–7]. Alarmingly, this rate of progression may increases in varying states of immunodeficiency with up to a 16% annual risk of progression of TB infection into active TB disease in HIV patients [8] that has led to the emergence of drug-resistant strains of *Mtb*. Therefore, the World Health Organization (WHO) acknowledged this resurgence of the global TB burden, leading to the initiation of the End TB initiative in 2016. This serves as a blueprint and an effective strategy for countries to reduce incidence, morbidity, and mortality associated with TB and to reduce costs for TB-affected households by improving diagnostic and therapeutic practices,

D. Yousif · R. Mesilhy · R. Aly · S. Hegazi · Z. Yousif · F. S. Cyprian · A. M. Abdallah (✉)
College of Medicine, QU Health, Qatar University, Doha, Qatar
e-mail: dy1904726@qu.edu.qa; rm1903550@qu.edu.qa; ra1903390@qu.edu.qa; sh1905249@qu.edu.qa; zy1802662@qu.edu.qa; fcyprian@qu.edu.qa; abdallah.musa@qu.edu.qa

M. E. H. Chowdhury, S. Kiranyaz (eds.), *Surveillance, Prevention, and Control of Infectious Diseases*, https://doi.org/10.1007/978-3-031-59967-5_5

and developing preventative strategies along with innovative research and patient education.

Every year approximately 4 million cases of TB are unreported by national health organizations, with a pronounced impact in underdeveloped countries. Moreover, cases under scrutiny for TB diagnosis experience delays in receiving test results, which not only worsen disease outcomes but also augment the transmission of *Mtb* pathogen [9]. Hence, there is a need for improving diagnostic technology to fast-track accurate TB diagnosis. Several TB screening programs involve the active identification of people who are at risk of developing active TB disease to facilitate early detection of TB cases.

2 Current TB Screening Methods

In relevant communities, screening for *Mtb* infection is vital due to the high prevalence of TB and the risk of latent TB progressing to active disease. High-risk individuals, including those in close contact with pulmonary TB (PTB) patients, people from endemic countries, healthcare workers dealing with at-risk patients, and those in a vulnerable setting (long-term care facilities or nursing homes, and homeless shelters), must be screened including infants, children, and adolescents exposed to TB risk. Current methods for TB screening include the tuberculin skin tests (TST)/TB skin test also known as the Mantoux test and the interferon-gamma release assay (IGRA) or TB blood test, both of which rely on measurement of *Mtb* specific cell-mediated immune responses [10–12] directed against *Mtb* in the infected individual. However, a positive TST test or IGRA test does not indicate whether the individual has a latent TB infection or has progressed to active TB disease. These tests only suggest that a person has been infected with TB bacteria. Therefore, additional tests, such as a chest x-ray (CXR) and sputum sample, are needed to see whether the individual has active TB disease. However, the definitive diagnosis of PTB is achieved through the isolation of Mtb from bodily secretions, fluids, or tissues [13].

2.1 Tuberculin Skin Test (TST)

The classical TST based on purified protein derivative (PPD) has been in use for the last 90 years to support TB diagnosis in the clinic as well as for screening in national TB programs and epidemiological studies [14]. This test assesses cell-mediated immunity towards *Mtb*, necessitating two healthcare center visits. During the initial visit, 0.1 ml/5-tuberculin units are administered intradermally, forming a 4–6 mm wheal on the forearm's anterior surface. A follow-up visit is scheduled at 48–72 h to measure the area of induration. Interpretation of the test results depends on the induration size and the patient's status. If the test result is negative, it indicates that the person's immune system did not react to the test and that a latent or active TB is unlikely. However, if the test result is positive it indicates that a person was infected previously with TB, is infected with active TB, has a latent TB infection, is infected with nontuberculous mycobacteria (NTM), or was vaccinated with bacille Calmette-Guerin (BCG) vaccine at birth. Thus, additional tests and clinical evaluation are required to identify the person's status. A positive test requires at least 5 mm of induration in high-risk individuals (HIV infection, close contact with an active TB patient, abnormal CXR with fibrotic abnormalities, recipient of an organ transplant, and immunosuppressed patients who take more than 15 mg of prednisone per day, TNF antagonists, and other biologics). Among individuals at elevated risk of reactivation, an induration measurement of 10 mm or greater signifies a positive result. High-risk category encompasses those with conditions such as; chronic kidney disease (CKD) requiring dialysis, diabetes mellitus, malignancy, underweight, post-gastrectomy, complicated pregnancy, post-organ transplantation, a history of injection drug abuse, age below 4 years, foreign-born individuals from TB-endemic countries who have immigrated within the last 5 years, as well as residents or workers in settings like prisons, jails, healthcare facilities, mentally challenged individuals and those in homeless or refugee shelters. In low-risk individuals, induration of 15 mm or larger is considered positive (ages four and above, with minimal risk of TB infection). TST is the preferred test for children under the age of five. In addition, it is the preferred test for people who require yearly testing such as health care professionals [15].

2.2 *Interferon-Gamma Release Assay (IGRA)*

IGRA measures the individual's cell-mediated immune response to *Mtb* infection. As an alternative to *in vivo* skin testing, PPD has also been used for the *in vitro* detection of specific interferon-gamma (IFN-γ) secreting lymphocytes from donors sensitized against mycobacterial antigen [16]. In this test, 1 patient's lymphocytes are stimulated with PPD, most conveniently in direct whole blood cultures during a period of 24 h, followed by ELISA detection of IFN-γ production as sensitive readout for lymphocyte activation. A commercial assay was originally developed for the diagnosis of bovine TB [17] and a similar test, called the *Quanti*FERON® test, was later shown to have a potential for the diagnosis of human TB [18]. Results of this test demonstrated that whole blood IFN-γ production following *Mtb* PPD stimulation in vitro correlated well with TST [19]. Today, the two assays that are approved by the United States Food and Drug Administration (US FDA) are QuantiFERON-TB Gold In-Tube (QFT-GIT) and the T-SPOT, TB (T-Spot) test. As the immune reaction is performed *ex vivo* in the laboratory, only one visit will be needed for a single blood draw, and the results are made available in 24–48 h. In contrast to TST, These tests can be used if the person does not want to get back again to the health care facility, or if the person was immunized with BCG vaccine as there is no chance of a cross-reaction with antigens of BCG vaccine [15].

2.3 Chest X-Ray (CXR) in Diagnosing and Screening for TB

According to WHO, around 10.6 million people were diagnosed with TB in 2021 with an incidence rate of 134 cases per 100,000 globally [20]. CXR is an essential tool to diagnose PTB and it can be used as an assistant tool for the screening of PTB. A posterior-anterior view is usually used to detect any abnormalities within the chest. These abnormalities may suggest active TB disease and can differ in size, shape, density, and cavitation. Although CXR cannot give a definite diagnosis of PTB, it can help in ruling out PTB in those patients with a positive TST or IGRA and have no symptoms [21]. In active case-finding setting, CXR alone has low specificity. The CXR outperforms symptoms alone in screening for TB cases in community settings, with a sensitivity of 93% and specificity of 97%. Combining CXRs and symptoms increased TB case detection. Integration of AI improved the sensitivity to 100% by compromising on the specificity adding value to TB diagnosis [22]. Nevertheless, it is recommended that CXR should be performed in conjunction with a bacteriological confirmatory test (TST, IGRA) that is both sensitive and specific for tuberculosis [23]. Available AI products show variable diagnostic accuracy, generally featuring high sensitivity and improving but modest specificity. Limited studies exist, especially for low TB burden areas. Although more research is needed to establish AI performance in TB diagnosis that is improving with time [24].

2.4 Limitations and Challenges of the Current TB Screening Methods

Despite the global usage of IGRA and TST to screen for TB, there are some limitations and challenges that impact the quality of healthcare. TST carries a risk of false-positive and false-negative results due to several factors [25]. Operator's variation in test technique, poor follow-up and patient compliance after 48–72 h [26], inter-observer variation in reading the results [15], the impact of BCG vaccination, cross-reactivity with nontuberculous mycobacteria (NTM) infections in specific geographic areas as well as unidentified HIV cases. Although PPD is a purified mixture of proteins from *Mtb*, its greatest drawback is the fact that the majority of protein components in PPD is known to be shared with other, NTM (which are abundantly present in the environment), and with unrelated species of bacteria. This fact significantly decreases the specificity of the TST as individuals sensitized by prior exposure to NTM or vaccinated with BCG; respond immunologically to PPD from *Mtb* often as well or better than individuals infected with *Mtb* itself. This fact has been used in many countries as an argument against BCG vaccination since retention of the diagnostic potential of the TST has been considered a priority. This situation is further complicated by the temporary depression of the cell-mediated immune response often seen in active TB patients, which can lead to false negative PPD skin test results. Furthermore, TST showed the lowest sensitivity in younger children, as up to 10% of children with positive TB culture do not react with tuberculin skin test giving a false negative result. False-negative TST results are also seen in children with severe or milliary TB, as well as those with immunosuppressive diseases, malnutrition, recent live virus vaccination status (measles, mumps, polio, smallpox), recent viral infections, and other concomitant bacterial infections [15, 25].

Similarly to the limitation of PPD's performance *in vivo* skin testing, the weakness of the PPD-based whole blood test is the lack of defined and highly *Mtb*-specific antigens, thus hampering specific TB diagnosis. Therefore, IGRA exhibits inherent limitations and drawbacks, encompassing potential errors in collecting or transporting blood specimens, along with the possibility of diminished accuracy stemming from challenges in conducting and interpreting the test [27]. Furthermore, healthcare practitioners grapple with the intricate clinical implications of QFT-GIT conversions during serial testing. The application of a singular cutoff criterion for IGRA also bears the potential risk of TB misdiagnosis [28]. There is limited data on the utility of IGRA to predict the progression of TB from latent to active infection, its use in children under the age of five; those recently exposed to *Mtb*, immunocompromised individuals, and in serial testing [27].

TST and IGRAs are ineffective at distinguishing latent TB infection from active TB disease, especially in the case of immune-compromised patients. In addition, TST and IGRAs cannot determine the disease duration nor the viability of the infecting *Mtb* strain [29]. Hence, it becomes imperative to tackle these limitations and enhance existing methodologies for TB screening and diagnosis, constituting a dynamic domain of ongoing research.

3 Innovations in TB Screening

Worldwide, the screening for PTB is clinical, depending on the signs and symptoms of infected individuals. Nowadays, several innovations are in evaluation to screen for TB. Recent advances aim to bring PTB effective screening closer to communities, particularly in resource-limited settings. These innovations include:

3.1 Mobile Health Application for TB Screening

Google Sheets developed a new "TB- screen" application based on a previously published algorithm [30]. The application calculates the risk of PTB progression in patients based on their sociodemographic characteristics and clinical history. The application suggests whether this person should undergo a CXR to screen for PTB infection. Following the resolution of COVID-19 outbreak, this application was launched in urban areas and its utility was evaluated. CXR compliance was assessed by scanning a QR code in the application. This study involved 453 individuals utilizing the application for which 322 individuals were identified as potential TB cases, with 24 cases subsequently confirmed to have active PTB disease [30]. This application needs further testing in larger cohorts for validation.

3.2 *Imaging Technologies for TB Screening*

Imaging's significance in TB has experienced remarkable expansion, mirroring the broader trends in the field of medicine. Imaging studies frequently serve as the initial indicator of a potential tubercular origin, especially in anatomically challenging locations. When dealing with a confirmed TB case, imaging is commonly utilized to gauge the disease's extent, monitor treatment progress, and identify any lingering infection post-treatment completion. Additionally, imaging serves as a critical tool for directing aspirations and biopsies, as well as offering guidance for therapeutic drainage of abnormal fluid accumulations [31]. Traditional radiography continues to be the primary choice for the initial assessment of suspected pulmonary tuberculosis or for mass screening applications, and its significance in musculoskeletal imaging remains undisputed [31]. Recently, the WHO issued a recommendation endorsing the use of computer-aided detection (CAD) software programs to interpret digital CXRs for TB screening and triage purposes [32]. CAD software assists healthcare professionals in overcoming challenges related to interpreting CXRs, leading to more efficient patient screening. Studies indicate that CAD programs serve as a viable and effective substitute for clinical radiologists, offering a significant benefit for countries aiming to enhance PTB diagnoses but facing a shortage of trained radiologists. Moreover, ultra-portable digital X-ray systems, characterized by their small size, wireless nature, and easy mobility, prove to be invaluable assets in delivering healthcare services to remote geographical localities. When incorporated into the PTB care process, these technologies have the potential to enhance case detection, progression, and treatment outcomes, improving overall patient care [33]. Although traditional chest X-rays are the usual choice for diagnosing pulmonary tuberculosis, alternative imaging techniques such as CT, PET-CT, and MRI prove valuable in evaluating both pulmonary and extrapulmonary tuberculosis [31]. The adoption of digital or computed radiography has increased efficiency, improved image quality, and reduced radiation exposure for patients [31]. Due to its rapid scanning capabilities and superior image quality, CT has become the preferred method for assessing thoracic, gastrointestinal, and urogenital tuberculosis. Multislice CT has largely supplanted traditional barium studies and intravenous pyelography. The potential nephrotoxicity associated with contrast agents used in CT remains a concern, particularly in patients with impaired kidney function. MRI, with its exceptional soft tissue contrast resolution and ability to provide images in multiple planes, is the preferred choice for evaluating TB in the central nervous system (CNS). Advances in MRI technology have expanded its role in examining other regions of the body as well [31].

3.3 *Other Emerging Digital Technologies*

There are recently developed technologies that can be used alongside imaging to screen for TB. Overall, the choice of modality depends on clinical context, cost effectiveness and patient needs [31]. Digital applications leverage Artificial Intelligence (AI) to analyze mobile phone recorded cough sounds, furnishing a standardized, efficient, and high-caliber approach for screening respiratory issues, encompassing pulmonary TB [34]. The expensive CXR hardware and a shortage of certified radiologists present significant hurdles for its use in PTB screening, particularly in resource-limited settings. Fortunately, recent advancements in AI and the availability of vast medical image datasets open up new possibilities and incorporation of CAD systems, especially leveraging deep learning (DL) technology in medical applications [32]. The technological advancements in CAD software hold significant promise for supporting cost-effective, large-scale screening programs in high TB-burden countries. CAD software in context of CXR demonstrated the capability to identify twice as many patients with undiagnosed TB compared to relying solely on symptom-based investigations. This integrated approach not only increases efficiency but reduces costs significantly [35, 36].

4 Role of Artificial Intelligence (AI) in TB

4.1 *AI-Based Algorithms for Interpreting Radiographic Images*

Machine Learning (ML) has been tested successfully in the diagnosis of TB. Today, several prediction algorithms relying on multilayer neural networks, decision trees, fuzzy algorithms, support vector machines, Bayesian classifiers, and genetic algorithms have been effectively tested in the diagnosis of PTB. Convolutional Neural Networks (CNNs), which are deep learning methods have emerged as a particularly promising approach in recent years. Through feed-forward learning, CNNs are meant to analyze visual images. They are ideal for classifying medical images and providing precise predictions based on digital inputs as they are composed of several layers, including input, convolutional, pooling, fully connected, and output layers [37, 38]. CNNs have demonstrated extraordinary performance in analyzing medical images and identifying patterns associated with PTB [37]. A recent study introduced TB-Net, a specialized Deep Convolutional Neural Network for detecting tuberculosis in chest X-ray images [39]. In experiments involving a multinational patient dataset, TB-Net achieved outstanding accuracy, sensitivity, and specificity rates of 99.86%, 100.0%, and 99.71%, respectively [39]. The study also tested TB-Net's decision-making through explainability-driven and radiologist validations which confirmed TB-Net's exceptional performance and clinical relevance in tuberculosis case detection [39].

CXRs and computed tomography (CT) scans are widely used to diagnose PTB-related abnormalities in the lungs, and AI algorithms have demonstrated accuracy and efficiency in analyzing these images for the extent of PTB infection [38]. By learning from vast datasets of annotated images, AI algorithms can detect complex patterns and features indicative of PTB, enabling a faster, cheaper, and more accurate diagnosis [40]. These algorithms can assist radiologists and clinicians to accurately identify PTB cases, particularly in resource-constrained regions with limited access to specialized healthcare providers.

Several studies have shown that AI-based image interpretation is efficient in PTB detection. Through a systematic review and meta-analysis, it was demonstrated that AI exhibits efficacy in diagnosing PTB based on medical imaging [41]. This AI system demonstrated excellent sensitivity and specificity, signifying the promise of AI in diagnosing PTB from CXR and providing a vital aid in screening programs [40]. In a retrospective study, researchers developed a deep learning algorithm called CheXNeXt to detect 14 different pathologies in CXR. The algorithm's performance was compared to that of practicing radiologists. The results demonstrated that the algorithm performed similarly to practicing radiologists on pulmonary pathologies of infectious origin. This suggests that deep learning algorithms can aid in the diagnosis of specific illnesses in chest radiographs at a level comparable to practicing radiologists [42]. The application of AI-based algorithms for radiographic image analysis facilities early diagnosis and enables timely interventions, ultimately resulting in improved patient outcomes. There is a pressing requirement for standardized reporting guidelines concerning AI-specific trials and multicenter clinical trials, in order to facilitate the genuine integration of this advanced technology into clinical practice.

4.2 Machine Learning (ML) for Improved Accuracy and Efficiency in TB Diagnosis

ML, a subset of AI, can increase the accuracy and efficiency of TB diagnosis following the training of a network model by analyzing massive datasets. Today, there are numerous ML models that have been used in health systems to improve TB diagnosis include naive Bayes, decision or classification trees, SVM, and Artificial Neural Networks (ANNs) [43, 44]. ANNs have proven particularly useful in incorporating ML into TB diagnosis via various architectures such as MultiLayer Perceptrons (MLP), Self-Organizing Maps, and adaptive resonance theory (ART) combined with fuzzy models in the Fuzzy-ART approach to support detection and clustering in risk groups for pulmonary TB and pleural TB [45–47]. It was found that ML can increase the accuracy and efficiency of TB diagnosis following the training of the model by analyzing massive data sets. By combining clinical information, patient history, and laboratory results, ML algorithms can find detailed patterns and subtle indicators of PTB infection that conventional diagnostic methods may fail to detect [48].

In a comprehensive review aimed at evaluating the effectiveness of ML and DL approaches for TB detection using CXR, it was observed that ML demonstrated a higher average accuracy, approximately around 93.71%, and increased sensitivity, averaging about 92.55% [49]. Conversely, DL yielded average accuracy of around 92.12%, as well as specificity, which averaged approximately 91.54%. Drawing from the findings of 10 studies that provided confusion matrix data, the combined sensitivity and specificity for ML and DL were calculated to be 0.9857 and 0.9805 respectively [49]. These results significantly surpass the accuracy levels typically achieved by conventional methods, which typically range from 60% to 80% [49].

ML algorithms do not only identify PTB but also forecast disease progression and estimate drug resistance risk [50]. A ML model was created to forecast multidrug-resistant tuberculosis using images of drug-sensitive TB obtained from CT scans. This model achieved a commendable accuracy rate of 91.11% [51]. Furthermore, ML has made significant strides in the field of TB diagnosis, encompassing the prediction of TB severity from CT pulmonary images, rapid screening, and chest radiography assessment. It has also been utilized in the creation of cutting-edge tools such as CAD4TB, Lunit INSIGHT, qXR, and others, designed to facilitate early and efficient diagnosis of TB [52].

Studies have shown that ML-based system greatly improves PTB detection with an accuracy of around 90%. This is significantly higher than the accuracy of traditional methods (typically ranging from 60% to 80%) [40]. In addition to accuracy, ML improves diagnostic efficiency in PTB cases. These findings underscore the considerable promise of ML and DL for TB detection via CXR. Notably, CNNs are more commonly employed than traditional ML approaches. Furthermore, DL methods often exhibit greater stability and consistency in their performance results compared to ML techniques [49]. Automated analysis of medical imaging and gene expression profiles speeds up the diagnostic process, enabling rapid and efficient identification of PTB cases. ML algorithms do not only identify PTB but also forecast disease progression and estimate drug resistance risk [50].

4.2.1 Gene Expression Analysis

ML is crucial in analyzing the gene expression profiles of patients with TB. Data on gene expression can provide insights into the host immune response and disease progression. ML algorithms can detect unique gene expression patterns associated with active TB, assisting the identification of reliable biomarkers for diagnosis and prognosis [53]. A systematic review revealed that ML-based biomarkers for PTB diagnosis could offer significant assistance in high-burden settings where access to conventional sputum-based diagnosis might be limited as well as in low-burden settings. Such a decision support system relying on biomarkers could prove invaluable when obtaining microbiological evidence of TB infection becomes challenging, particularly in cases of smear-negative PTB and extra-pulmonary TB [54].

4.3 Role of AI in Estimating TB Severity and Treatment Monitoring

The detection of PTB using AI goes beyond initial diagnosis and extends to treatment monitoring and estimation of disease severity. A model of DL demonstrated its ability to detect PTB with high accuracy [55]. This model's performance improved as the degree of smear positivity increased, as it tracked changes in patients' conditions throughout treatment [55]. Additionally, CT images, with their higher resolution and detailed presentation, have proven to be valuable in the diagnosis of PTB [56]. An AI model has been developed that not only detects PTB but also quantitatively evaluates the disease burden [57]. The model's quantified TB scores are significantly higher in severe patients compared to non-severe cases and demonstrate a strong correlation with CT scores assessed by radiologists [57]. The model also demonstrates high accuracy in classifying various pulmonary lesion types and effectively distinguishing between active PTB patients and inactive individuals [57]. These studies represent valuable advancements in utilizing AI for PTB diagnosis, treatment monitoring, and severity estimation.

4.4 AI-Driven Tools for Risk Prediction and Stratification

ML algorithms excel in processing immense amounts of epidemiological data, such as demographic information, geographic location, medical history, exposure to TB patients, and genetic susceptibility. By analyzing this data, ML models can forecast the likelihood of TB outbreaks, assess disease transmission patterns, and stratify individuals depending on their risk of contracting TB or developing severe forms of the disease [58]. Utilizing AI-driven risk prediction tools such as decision trees, Fuzzy Algorithms (FA) and Multilayer neural networks can aid public health efforts by identifying high-risk populations and enabling targeted interventions such as contact tracing or preventive therapy [48]. In this context, an AI-driven risk prediction model facilitated personalized PTB screening strategies and improved overall screening efficiency in 944 participants [59].

4.5 Role of AI in Differentiating TB from Non-Tuberculous Mycobacterium Lung Disease

The discrimination between TB and Non-Tuberculous Mycobacterium Lung Disease (NTM-LD) is crucial due to their increasing incidence and similar clinical symptoms and CT imaging characteristics [60]. To address this a DL framework was developed to differentiate between NTM-LD and PTB on chest CT images. The model achieved high performance, with an AUC of 0.86 in the internal test set and 0.78 in the external test cohort. Interestingly, the model outperformed three radiologists in various metrics, with higher diagnostic efficiency (1000 times faster) and output class activation maps that identified abnormal lung areas without requiring manual annotation [61]. These advanced AI approaches show promising potential in discriminating between PTB and NTM-LD, enabling faster and more accurate diagnosis to implement appropriate treatment strategies.

5 Implementation Challenges and Considerations

5.1 Cost-Effectiveness and Scalability of Innovative Screening Methods

AI has the potential to revolutionize TB screening, but it also brings challenges concerning cost and scalability. While AI can enhance the accuracy and efficiency of diagnosis it requires investments in technology and infrastructure. The costs associated with developing, integrating, and maintaining AI algorithms and software platforms can burden healthcare systems in regions where TB is prevalent, and resources are limited [62]. To address cost-effectiveness, it is important to evaluate the return on investment, long-term benefits, and potential cost savings that come from improved diagnosis accuracy and reduced treatment delays. Collaborations among governments, international organizations, and private sectors can help secure funding for implementing AI-powered screening programs. Additionally utilizing cloud-based solutions offers a cost-effective way to access AI tools without requiring upfront investments. Scalability is another consideration. Given the impact of TB, it is vital to ensure that AI screening methods can be widely adopted across various healthcare settings. Finding the balance, between the complexity of AI tools and their ease of use is crucial. It is important to make sure that even simple healthcare facilities can effectively utilize these technologies.

5.2 Addressing Barriers to Access and Adoption of New Technologies

To successfully integrate AI in TB screening, we must overcome obstacles that hinder access and adoption. These challenges include the lack of infrastructure limited digital literacy among healthcare professionals and resistance to change within healthcare systems [62]. To overcome these challenges, it is crucial to implement targeted initiatives aimed at enhancing capabilities in healthcare facilities. This objective can be realized by implementing training programs and providing support to healthcare professionals, empowering them to effectively employ AI tools for TB screening. Moreover, fostering partnerships between private sectors can contribute significantly to ensuring the accessibility of AI technologies, especially within resource-constrained contexts. Such collaborations encompass providing valuable assistance and allocating essential resources to healthcare facilities. Additionally, the active involvement of communities and stakeholders remains a pivotal component for the successful implementation of AI-driven screening initiatives [62]. Engaging patients' community leaders and healthcare providers in decision-making processes can build trust in AI technology while garnering support.

5.3 Ensuring Quality Assurance and Standardization in Innovative Screening Approaches

Maintaining quality assurance and standardization is paramount when adopting screening approaches driven by AI [62]. Consistency and reliability must be ensured throughout the PTB screening process to deliver results. This requires developing standardized guidelines that outline how AI algorithms should be trained and validated using high-quality data. Collaboration between experts, AI developers, and regulatory authorities is necessary to establish these guidelines. Furthermore, it is crucial to conduct audits and evaluations of AI systems to monitor their performance and identify any biases or inaccuracies. Ensuring the quality of AI algorithm training is also important. It should involve learning from data combined with effective feedback loops allowing the models to adapt to changes, in disease patterns and remain relevant over time. Given that AI assistance will be employed for screening purposes, and confirmatory diagnosis will remain essential, this approach will introduce a protective measure against overdiagnosis.

5.4 Ethical Considerations in the Use of AI and New Technologies

Ethical considerations play a role when integrating AI into TB screening. One key concern is the risk of exacerbating health disparities. If AI-based screening primarily benefits resourced healthcare settings, it may further marginalize underserved populations who lack access to technologies [62]. To prevent widening existing health inequities efforts must be made to ensure that AI-driven screening programs are accessible and available to all. Safeguarding patient privacy and data protection are considerations as well [62]. The use of AI requires data, including sensitive health information. Therefore, it is essential to establish data protection protocols and comply with privacy regulations in order to maintain patient confidentiality and prevent any potential breaches. Transparency and explainability of AI algorithms are considerations that need careful attention. It is important, for AI models used in TB screening to be understandable, by healthcare professionals. They should provide explanations of how the algorithms make their decisions. This helps to establish trust among practitioners and allows for validation and accountability. Additionally, it is crucial to view AI as a tool that complements expertise rather than replacing it. Healthcare providers should continue to play a role in care with AI acting as a valuable support system that enhances diagnostic accuracy, and efficiency while enhancing cost-effectiveness. This approach ensures that we can harness the benefits of AI while maintaining the patient nature of healthcare.

6 Conclusion

TB remains a significant global health challenge, with considerable morbidity and mortality. In order to control the TB pandemic, early and accurate TB screening is crucial for timely diagnosis, treatment, and limiting disease transmission. Traditional screening methods, such as the TST and IGRA, have limitations in terms of costs, accuracy, and efficiency, necessitating the development of innovative screening approaches. Recent innovations in PTB screening leverages the power of AI and digital technologies to enhance the detection and management of TB cases. AI-driven algorithms offer the potential to analyze radiographic images, including CXRs, with high accuracy, aiding in the early detection of PTB and differentiation from other lung diseases. Currently, ML also improves TB diagnosis by processing large datasets and predicting disease progression, drug resistance risk, and outbreak patterns.

While these innovations show promise, their successful implementation faces challenges such as cost-effectiveness, scalability, access barriers, patient confidentiality, and ethical considerations. Investing in technology, infrastructure, and training is essential to ensure that AI-powered screening is widely available and beneficial across different healthcare settings, including resource-limited areas. Collaborations between governments, international organizations, and private sectors can help secure funding and resources. To address access barriers, targeted initiatives should enhance the capabilities of healthcare professionals and involve communities in decision-making processes. Quality assurance and standardization are critical to maintain consistency and reliability in AI-based screening, and ethical considerations must safeguard patient privacy, data protection, and prevent exacerbating health disparities.

In conclusion, AI-driven innovations hold promise in revolutionizing PTB screening, diagnosis, and management. By overcoming implementation challenges and ethical considerations, these technologies can significantly enhance the early detection of TB cases, reduce transmission, and mortality while remaining cost-effective. Continuous research, collaboration, and efforts to make these technologies accessible to all will be essential in the global fight against tuberculosis.

References

1. A.G. Nerlich, C.J. Haas, A. Zink, U. Szeimies, H.G. Hagedorn, Molecular evidence for tuberculosis in an ancient Egyptian mummy. Lancet **350**, 1404 (1997). https://doi.org/10.1016/S0140-6736(05)65185-9
2. P. Demaeyer, Not available. Rev. Med. Brux. **37**, 52–56 (2016)
3. I. Hershkovitz et al., Detection and molecular characterization of 9,000-year-old Mycobacterium tuberculosis from a Neolithic settlement in the Eastern Mediterranean. PLoS One **3**, e3426 (2008). https://doi.org/10.1371/journal.pone.0003426
4. WHO, *Global tuberculosis report 2022* (Geneva, 2022)
5. L.C. Kahwati et al., Primary care screening and treatment for latent tuberculosis infection in adults: Evidence report and systematic review for the US Preventive Services Task Force. JAMA **316**, 970–983 (2016). https://doi.org/10.1001/jama.2016.10357
6. S.M. Marks et al., Outcomes of contact investigations of infectious tuberculosis patients. Am. J. Respir. Crit. Care Med. **162**, 2033–2038 (2000). https://doi.org/10.1164/ajrccm.162.6.2004022
7. L.C. Kahwati et al., *Screening for Latent Tuberculosis Infection in Adults: An Evidence Review for the U.S. Preventive Services Task Force U.S. Preventive Services Task Force Evidence Syntheses, formerly Systematic Evidence Reviews* (2016)
8. P.A. Selwyn et al., A prospective study of the risk of tuberculosis among intravenous drug users with human immunodeficiency virus infection. N. Engl. J. Med. **320**, 545–550 (1989). https://doi.org/10.1056/NEJM198903023200901
9. C.T. Sreeramareddy, K.V. Panduru, J. Menten, J. Van den Ende, Time delays in diagnosis of pulmonary tuberculosis: A systematic review of literature. BMC Infect. Dis. **9**, 91 (2009). https://doi.org/10.1186/1471-2334-9-91
10. R. Rajput, P. Singh, R. Sarin, P. Sethi, S. Sharma, Diagnostic accuracy of loop-mediated isothermal amplification assay for extra-pulmonary tuberculosis in Indian population. J. Microbiol. Methods **158**, 59–65 (2019). https://doi.org/10.1016/j.mimet.2019.01.016
11. S. Kedia et al., Differentiating Crohn's disease from intestinal tuberculosis. World J. Gastroenterol. **25**, 418–432 (2019). https://doi.org/10.3748/wjg.v25.i4.418
12. X. Yang et al., Challenges in diagnosis of spinal epidural abscess: A case report. Medicine (Baltimore) **98**, e14196 (2019). https://doi.org/10.1097/MD.0000000000014196
13. M. Pai, M.P. Nicol, C.C. Boehme, Tuberculosis diagnostics: State of the art and future directions. Microbiol. Spectr. **4** (2016). https://doi.org/10.1128/microbiolspec.TBTB2-0019-2016
14. B. Kestler, S.K. Tyler, Latent tuberculosis testing through the ages: The search for a sleeping killer. Am. J. Physiol. Lung Cell. Mol. Physiol. **322**, L412–L419 (2022). https://doi.org/10.1152/ajplung.00217.2021
15. D.F. de Lima Corvino, S. Shrestha, A.R. Kosmin, *StatPearls* (2023)
16. P. Andersen, M.E. Munk, J.M. Pollock, T.M. Doherty, Specific immune-based diagnosis of tuberculosis. Lancet **356**, 1099–1104 (2000). https://doi.org/10.1016/s0140-6736(00)02742-2
17. A. Pugsley, M. Maxime Schwartz, Export and secretion of proteins by bacteria. FEMS Microbiol. Rev. **1** (1985). https://doi.org/10.1111/j.1574-6968.1985.tb01180.x
18. S.J. Hubbard, S.F. Campbell, J.M. Thornton, Molecular recognition., Conformational analysis of limited proteolytic sites and serine proteinase protein inhibitors. J. Mol. Biol. **220**, 507–530 (1991). https://doi.org/10.1016/0022-2836(91)90027-4
19. S. Pottumarthy, A.J. Morris, A.C. Harrison, V.C. Wells, Evaluation of the tuberculin gamma interferon assay: Potential to replace the Mantoux skin test. J. Clin. Microbiol. **37**, 3229–3232 (1999). https://doi.org/10.1128/JCM.37.10.3229-3232.1999
20. WHO, *TB incidence*, https://www.who.int/teams/global-tuberculosis-programme/tb-reports/global-tuberculosis-report-2022/tb-disease-burden/2-1-tb-incidence#:~:text=The%20estimated%2010.6%20million%20people,2.1 (2022)

21. CDC., C. f. D. C. a. P. *Diagnosing latent TB Infection & TB Disease*, https://www.cdc.gov/tb/topic/testing/diagnosingltbi.htm#:~:text=Chest%20Radiograph,used%20to%20definitively%20diagnose%20TB. (2016)
22. J. Nalunjogi et al., Accuracy and incremental yield of the chest X-ray in screening for tuberculosis in Uganda: A cross-sectional study. Tuberc. Res. Treat. **2021**, 6622809 (2021). https://doi.org/10.1155/2021/6622809
23. WHO, *Chest Radiography in Tuberculosis Detection* (2016)
24. D. Hua et al., Benchmarking the diagnostic test accuracy of certified AI products for screening pulmonary tuberculosis in digital chest radiographs: Preliminary evidence from a rapid review and meta-analysis. Int. J. Med. Inform. **177**, 105159 (2023). https://doi.org/10.1016/j.ijmedinf.2023.105159
25. D. Shingadia, V. Novelli, The tuberculin skin test: A hundred, not out? Arch. Dis. Child. **93**, 189–190 (2008). https://doi.org/10.1136/adc.2007.129585
26. S.H.R. Schaaf, Chapter 22: Helmuth, in *Tuberculosis*, (2009), pp. 216–226
27. Prevention., C. f. D. C. a. *IGRAs– Blood Tests for TB Infection Fact Sheet*, https://www.cdc.gov/tb/publications/factsheets/testing/igra.htm (2016)
28. K.S. Fong et al., Challenges of interferon-gamma release assay conversions in serial testing of health-care workers in a TB control program. Chest **142**, 55–62 (2012). https://doi.org/10.1378/chest.11-0992
29. E.C. Jones-Lopez, J.J. Ellner, *Chapter 35: Tropical Infectious Diseases: Principles, Pathogens and Practice* (2011), pp. 228–247
30. K.K.K. Htet, A.N. Phyu, T. Thwin, V. Chongsuvivatwong, Mobile health app for tuberculosis screening and compliance to undergo chest X-ray examination among presumptive cases detected by the app in Myanmar: Usability study. JMIR Form. Res. **6**, e37779 (2022). https://doi.org/10.2196/37779
31. J.B. Bomanji, N. Gupta, P. Gulati, C.J. Das, Imaging in tuberculosis. Cold Spring Harb. Perspect. Med. **5** (2015). https://doi.org/10.1101/cshperspect.a017814
32. X.F. Cao et al., Application of artificial intelligence in digital chest radiography reading for pulmonary tuberculosis screening. Chronic Dis. Transl. Med. **7**, 35–40 (2021). https://doi.org/10.1016/j.cdtm.2021.02.001
33. L.N.Q. Vo et al., Early evaluation of an ultra-portable X-ray system for tuberculosis active case finding. Trop. Med. Infect. Dis. **6** (2021). https://doi.org/10.3390/tropicalmed6030163
34. K.S. Alqudaihi et al., Cough sound detection and diagnosis using artificial intelligence techniques: Challenges and opportunities. IEEE Access **9**, 102327–102344 (2021). https://doi.org/10.1109/ACCESS.2021.3097559
35. K. Velen et al., Digital chest X-ray with computer-aided detection for tuberculosis screening within correctional facilities. Ann. Am. Thorac. Soc. **19**, 1313–1319 (2022). https://doi.org/10.1513/AnnalsATS.202103-380OC
36. S. Bashir et al., Economic analysis of different throughput scenarios and implementation strategies of computer-aided detection software as a screening and triage test for pulmonary TB. PLoS One **17**, e0277393 (2022). https://doi.org/10.1371/journal.pone.0277393
37. S.S. Meraj, R. Yaakob, A. Azman, S.N.M. Rum, A.S.A. Nazri, Artificial intelligence in diagnosing tuberculosis: A review. Int. J. Adv. Sci. Eng. Inf. Technol. **9**, 81 (2019). https://doi.org/10.18517/ijaseit.9.1.7567
38. J. Schmidhuber, Deep learning in neural networks: An overview. Neural Netw. **61**, 85–117 (2015). https://doi.org/10.1016/j.neunet.2014.09.003
39. A. Wong et al., TB-Net: A tailored, self-attention deep convolutional neural network design for detection of tuberculosis cases from chest X-ray images. Front. Artif. Intell. **5**, 827299 (2022). https://doi.org/10.3389/frai.2022.827299
40. P. Lakhani, B. Sundaram, Deep learning at chest radiography: Automated classification of pulmonary tuberculosis by using convolutional neural networks. Radiology **284**, 574–582 (2017). https://doi.org/10.1148/radiol.2017162326

41. Y. Zhan, Y. Wang, W. Zhang, B. Ying, C. Wang, Diagnostic accuracy of the artificial intelligence methods in medical imaging for pulmonary tuberculosis: A systematic review and meta-analysis. J. Clin. Med. **12** (2022). https://doi.org/10.3390/jcm12010303
42. P. Rajpurkar et al., Deep learning for chest radiograph diagnosis: A retrospective comparison of the CheXNeXt algorithm to practicing radiologists. PLoS Med. **15**, e1002686 (2018). https://doi.org/10.1371/journal.pmed.1002686
43. A. Awaysheh et al., Review of medical decision support and machine-learning methods. Vet. Pathol. **56**, 512–525 (2019). https://doi.org/10.1177/0300985819829524
44. M.K. Yu et al., Visible machine learning for biomedicine. Cell **173**, 1562–1565 (2018). https://doi.org/10.1016/j.cell.2018.05.056
45. A.D. Orjuela-Canon, J.E. Camargo Mendoza, C.E. Awad Garcia, E.P. Vergara Vela, Tuberculosis diagnosis support analysis for precarious health information systems. Comput. Methods Prog. Biomed. **157**, 11–17 (2018). https://doi.org/10.1016/j.cmpb.2018.01.009
46. F.S. Aguiar et al., Development of two artificial neural network models to support the diagnosis of pulmonary tuberculosis in hospitalized patients in Rio de Janeiro, Brazil. Med. Biol. Eng. Comput. **54**, 1751–1759 (2016). https://doi.org/10.1007/s11517-016-1465-1
47. J.M. Seixas et al., Artificial neural network models to support the diagnosis of pleural tuberculosis in adult patients. Int. J. Tuberc. Lung Dis. **17**, 682–686 (2013). https://doi.org/10.5588/ijtld.12.0829
48. A.D. Orjuela-Canon, A.L. Jutinico, C. Awad, E. Vergara, A. Palencia, Machine learning in the loop for tuberculosis diagnosis support. Front. Public Health **10**, 876949 (2022). https://doi.org/10.3389/fpubh.2022.876949
49. S. Hansun, A. Argha, S.T. Liaw, B.G. Celler, G.B. Marks, Machine and deep learning for tuberculosis detection on chest X-rays: Systematic literature review. J. Med. Internet Res. **25**, e43154 (2023). https://doi.org/10.2196/43154
50. S. Liang et al., The application of artificial intelligence in the diagnosis and drug resistance prediction of pulmonary tuberculosis. Front. Med. (Lausanne) **9**, 935080 (2022). https://doi.org/10.3389/fmed.2022.935080
51. X.W. Gao, Y. Qian, Prediction of multidrug-resistant TB from CT pulmonary images based on deep learning techniques. Mol. Pharm. **15**, 4326–4335 (2018). https://doi.org/10.1021/acs.molpharmaceut.7b00875
52. M. Singh et al., Evolution of machine learning in tuberculosis diagnosis: A review of deep learning-based medical applications. Electronics-Switz **11**, ARTN 2634 (2022). https://doi.org/10.3390/electronics11172634
53. T.E. Tavolara et al., Deep learning predicts gene expression as an intermediate data modality to identify susceptibility patterns in Mycobacterium tuberculosis infected diversity outbred mice. EBioMedicine **67**, 103388 (2021). https://doi.org/10.1016/j.ebiom.2021.103388
54. V. Balakrishnan, Y. Kherabi, G. Ramanathan, S.A. Paul, C.K. Tiong, Machine learning approaches in diagnosing tuberculosis through biomarkers – A systematic review. Prog. Biophys. Mol. Biol. **179**, 16–25 (2023). https://doi.org/10.1016/j.pbiomolbio.2023.03.001
55. S. Lee et al., Deep learning to determine the activity of pulmonary tuberculosis on chest radiographs. Radiology **301**, 435–442 (2021). https://doi.org/10.1148/radiol.2021210063
56. A.C. Nachiappan et al., Pulmonary tuberculosis: Role of radiology in diagnosis and management. Radiographics **37**, 52–72 (2017). https://doi.org/10.1148/rg.2017160032
57. C. Yan et al., A fully automatic artificial intelligence-based CT image analysis system for accurate detection, diagnosis, and quantitative severity evaluation of pulmonary tuberculosis. Eur. Radiol. **32**, 2188–2199 (2022). https://doi.org/10.1007/s00330-021-08365-z
58. R. Doshi et al., Tuberculosis control, and the where and why of artificial intelligence. ERJ Open Res. **3** (2017). https://doi.org/10.1183/23120541.00056-2017
59. L.S. Peetluk et al., A clinical prediction model for unsuccessful pulmonary tuberculosis treatment outcomes. Clin. Infect. Dis. **74**, 973–982 (2022). https://doi.org/10.1093/cid/ciab598

60. N. Kwak et al., Non-tuberculous mycobacterial lung disease: Diagnosis based on computed tomography of the chest. Eur. Radiol. **26**, 4449–4456 (2016). https://doi.org/10.1007/s00330-016-4286-6
61. L. Wang et al., Distinguishing nontuberculous mycobacteria from Mycobacterium tuberculosis lung disease from CT images using a deep learning framework. Eur. J. Nucl. Med. Mol. Imaging **48**, 4293–4306 (2021). https://doi.org/10.1007/s00259-021-05432-x
62. K. Tachkov et al., Barriers to use artificial intelligence methodologies in health technology assessment in central and east European countries. Front. Public Health **10**, 921226 (2022). https://doi.org/10.3389/fpubh.2022.921226

A Framework to Identify the Children Who Missed Basic Vaccines in Developing Countries

Ayesha Siddiqua, Muhammad Ashad Kabir, and Muhammad E. H. Chowdhury

1 Introduction

Basic vaccines, also known as routine or childhood vaccines, are a set of immunizations that are recommended or required for all children as part of their standard healthcare. These vaccines play a crucial role in bolstering a child's immune system, paving the way for the establishment of herd immunity, a collective shield against severe and potentially life-threatening diseases. When a high proportion of individuals receive basic vaccines, outbreaks of the illness are prevented. Conversely, regions with a high proportion of unvaccinated individuals are at risk of epidemics, underscoring the paramount importance of vaccination coverage in our global health landscape [1, 2].

However, a disconcerting reality persists as a substantial number of children continue to miss their vaccinations, either in part or entirely. Such children, classified as either "missed vaccines" or "zero vaccines," are left more vulnerable to a spectrum of illnesses [3–6]. Alarming statistics reveal that one in every five children across the globe lacks access to life-saving vaccinations [7], with the onslaught of epidemics further exacerbating this issue. During the recent epidemic,

A. Siddiqua
Department of Computer Science and Engineering, Central Women's University, Dhaka, Bangladesh
e-mail: ayesha.siddiqua@cwu.edu.bd

M. A. Kabir (✉)
School of Computing, Mathematics and Engineering, Charles Sturt University, Bathurst, NSW, Australia
e-mail: akabir@csu.edu.au

M. E. H. Chowdhury
Department of Electrical Engineering, Qatar University, Doha, Qatar
e-mail: mchowdhury@qu.edu.qa

M. E. H. Chowdhury, S. Kiranyaz (eds.), *Surveillance, Prevention, and Control of Infectious Diseases*, https://doi.org/10.1007/978-3-031-59967-5_6

a staggering 67 million children were deprived of their routine vaccines. These grim figures are mirrored in the World Health Organization's report, which indicates that 14.3 million newborns in 2022 missed their first dose of diphtheria, tetanus, and pertussis (DTP) vaccination, while 6.2 million only received a partial dose. Notably, the burden of these missed vaccinations disproportionately affects ten nations, including Angola, Brazil, the Democratic Republic of the Congo, Ethiopia, India, Indonesia, Mozambique, Nigeria, Pakistan, and the Philippines [8].

Many studies [5, 9–23] have explored why some children miss their vaccine doses or receive none at all, particularly in one or a few developing countries. These investigations have often uncovered common reasons for missed vaccinations. Some studies [5, 24–35] have even offered potential solutions after analyzing the factors contributing to vaccine gaps. However, an important aspect remains largely unaddressed—the identification of children who have missed crucial vaccinations in impoverished nations.

This chapter endeavors to fill this gap by proposing a framework to identify these children who have missed basic vaccines in developing countries. This framework aims to improve our ability to locate and assist these vulnerable children, ultimately contributing to more comprehensive vaccination coverage in underprivileged regions. By synthesizing the extensive research on both the reasons behind these gaps and the strategies to identify and intervene in such cases using advanced technologies, this framework offers a holistic approach to a complex problem. It recognizes that understanding the root causes, as well as implementing effective identification and intervention measures, is crucial to achieving comprehensive vaccination coverage. Drawing from state-of-the-art studies, this framework provides a practical guide for healthcare professionals, policymakers, and organizations working in the field of public health to systematically locate and support children who have missed essential vaccinations. In doing so, it not only contributes to the global effort to combat vaccine-preventable diseases but also underscores the imperative of equitable access to life-saving immunizations for all children, regardless of their socioeconomic background or geographic location.

2 Reasons for Missing Basic Vaccination

In this section, we undertake an in-depth analysis of the causal factors contributing to the phenomenon of missed basic vaccination within developing countries. Utilizing a comprehensive synthesis of state-of-the-art research studies, we have distilled these intricate factors into ten discrete categories with insights drawn from nineteen distinct developing countries. A summary of these categories is presented in Table 1. A brief description of those categories is provided below.

Mother's Implications The willingness to receive vaccinations is significantly influenced by a mother's level of education and occupational status [20, 36–38]. Mothers with higher levels of education are more likely to adhere to their children's

Table 1 Reasons for zero-dose or missed-dose children in developing countries

Category	Factors	Reference	County
Mother's implications	Education	[20, 36–48]	Nigeria, Peru, Bangladesh, India, Ethiopia
	Age	[5, 20, 43–46, 48, 49]	Ethiopia, Lao, Nigeria, Bangladesh
	Marital status	[5, 20, 43, 45]	Ethiopia, Nigeria
	Service type	[43, 45, 46]	Lao, Ethiopia
	Empowered	[5, 43, 45, 50–52]	India, Bangladesh, Nigeria, Ethiopia
	Mother's mobility	[48]	Bangladesh
	Health consciousness	[5, 36]	India, Nigeria
	Health insurance	[45]	Nigeria
	Antenatal care	[5, 20, 53–57]	Egypt, Ethiopia, Zimbabwe, Nigeria, Kenya
	Health facility birth	[5, 46]	Lao, Nigeria
	Social activity participation	[5, 48]	Bangladesh, Nigeria
	Race	[45]	Nigeria
Child's implications	Birth order	[5, 48]	Bangladesh, Nigeria
	Underweight birth	[5, 58, 59]	India, Bangladesh, Uganda, Indonesia, Nepal, Ghana, Nigeria
	Birthplace	[43, 44, 46]	Ethiopia, Lao
	Sex	[20, 43, 44, 46, 48]	Bangladesh, Ethiopia, Lao
	Place of delivery	[20, 43, 44]	Peru, Ethiopia
Paternal/caregiver's influences	Encouraging vaccination	[5, 10]	Zimbabwe, Nigeria
	Permission for vaccination	[5, 45, 46]	Lao, Nigeria
	Father's education	[50, 60–63]	Cambodia, Pakistan, Bangladesh, Kenya
	Connection with media	[5, 20, 44, 48]	Nigeria
	Number of kids	[46]	Lao
	Family size	[5, 20, 43, 44]	Nigeria, Ethiopia
Socioeconomic status	Poor/Well-off	[5, 9, 18, 20, 43–45, 48, 64–66]	Ghana, Brazil, Ethiopia, Bangladesh, Nigeria, India
Cultural effects	Religious observance	[5, 20, 45]	Nigeria
	Ethnicity	[5, 43, 46]	Ethiopia, Nigeria, Lao
Geographical differences	Region (North vs South)	[5, 45]	Nigeria
	Setting (rural vs urban)	[5, 44, 48]	Nigeria

(continued)

Table 1 (continued)

Category	Factors	Reference	County
Approach towards vaccination	Fears and misconceptions	[5, 67, 68]	Malaysia, Nigeria
	Community refusal of vaccination	[5, 69]	Nigeria
	Long queue	[5, 43, 45]	Ethiopia, Nigeria
	Mismanagement	[5, 70, 71]	South Africa, Nigeria
Health system conditions	Access to health facilities	[5, 72]	Nigeria, Rural South Africa
	Available vaccine	[5, 73]	Nigeria
	Available vaccine provider	[5, 74]	Nigeria
	Cost of vaccination	[5, 22, 75, 76]	Africa, Nigeria
	Queues at vaccine centre	[5]	Nigeria
Awareness of vaccination	Awareness need for vaccination	[5, 45, 77, 78]	India, Bangladesh, Nigeria
	Awareness of vaccination schedules	[5, 45, 79–81]	Nigeria
	Vaccination record keeping	[5, 82]	Indonesia, Nigeria
Miscellaneous	COVID-19 pandemic	[5, 83]	Bangladesh, Nigeria
	Vaccination campaign	[5, 84]	Nigeria
	Campaign worker capability	[5, 85]	Nigeria
	Healthcare worker	[5, 86, 87]	Africa, Nigeria
	Health system governance	[5, 75, 88]	Nigeria
	Community engagement	[5]	Nigeria
	Insurgency and conflict	[5]	Nigeria
	Migration and refugee	[5, 9, 45, 89]	Istanbul, Nigeria
	Transportation	[20, 43, 46, 48]	Ethiopia, Lao

recommended vaccination regimens. In contrast, mothers with lower levels of education may have limited knowledge about vaccinations and their safety [39–48]. Additionally, older mothers tend to have a higher likelihood of having their children fully vaccinated [5, 20, 43–46, 48, 49].

Compared to unmarried mothers, married mothers are significantly more likely to have their children fully immunized [5, 20, 43, 45]. Mothers who have the opportunity to leave the house for employment are often seen as more powered and are more inclined to ensure their children receive the appropriate immunizations [5, 43, 45, 50–52]. According to multiple studies [43, 45, 46], mothers working in agricultural or household jobs may exhibit lower levels of caution and enthusiasm toward vaccinating their children compared to those working in office or institutional settings.

Freedom of movement fosters independence, awareness, and stability in individuals, enabling them to make more informed life decisions. Consequently, mothers who feel comfortable visiting hospitals or clinics are more likely to ensure their children are vaccinated compared to mothers who face difficulties leaving their homes [48].

Moreover, maternal awareness of immunization plays a pivotal role in children's vaccination. Health-conscious mothers possess knowledge about the benefits, safety, and vaccination schedules, staying informed about where and how to access immunization services [5, 36]. Parents with health insurance tend to have a positive attitude towards vaccinating their children [45].

Receiving antenatal care and having a skilled delivery significantly benefit both maternal and child health. Increased antenatal care visits correlate with substantially higher vaccination rates. Children born to mothers who had four or more antenatal care appointments are three times more likely to be immunized than infants whose mothers received no antenatal care [5, 20, 53–57].

A strong correlation exists between immunization and giving birth in a medical facility, particularly regarding birth doses [5, 46]. Conversely, factors hindering the completion of children's immunizations include mothers attending social engagements, maternal or child illness, and competing demands on their time, such as agricultural labor or caring for other children. Highly active social lives can often leave mothers too occupied to provide their children with the necessary time and attention [5, 48].

Child's Implications Vaccination rates are influenced by factors such as birth order and the age of the child. Children with higher birth orders and older siblings tend to have higher vaccination rates [5, 48]. Conversely, children with low birth weights often experience delays or missed vaccinations for their birth-dose shots [5, 58, 59]. Additionally, the child's birthplace, gender, and place of delivery, as well as the overall environment, significantly impact the vaccination schedule [20, 43, 44, 46, 48].

Paternal or Caregiver's Influences Higher childhood vaccination rates are closely tied to paternal or caregiver awareness and their active support for immunization [5, 10]. In contrast, fathers with lower levels of education may not prioritize vaccination [50, 60–63]. When fathers decline to give consent for vaccination, participation in immunization programs decreases [5, 45, 46].

Access to information about the benefits of vaccination, healthcare services, and the locations of medical facilities is often facilitated through media channels such as television, radio, and the Internet. Homes with access to such media, especially in rural areas, tend to have higher childhood immunization rates [5, 20, 44, 48]. Parents with fewer children, typically those with fewer than three children, also tend to have higher vaccination rates [46]. Smaller family sizes allow for greater attention to each child's vaccination needs compared to larger families [5, 20, 43, 44].

Socioeconomic Status Vaccination rates tend to increase with family wealth and privilege, while children from low-income families are more likely to remain unvaccinated (zero-dose) [3, 4, 90, 91]. However, progress in this regard has been slow, and the most significant disparities in vaccination rates are observed in the poorest nations. Children who have received zero doses of vaccines are often found in impoverished conditions [5, 9, 18, 20, 43–45, 48, 64–66].

Cultural Effects Christian households are more likely to have received vaccinations compared to households of other religions [5, 20, 45]. Additionally, when compared to ethnic groups such as Igbo or Yoruba, the Hausa/Fulani ethnic groups, who are typically nomadic or semi-nomadic pastoralists, tend to have lower vaccination rates [5, 43, 46].

Geographical Differences Vaccination rates in Northern Nigerian villages are lower when compared to Southern Nigerian areas. This disparity has been attributed to factors such as the higher levels of insecurity in the North and the better income and education levels in the South [5, 45]. Additionally, rural communities, in contrast to metropolitan regions, often exhibited lower immunization rates and higher dropout rates [5, 44, 48].

Approach Towards Vaccination The refusal to undergo immunization and the occurrence of missed or omitted immunization dates have been associated with concerns and misconceptions regarding the effectiveness and safety of vaccines [5, 67, 68]. Instances of immunization rejection are commonly observed in communities with similar racial and religious demographics [5, 69]. Additionally, some individuals may be disinclined to vaccinate their children due to factors such as long waiting times and mismanagement at healthcare clinics [5, 43, 45, 70, 71].

Health System Conditions The absence of or incomplete immunization is associated with factors such as long travel distances, challenging environmental conditions, poor or nonexistent road infrastructure, and the perception of healthcare facilities being geographically distant, especially for rural and low-income populations [5, 72]. Lower vaccination rates are often linked to vaccine shortages and procurement delays, including delays in acquiring related supplies such as Adverse Events Following Immunization (AEFI) kits [5, 73]. Inadequate staffing of immunizers in maternity units and health centers, along with factors like limited funding, restricted access to healthcare facilities, and reluctance to provide vaccinations, are additional contributing factors [5, 74]. There are instances where immunization personnel did not visit households during vaccination campaigns [5]. Furthermore, the cost associated with vaccination posed a barrier to immunization, along with the perceived expenses associated with traveling to healthcare facilities [5, 22, 75, 76]. Moreover, some healthcare facilities were reported to demand money or bribes in exchange for what was supposed to be "free" vaccinations. Long waiting times at healthcare institutions also significantly hindered the uptake of vaccines [5].

Awareness of Vaccination Low vaccination coverage rates have been associated with inadequate knowledge about vaccinations [5, 45, 77, 78]. Incomplete coverage often results from a lack of understanding regarding the timing and necessity of additional vaccine doses, primarily due to parents' limited awareness of vaccination schedules [5, 45, 79–81].

Maintaining residence-based data and vaccination cards has been linked to successful immunization. The retention of vaccination cards may signify a deeper appreciation of the importance of vaccinations and a better understanding of the recommended immunization schedule [5, 82].

Miscellaneous The COVID-19 pandemic disrupted vaccination efforts due to health system disruptions, facility closures, transportation restrictions, stay-at-home orders, and concerns about disease transmission [5, 83]. Lower vaccination coverage resulted from inadequate preparation for immunization campaigns, including outdated population estimates, limited community engagement, and underutilization of data [5, 84]. Campaign-related factors, such as finger marking without administering vaccines, exaggeration of the number of vaccinated children, failure to adhere to microplans, and neglect of residence-based records/vaccination certificates, contributed to lower campaign coverage rates [5, 85].

The attitude of healthcare professionals towards vaccine consumers is very important. People are more likely to take vaccines if vaccine providers are helpful in centers. Among healthcare professionals, reduced coverage has been associated with poor interpersonal skills, lack of motivation, community hostility toward healthcare workers, and unfavorable clinical conditions for vaccine administration [5, 86, 87].

Moreover, weak governance within healthcare systems in developing countries has also led to lower coverage rates, stemming from issues like inefficient administration, a shortage of qualified healthcare personnel, poor data management, unequal financial resource allocation, and limited budgets [5, 75, 88]. Insufficient community mobilization, awareness campaigns, and community participation have hindered vaccination uptake [5].

In regions like Northern Nigeria, internal displacement resulting from insurgency and violence posed significant challenges for vaccination and monitoring teams to access communities, leading to reduced immunization rates [5]. Specific populations, such as rural-to-urban migrants, internally displaced individuals, and recent migrants, were less likely to receive vaccinations, often due to difficulties in conducting follow-ups for missing children and delayed return visits [5, 9, 45, 89]. Transportation constraints also impacted the willingness to visit clinics or vaccination centers for children's vaccinations [20, 43, 46, 48].

3 Strategies to Identify and Intervene Children Missing Basic Vaccination

This section explores various methods to identify children who have either not received any vaccinations or have missed some of their scheduled vaccinations. Several of these strategies have been successfully employed in developed nations such as the USA, UK, Australia, and others, resulting in improved vaccination rates and outcomes. The knowledge and experiences gained from these approaches in developed countries can offer valuable insights for identifying children who may have missed vaccinations in underdeveloped or resource-constrained nations and intervening accordingly.

3.1 Verification of Children's Vaccination Records at School Admission

Education is a fundamental human right, and the progress and development of a nation are intricately tied to education. It is the key to propelling a nation towards prosperity and excellence. Primary education, in particular, serves as the cornerstone of the education system, playing a pivotal role in equipping individuals with the skills they need to secure employment, become literate, and gain numeracy skills, enabling them to address challenges across various contexts. In many developing nations like Bangladesh and India, the provision of primary education is a universal commitment [92, 93].

In developed countries such as the USA, Italy, and Australia, some schools have enforced a variety of rules to ensure child vaccination. For instance, in 2019, Italy implemented legislation mandating that children must provide proof of immunization before enrolling in schools. This law requires children to be immunized against measles, mumps, rubella, polio, chickenpox, and tetanus under the Lorenzin legislation. Children up to the age of six without confirmation of immunization are not permitted to attend nursery and kindergarten. While children between six and sixteen are not prohibited from attending school, their parents may face fines if they do not adhere to the prescribed vaccination schedule [94, 95].

In Australia, enrolling in primary school requires children to present an immunization history statement from the Australian Immunization Register (AIR). Ensuring that children are up-to-date on their vaccines is a legal obligation, as it safeguards them from potentially harmful diseases. Schools retain copies of the AIR to identify unvaccinated students in the event of disease outbreaks [96, 97].

To identify unvaccinated children in developing countries, a practical approach is to inspect vaccine cards when admitting children to school. This practice should be repeated each time a child advances to a new class. By implementing this annual check, parents are continually reminded about their child's vaccination status and may become more engaged in the vaccination process. Schools can also serve as vaccination centers when school authorities are diligent. On such occasions, all unvaccinated children can be required to receive vaccinations at the school, contributing to improved vaccination coverage rates.

3.2 *Verifying Vaccination Card During Each Doctor Visit*

Numerous countries place a high value on preserving vaccination records. Having vaccination cards makes parents more aware and promotes timely immunization. In Jordan, as reported in a study [98], a remarkable 97.2% of women maintain vaccination cards for their children, which they readily provide to hospitals or health centers in cases where a vaccine dose may be missing or delayed. This practice is recommended not only in Jordan but also in numerous countries, including Brazil, Pakistan, Nigeria, and India, to ensure the consistent administration of essential vaccines for children [99–102].

Although mothers typically maintain accurate records of their children's vaccinations, the Egyptian government recommends keeping health cards to ensure proper documentation of vaccinations [103]. In Vietnam, project workers visit households regularly to review immunization records and keep track of vaccinated children [104]. In developing countries such as India, vaccination cards are commonly employed to track vaccination status [105–107].

Moreover, five countries provide personal immunization cards to migrants, while Malta and Portugal maintain digitized vaccine registries. Slovenia maintains a paper-based registry for vaccinated asylum applicants. Both Malta and Croatia provide digitized individual and aggregated data to their National Public Health Institutes (NPHI) [108]. In industrialized nations like the USA, communities with lower socioeconomic status maintain vaccination records and contact parents to promote childhood vaccine coverage [24, 109–111].

Hospitals can play an active role in increasing awareness about child vaccination. When a child is visited to the hospital for any reason, healthcare authorities should assess the child's vaccination status and interest in receiving any required vaccinations before proceeding with other treatments. This proactive approach encourages parents to prioritize vaccinations for their children, reducing the risk of missed vaccinations.

Moreover, it is common for families to relocate due to changes in their parents' workplaces or for better educational opportunities. Regardless of where the child receives medical care, healthcare providers should routinely check the child's vaccination card whenever they visit a new healthcare facility. This practice ensures the continuity of vaccinations and facilitates the identification of children who may have missed a vaccination dose.

3.3 Hospital's Record-Keeping, Follow-up, and Parent Education

In developing countries, hospitals can play a vital role in identifying and ensuring that children born within their facilities receive the basic vaccinations they need [112]. Hospitals can maintain comprehensive records of all births and medical procedures, including vaccinations administered to newborns. This meticulous record-keeping allows healthcare providers to track the vaccination status of each child. These records serve as valuable references to determine which vaccines a child has received, which ones are pending, and when the next doses are due. This data-driven approach has enabled timely identification of missed vaccinations and contributed to high vaccination coverage rates in developed nations such as Canada [113].

In addition, hospitals can facilitate the transition of newborns to primary care and vaccination services after discharge [114]. They can provide parents with vaccination cards or documentation detailing the vaccines administered during the hospital stay. This documentation serves as a crucial link between hospital-based care and ongoing vaccination services, ensuring that children continue to receive their vaccines according to the recommended schedule. This approach has resulted in sustained high vaccination coverage rates in developed nations [115].

Furthermore, hospitals can also serve as platforms for educating parents and caregivers about the importance of vaccinations. Sometimes, misconceptions are a prime cause of unimmunized children in developed countries, for example, Turkey [116]. So, healthcare providers can engage with parents during the hospital stay, explaining the significance of vaccines, the vaccination schedule, and the potential consequences of missed vaccinations. This educational component helps raise awareness and encourages parents to prioritize their children's immunization in developed countries [117].

3.4 Government Verification During Birth Registration

Government verification of vaccination records during birth registration is a powerful strategy to identify children who have missed basic vaccinations. This approach ensures that vaccination records are systematically integrated into official birth registration processes, allowing for the timely identification of children who are behind schedule or have not received basic vaccines. Developed countries have successfully implemented such systems, showcasing the benefits of this approach [118].

In countries like the USA, the birth registration process often includes the collection of vaccination information [119]. The birth certificate typically includes details about the child's vaccination status, ensuring that this crucial information is recorded alongside other essential birth details [120, 121]. This information can be used to trigger alerts or notifications when a child's vaccination schedule is due [95, 122].

For instance, in countries like Sweden, the national vaccination registry sends reminders to parents and healthcare providers when vaccinations are scheduled, ensuring that children do not miss basic vaccines [123]. In developed countries like the USA and Canada, vaccination records are often accessible to healthcare providers, schools, and public health authorities [113, 124]. This accessibility ensures that vaccination data can be easily shared and verified when necessary. Seamless data sharing among relevant stakeholders and data-driven approaches to tracking and monitoring vaccine coverage have led to high vaccination rates in developed countries [124].

3.5 *Healthcare Professionals for Enhanced Vaccination Awareness and Coverage*

To enhance vaccination awareness, it is crucial for healthcare professionals at various levels, including district, upazila, and union levels, to collaborate more closely [125–127]. Typically, health workers are provided with a set quantity of vaccines for distribution and administration within a given area [128–130].

In many instances, government elementary schools are designated as vaccination sites, where children receive their immunizations at scheduled times. A useful method for determining the vaccination coverage in a specific region is to calculate the number of vaccinated children and the remaining unvaccinated ones. This approach simplifies the identification of children who have not yet received their vaccinations. For instance, developed countries such as Canada, maintain comprehensive vaccination registries that allow for real-time tracking and monitoring of vaccine coverage. This system enables healthcare authorities to identify geographic areas or populations with lower vaccine coverage rates and implement targeted interventions [117].

Immunization information should be included in a unique number after the birth of the child [120, 121, 131]. It will remind us about vaccination after a certain period of time [95, 122]. Each child is given a distinctive ID in several countries, such as Denmark, Bangladesh, Montana, and Iran, to keep track of essential vaccines. They stay up to date on immunizations and can remind or remember their participants to receive the required vaccinations by utilizing this specific ID.

3.6 *Proactive Measures to Ensure Vaccination Compliance*

To ensure vaccination, several proactive steps have been taken in different developed countries. For example, in the wake of a chickenpox epidemic, a high school in

Michigan took decisive action by implementing a policy that banned unvaccinated students from attending classes. The St. Clair County Health Department identified 37 students who could not provide proof of immunization, prompting parents to be urged to verify their children's vaccination status. The health department had communicated that these affected children would only be permitted to return to school once they could demonstrate that their chickenpox immunizations had been up to date [132, 133].

Similarly, Rockland county in the USA responded to a six-month measles outbreak by declaring a state of emergency and issuing a prohibition on unvaccinated children under the age of 18 from entering educational institutions, grocery stores, restaurants, and places of worship. Playgrounds and outdoor areas had been excluded from the restriction. This measure had been set to last for 30 days or until minors who had not received the measles, mumps, and rubella vaccine did so. The county executive emphasized the urgency of halting the epidemic's spread. While authorities had not actively sought unvaccinated children, they had expected parents and legal guardians to ensure their children were vaccinated [134–136].

As developed countries have gained success in vaccinating children by enforcing such laws, developing countries can also apply these policies to identify unvaccinated children. Enforcing laws that restrict unvaccinated children from accessing public spaces, such as malls, restaurants, book fairs, and social events, plays a critical role in identifying unvaccinated children or those who have missed vaccine doses. By diligently following these regulations in both developed and underdeveloped nations, it becomes easier to identify children who have not received recommended vaccinations, ultimately fostering greater willingness among parents to vaccinate their children.

4 Advanced Technologies to Enhance Vaccination Coverage

Advanced technologies, including Artificial Intelligence (AI), blockchain, and smartphone apps, have the potential to play a significant role in identifying and intervening in cases of children who have missed basic vaccines in developing countries [137, 138]. Through the utilization of these technologies, healthcare systems and organizations can enhance their capacity to locate and support underserved populations, ultimately improving vaccination coverage [139–142]. Below we briefly discuss several potential applications of these technologies.

4.1 Data Analytics for Targeted Interventions

AI-driven data analytics can process vast amounts of healthcare data, including electronic health records, immunization registries, and demographic information. Machine learning algorithms can identify trends and patterns related to vaccination gaps in specific regions or populations. For instance, AI can detect areas with consistently low vaccine coverage rates or pinpoint communities with a high number of unvaccinated children. By analyzing these data, healthcare authorities can strategically allocate resources and launch targeted vaccination campaigns in areas with the greatest need [143].

Predictive modeling using AI can forecast vaccination gaps and identify factors contributing to missed doses. Machine learning algorithms can analyze historical vaccination data, socioeconomic indicators, and healthcare infrastructure to predict areas or populations at higher risk of missing vaccines. Such predictive analytics can guide proactive interventions, allowing healthcare systems to allocate resources and manpower efficiently to areas expected to face vaccination challenges [144, 145].

Natural language processing (NLP), a branch of AI, can analyze social media, online forums, and local languages to gain insights into public sentiment and vaccine-related discussions [146, 147]. This information can be used to tailor public health messaging and interventions to address specific concerns or misinformation within communities. AI-powered NLP can also assist healthcare workers in communicating effectively with caregivers and parents, especially in regions with diverse languages and dialects [148].

4.2 AI-Enhanced Mobile Apps and Chatbots

Mobile applications and chatbots powered by AI can serve as valuable tools to engage with caregivers and parents [149]. These AI-driven platforms can send automated reminders for upcoming vaccinations, provide information about vaccine schedules, and address common concerns or misconceptions about vaccines. Additionally, they can enable parents to schedule vaccination appointments conveniently. AI chatbots can offer a personalized approach, answering specific questions [150] and providing real-time support to hesitant or unsure caregivers [151, 152].

Mobile apps can provide easily accessible information about vaccines, their importance, and their safety [153]. These apps can include educational materials, videos, and frequently asked questions to address any concerns or misconceptions that parents may have about vaccines. Well-informed parents are more likely to prioritize vaccination for their children [33].

Mobile apps can incorporate geo-tagging functionality to identify areas with low vaccination coverage rates [154]. Healthcare workers can use these apps to plan targeted vaccination outreach campaigns in specific communities or regions. Geo-tagging can also help locate mobile vaccination clinics closer to underserved populations [155, 156].

Mobile apps can provide real-time data on vaccination coverage [156] and adherence [157]. Healthcare workers can use these apps to input vaccination data directly into a centralized database. This real-time reporting allows authorities to monitor progress, identify areas of concern, and take timely action to address vaccination gaps.

Apps can implement incentive and reward systems to motivate parents to vaccinate their children. Parents can earn points, discounts, or other incentives for adhering to vaccination schedules. Such gamification strategies can encourage parents to prioritize vaccination and stay engaged with the vaccination process [158]. Additionally, healthcare workers can receive rewards for reaching vaccination targets, fostering motivation and accountability [30].

4.3 Blockchain-Based Patient Records and Vaccine Supply Chain Management

Blockchain can be used to create secure and interoperable digital health records for children, including vaccination histories [159]. Each child can have a digital identity on the blockchain, and their vaccination records can be securely stored and updated by healthcare providers. This decentralized approach ensures that children's health information is accessible across different healthcare facilities and regions, reducing the chances of missed vaccinations due to incomplete or lost paper records.

Blockchain can provide an immutable and transparent ledger for tracking vaccines throughout the supply chain. Each vaccine batch can be assigned a unique digital identity that is recorded on the blockchain. This ensures the authenticity and integrity of vaccines, reducing the risk of counterfeit or substandard products entering the system. By enhancing the transparency of vaccine distribution, healthcare authorities can better manage the availability of vaccines in remote areas and minimize stockouts, ensuring that children receive their doses on time [160].

5 Conclusion

The immunization of children is crucial for the healthy development of a country. However, in the majority of underdeveloped nations, children either skip routine vaccinations or begin vaccinations but do not finish the program. Much research has been done to determine the cause of missing or zero-dosage vaccines. In this chapter, we have synthesized the reasons for missing basic vaccination and potential strategies to identify and intervene in children who missed or received zero doses. We have summarized several critical aspects of vaccination programs, emphasizing the significance of comprehensive and proactive approaches. The evidence presented underscores that identifying and addressing missed vaccinations is not only feasible but also imperative for ensuring that every child receives the protection they deserve against preventable diseases. We have synthesized a range of strategies and interventions, drawing inspiration from successful practices in developed countries. From government verification of vaccination records during birth registration to collaboration among healthcare professionals and educational institutions, the evidence shows that a concerted effort can significantly boost vaccination awareness and coverage. Moreover, we have highlighted the crucial role played by healthcare professionals in delivering accurate information and promoting vaccination. Their involvement is pivotal in dispelling vaccine hesitancy and increasing parental confidence in immunization. Furthermore, we have discussed the application of advanced technologies in this context, demonstrating their potential to revolutionize immunization efforts and enhance vaccination outreach and coverage.

While challenges persist, particularly in developing countries, the evidence suggests that these challenges can be overcome. Targeted interventions, data-driven approaches, and legal measures have proven effective in increasing vaccination rates and reducing the risk of vaccine-preventable diseases. This chapter reinforces the notion that immunization is a cornerstone of public health. It is a collective responsibility to ensure that children receive the vaccines they need to lead healthy lives. By implementing the strategies and lessons learned from this chapter, we can work towards achieving higher vaccination coverage rates and a brighter, healthier future for all children, regardless of their place of birth or socioeconomic background.

References

1. R.K. Chandra, Nutrition and the immune system: an introduction. Am. J. Clin. Nutr. **66**(2), 460S–463S (1997)
2. K.Y. Cheung, L. Petrou, B. Helfer, E. Porubayeva, E. Dolgikh, S. Ali, I. Ali, L. Archibald-Durham, M.M. Brockway, P. Bugaeva, et al., Health and nutrition claims for infant formula: international cross sectional survey. BMJ **380**, e071075 (2023)
3. N. Fullman, G.C. Correa, G. Ikilezi, D.E. Phillips, H.W. Reynolds, Assessing potential exemplars in reducing zero-dose children: a novel approach for identifying positive outliers in decreasing national levels and geographic inequalities in unvaccinated children. Vaccines **11**(3), 647 (2023)
4. A. Wigley, J. Lorin, D. Hogan, C.E. Utazi, B. Hagedorn, E. Dansereau, A.J. Tatem, N. Tejedor-Garavito, Estimates of the number and distribution of zero-dose and under-immunised children across remote-rural, urban, and conflict-affected settings in low and middle-income countries. PLOS Glob. Public Health **2**(10), e0001126 (2022)
5. K. Mahachi, J. Kessels, K. Boateng, A.E.J.B. Achoribo, P. Mitula, E. Ekeman, L.N. Lochlainn, A. Rosewell, S.V. Sodha, B. Abela-Ridder, et al., Zero-or missed-dose children in Nigeria: contributing factors and interventions to overcome immunization service delivery challenges. Vaccine **40**, 5433–5444 (2022)
6. D.R. Feikin, B. Flannery, M.J. Hamel, M. Stack, P.M. Hansen, Vaccines for children in low- and middle-income countries, in *Reproductive, Maternal, Newborn, and Child Health: Disease Control Priorities*, vol. 2 (World Bank, Washington, 2006), pp. 187–204
7. UNICEF, The state of the world's children 2023 (2023). https://www.unicef.org/reports/state-worlds-children-2023. Accessed 4 Aug 2023
8. World Health Organization (WHO), Immunization coverage (2023). https://www.who.int/news-room/fact-sheets/detail/immunization-coverage. Accessed 04 Aug 2023
9. D. Hogan, A. Gupta, Why reaching zero-dose children holds the key to achieving the sustainable development goals. Vaccines **11**(4), 781 (2023)

10. T.M. Matsungo, F. Kamazizwa, T. Mavhudzi, S. Makota, B. Kamunda, C. Matsinde, D. Chagwena, K. Mukudoka, P. Chopera. The effect of care groups on infant and young child feeding, dietary diversity and wash behaviours in rural Zimbabwe: a case-control study. medRxiv (2023), pp. 2023-01
11. S.M.A. Hanifi, N. Jahan, N. Sultana, S.-A. Hasan, A. Paul, D.D. Reidpath, Millions of Bangladeshi children missed their scheduled vaccination amidst covid-19 pandemic. Front. Public Health **9**, 738623 (2022)
12. M.A. Eryurt, S.S. Yalçin, Zero-dose children in turkey: regional comparison of pooled data for the period 1990 to 2018. BMC Infect. Dis. **22**(1), 421 (2022)
13. G. Tracey, B. Olivia, M. Jean, H. Megan, S. Sagri, Why does gender matter for immunization? Vaccine (2022). https://doi.org/10.1016/j.vaccine.2022.11.071
14. C.E. Utazi, O. Pannell, J.M.K. Aheto, A. Wigley, N. Tejedor-Garavito, J. Wunderlich, B. Hagedorn, D. Hogan, A.J. Tatem, Assessing the characteristics of un-and under-vaccinated children in low-and middle-income countries: a multi-level cross-sectional study. PLOS Glob. Public Health **2**(4), e0000244 (2022)
15. A. Wendt, T.M. Santos, B.O. Cata-Preta, J.C. Costa, T. Mengistu, D.R. Hogan, C.G. Victora, A.J.D. Barros, Children of more empowered women are less likely to be left without vaccination in low-and middle-income countries: a global analysis of 50 dhs surveys. J. Glob. Health **12** (2022). https://doi.org/10.7189%2Fjogh.12.04022
16. T.M. Santos, B.O. Cata-Preta, A. Wendt, L. Arroyave, D.R. Hogan, T. Mengistu, A.J.D. Barros, C.G. Victora, Religious affiliation as a driver of immunization coverage: analyses of zero-dose vaccine prevalence in 66 low-and middle-income countries. Front. Public Health **10**, 977512 (2022)
17. N. Stoop, K. Hirvonen, J.-F. Maystadt, Institutional mistrust and child vaccination coverage in Africa. BMJ Glob. Health **6**(4), e004595 (2021)
18. M.F. Silveira, C.T. Tonial, A.G.K. Maranhão, A.M.S. Teixeira, P.C. Hallal, A.M.B. Menezes, B.L. Horta, F.P. Hartwig, A.J.D. Barros, C.G. Victora, Missed childhood immunizations during the covid-19 pandemic in Brazil: analyses of routine statistics and of a national household survey. Vaccine **39**(25), 3404–3409 (2021)
19. M. Dheresa, Y. Dessie, B. Negash, B. Balis, T. Getachew, G.M. Ayana, B.T. Merga, L.D. Regassa, Child vaccination coverage, trends and predictors in eastern Ethiopia: implication for sustainable development goals. J. Multidiscip. Healthcare **14**, 2657–2667 (2021)
20. T.M. Santos, B.O. Cata-Preta, C.G. Victora, A.J.D. Barros, Finding children with high risk of non-vaccination in 92 low-and middle-income countries: a decision tree approach. Vaccines **9**(6), 646 (2021)
21. M.M. Hossain, F. Abdulla, M. Karimuzzaman, A. Rahman, Routine vaccination disruption in low-income countries: an impact of covid-19 pandemic. Asia Pac. J. Public Health **32**(8), 509–510 (2020)
22. A.A. Adamu, A.M. Sarki, O.A. Uthman, A.B. Wiyeh, M.A. Gadanya, C.S. Wiysonge, Prevalence and dynamics of missed opportunities for vaccination among children in Africa: applying systems thinking in a systematic review and meta-analysis of observational studies. Expert Rev. Vaccines **18**(5), 547–558 (2019)
23. K. Attwell, M.C. Navin, Childhood vaccination mandates: scope, sanctions, severity, selectivity, and salience. Milbank Q. **97**(4), 978–1014 (2019)
24. A.A. Machado, S.A. Edwards, M. Mueller, V. Saini, Effective interventions to increase routine childhood immunization coverage in low socioeconomic status communities in developed countries: a systematic review and critical appraisal of peer-reviewed literature. Vaccine **39**(22), 2938–2964 (2021)
25. J.C. Jacobson Vann, R.M. Jacobson, T. Coyne-Beasley, J.K. Asafu-Adjei, P.G. Szilagyi, Patient reminder and recall interventions to improve immunization rates. Cochrane Database Syst. Rev. (1) (2018). https://doi.org/10.1002/14651858.CD003941.pub3
26. A. Kempe, M.S. Stockwell, P. Szilagyi, The contribution of reminder-recall to vaccine delivery efforts: a narrative review. Acad. Pediatr. **21**(4), S17–S23 (2021)

27. U. Yunusa, S.N. Garba, A.B. Umar, S.H. Idris, U.L. Bello, I. Abdulrashid, J. Mohammed, Mobile phone reminders for enhancing uptake, completeness and timeliness of routine childhood immunization in low and middle income countries: a systematic review and meta-analysis. Vaccine **39**(2), 209–221 (2021)
28. L.M. Gottlieb, H. Wing, N.E. Adler, A systematic review of interventions on patients' social and economic needs. Am. J. Prev. Med. **53**(5), 719–729 (2017)
29. J. Kaufman, R. Ryan, L. Walsh, D. Horey, J. Leask, P. Robinson, S. Hill, Face-to-face interventions for informing or educating parents about early childhood vaccination. Cochrane Database Syst. Rev. (5) (2018). https://doi.org/10.1002/14651858.CD010038.pub3
30. N.T. Brewer, G.B. Chapman, A.J. Rothman, J. Leask, A. Kempe, Increasing vaccination: putting psychological science into action. Psychol. Sci. Public Interest **18**(3), 149–207 (2017)
31. X. Huang, B. Wu, Impact of urban-rural health insurance integration on health care: evidence from Rural China. China Econ. Rev. **64**, 101543 (2020)
32. J.R. Cataldi, M.E. Kerns, S.T. O'Leary, Evidence-based strategies to increase vaccination uptake: a review. Curr. Opin. Pediatr. **32**(1), 151–159 (2020)
33. O. Olson, C. Berry, N. Kumar, Addressing parental vaccine hesitancy towards childhood vaccines in the united states: a systematic literature review of communication interventions and strategies. Vaccines **8**(4), 590 (2020)
34. S.C. Shen, V. Dubey, Addressing vaccine hesitancy: clinical guidance for primary care physicians working with parents. Can. Fam. Physician **65**(3), 175–181 (2019)
35. C. Mantel, T. Cherian, New immunization strategies: adapting to global challenges. Bundesgesundheitsblatt-Gesundheitsforschung-Gesundheitsschutz **63**(1), 25–31 (2020)
36. S. Paul, S. Paul, A. Kumar Gupta, K.S. James, Maternal education, health care system and child health: evidence from India. Soc. Sci. Med. **296**, 114740 (2022)
37. K. Vikram, R. Vanneman, S. Desai, Linkages between maternal education and childhood immunization in India. Soc. Sci. Med. **75**(2), 331–339 (2012)
38. B.A. Ushie, O.A. Fayehun, D.B. Ugal, Trends and patterns of under-5 vaccination in Nigeria, 1990–2008: What manner of progress? Child Care Health Dev. **40**(2), 267–274 (2014)
39. J.J. Rainey, M. Watkins, T.K. Ryman, P. Sandhu, A. Bo, K. Banerjee, Reasons related to non-vaccination and under-vaccination of children in low and middle income countries: findings from a systematic review of the published literature, 1999–2009. Vaccine **29**(46), 8215–8221 (2011)
40. D. Adeloye, W. Jacobs, A.O. Amuta, O. Ogundipe, O. Mosaku, M.A. Gadanya, G. Oni, Coverage and determinants of childhood immunization in Nigeria: a systematic review and meta-analysis. Vaccine **35**(22), 2871–2881 (2017)
41. R. Gunnala, I.U. Ogbuanu, O.J. Adegoke, H.M. Scobie, B.V. Uba, K.A. Wannemuehler, A. Ruiz, H. Elmousaad, C.J. Ohuabunwo, M. Mustafa, et al., Routine vaccination coverage in northern Nigeria: results from 40 district-level cluster surveys, 2014–2015. PLoS One **11**(12), e0167835 (2016)
42. S.A. Adedini, C. Odimegwu, E.N.S. Imasiku, D.N. Ononokpono, L. Ibisomi, Regional variations in infant and child mortality in Nigeria: a multilevel analysis. J. Biosoc. Sci. **47**(2), 165–187 (2015)
43. A.N. Mohamud, A. Feleke, W. Worku, M. Kifle, H.R. Sharma, Immunization coverage of 12–23 months old children and associated factors in Jigjiga district, Somali National Regional State, Ethiopia. BMC Public Health **14**(1), 1–9 (2014)
44. A. A.-k. Córdova, C. Mendez-Guerra, C. Silva-Perez, P. Herrera-Añazco, V.A. Benites-Zapata, Inequalities in covid-19 vaccination coverage in Peru: an ecological study. Public Health Pract. **5**, 100384 (2023)
45. O. Oleribe, V. Kumar, A. Awosika-Olumo, S.D. Taylor-Robinson, Individual and socioeconomic factors associated with childhood immunization coverage in Nigeria. Pan Afr. Med. J. **26** (2017). https://doi.org/10.11604%2Fpamj.2017.26.220.11453
46. T. Kitamura, K. Komada, A. Xeuatvongsa, M. Hachiya, Factors affecting childhood immunization in Lao People's Democratic Republic: a cross-sectional study from nationwide, population-based, multistage cluster sampling. Biosci. Trends **7**(4), 178–185 (2013)

47. K. Vikram, R. Vanneman, Maternal education and the multidimensionality of child health outcomes in India. J. Biosoc. Sci. **52**(1), 57–77 (2020)
48. K. Jamil, A. Bhuiya, K. Streatfield, N. Chakrabarty, The immunization programme in Bangladesh: impressive gains in coverage, but gaps remain. Health Policy Plan. **14**(1), 49–58 (1999)
49. C.C. Nwangwu, A.E. Chike, I.O. Eucharia Ijeoma, Cross-sectional survey on parental perception and attitude on measles vaccine: low hospital measles case presentation in rural area in Enugu Nigeria. J. Clin. Diagn. Res. **15**(2), EC14-EC19 (2021). https://doi.org/10.7860/JCDR/2021/45315.14574
50. S. Subhani, S. Anwar, M.A. Khan, G. Jeelani, Impact of mother's employment on child vaccination (a case study of Bangladesh). J. Finance Econ. **3**(4), 64–66 (2021)
51. S. Thorpe, K. VanderEnde, C. Peters, L. Bardin, K.M. Yount, The influence of women's empowerment on child immunization coverage in low, lower-middle, and upper-middle income countries: a systematic review of the literature. Matern. Child Health J. **20**, 172–186 (2016)
52. A. Ibrahim, S. Tripathi, A. Kumar, The effect of women's empowerment on child health status: study on two developing nations. Int. J. Sci. Res. Publications **5**(4), 1–8 (2015)
53. T. Mukungwa, Factors associated with full immunization coverage amongst children aged 12–23 months in Zimbabwe. Afr. Popul. Stud. **29**(2), 1761–1774 (2015). https://doi.org/10.11564/29-2-745
54. P. Eze, C.L. Aniebo, U.J. Agu, S.A. Agu, Y. Acharya, Validity of maternal recall for estimating childhood vaccination coverage–evidence from Nigeria. Vaccine **40**(1), 28–36 (2022)
55. Z.A. Mekonnen, K.A. Gelaye, M.C. Were, B. Tilahun, Timely completion of vaccination and its determinants among children in Northwest, Ethiopia: a multilevel analysis. BMC Public Health **20**, 1–13 (2020)
56. K. Elizabeth, K. George, N. Raphael, E. Moses, Factors influencing low immunization coverage among children between 12–23 months in East Pokot, Baringo Country, Kenya. Int. J. Vaccines **1**(2), 00012 (2015)
57. L. Benova, O.M.R. Campbell, G.B. Ploubidis, Socio-economic gradients in maternal and child health-seeking behaviours in Egypt: systematic literature review and evidence synthesis. PLoS One **9**(3), e93032 (2014)
58. I. Jahan, M. Muhit, D. Hardianto, F. Laryea, S. Kofi Amponsah, A.B. Chhetri, H. Smithers-Sheedy, S. McIntyre, N. Badawi, G. Khandaker, Epidemiology of malnutrition among children with cerebral palsy in low-and middle-income countries: findings from the global LMIC CP register. Nutrients **13**(11), 3676 (2021)
59. M.W. Godah, Z. Beydoun, R.A. Abdul-Khalek, B. Safieddine, A.M. Khamis, S. Abdulrahim, Maternal education and low birth weight in low-and middle-income countries: systematic review and meta-analysis. Matern. Child Health J. **25**(8), 1305–1315 (2021)
60. K.D. Kihara, I. Mwanzo, E. Gitonga, Immunization coverage among children aged between 12–23 months in West Pokot County, Kenya. J. Med. Nurs. Public Health **5**, 22–38 (2022)
61. M. Sreevatsava, A.L. Burman, A. Wahdan, R.M. Safdar, A. O'Leary, R. Amjad, A. Salam, M. Quershi, R. Ishaq, J. Khan, et al., Routine immunization coverage in Pakistan: a survey of children under 1 year of age in community-based vaccination areas. Vaccine **38**(28), 4399–4404 (2020)
62. E. Jimenez-Soto, J. Durham, A. Hodge, Entrenched geographical and socioeconomic disparities in child mortality: trends in absolute and relative inequalities in Cambodia. PLoS One **9**(10), e109044 (2014)
63. R. Hong, V. Chhea, Trend and inequality in immunization dropout among young children in cambodia. Matern. Child Health J. **14**, 446–452 (2010)
64. Y. Lakew, A. Bekele, S. Biadgilign, Factors influencing full immunization coverage among 12–23 months of age children in Ethiopia: evidence from the national demographic and health survey in 2011. BMC Public Health **15**, 1–8 (2015)
65. E. Zerhouni, Gavi, the vaccine alliance. Cell **179**(1), 13–17 (2019)

66. A.A. Bawah, J.F. Phillips, M. Adjuik, M. Vaughan-Smith, B. Macleod, F.N. Binka, The impact of immunization on the association between poverty and child survival: evidence from Kassena-Nankana district of Northern Ghana. Scand. J. Public Health **38**(1), 95–103 (2010)
67. H.K. Balbir Singh, V.B. Badgujar, R.S. Yahaya, S. Abd Rahman, F.M. Sami, S. Badgujar, S.N. Govindan, M.T. Ansari, Assessment of knowledge and attitude among postnatal mothers towards childhood vaccination in Malaysia. Hum. Vaccines Immunother. **15**(11), 2544–2551 (2019)
68. M. Vivion, C. Hennequin, P. Verger, E. Dubé, Supporting informed decision-making about vaccination: an analysis of two official websites. Public Health **178**, 112–119 (2020)
69. J.A. Reich, Neoliberal mothering and vaccine refusal: imagined gated communities and the privilege of choice. Gender Soc. **28**(5), 679–704 (2014)
70. W. Imran, F. Abbas, S.A. Javed, What is causing high polio vaccine dropout among Pakistani children? Public Health **164**, 16–25 (2018)
71. C. Bateman, Vaccines: Sa's immunisation programme debunked. S. Afr. Med. J. **106**(4), 318–319 (2016)
72. F. Tanser, B. Gijsbertsen, K. Herbst, Modelling and understanding primary health care accessibility and utilization in rural South Africa: an exploration using a geographical information system. Soc. Sci. Med. **63**(3), 691–705 (2006)
73. G.K. Shapiro, J. Kaufman, N.T. Brewer, K. Wiley, L. Menning, J. Leask, N. Abad, C. Betsch, V. Bura, G. Correa, et al., A critical review of measures of childhood vaccine confidence. Curr. Opin. Immunol. **71**, 34–45 (2021)
74. S.B. Omer, D.A. Salmon, W.A. Orenstein, M.P. Dehart, N. Halsey, Vaccine refusal, mandatory immunization, and the risks of vaccine-preventable diseases. N. Engl. J. Med. **360**(19), 1981–1988 (2009)
75. E.T. Tagoe, N. Sheikh, A. Morton, J. Nonvignon, A.R. Sarker, L. Williams, I. Megiddo, Covid-19 vaccination in lower-middle income countries: national stakeholder views on challenges, barriers, and potential solutions. Front. Public Health **9**, 709127 (2021)
76. U.J. Okenwa, M.D. Dairo, B. Uba, O. Ajumobi, Maternal reasons for non-receipt of valid hepatitis b birth dose among mother-infant pairs attending routine immunization clinics, south-east, Nigeria. Vaccine **37**(46), 6894–6899 (2019)
77. H.J. Larson, C. Jarrett, E. Eckersberger, D.M.D. Smith, P. Paterson, Understanding vaccine hesitancy around vaccines and vaccination from a global perspective: a systematic review of published literature, 2007–2012. Vaccine **32**(19), 2150–2159 (2014)
78. M. Rahman, S. Obaida-Nasrin, Factors affecting acceptance of complete immunization coverage of children under five years in rural Bangladesh. Salud pública de méxico **52**(2), 134–140 (2010)
79. O.G. Chido-Amajuoyi, C. Wonodi, D. Mantey, A. Perez, A. Mcalister, Prevalence and correlates of never vaccinated Nigerian children, aged 1–5 years. Vaccine **36**(46), 6953–6960 (2018)
80. P. Eze, U.J. Agu, C.L. Aniebo, S.A. Agu, L.O. Lawani, Y. Acharya, Factors associated with incomplete immunisation in children aged 12–23 months at subnational level, Nigeria: a cross-sectional study. BMJ Open **11**(6), e047445 (2021)
81. L.E. Smith, R. Amlôt, J. Weinman, J. Yiend, G.J. Rubin, A systematic review of factors affecting vaccine uptake in young children. Vaccine **35**(45), 6059–6069 (2017)
82. M. Hardhantyo, Y.-C. Chuang, Urban-rural differences in factors associated with incomplete basic immunization among children in Indonesia: a nationwide multilevel study. Pediatr. Neonatol. **62**(1), 80–89 (2021)
83. M.R. Islam, M. Hasan, W. Nasreen, M.I. Tushar, M.A. Bhuiyan, The covid-19 vaccination experience in Bangladesh: findings from a cross-sectional study. Int. J. Immunopathol. Pharmacol. **35**, 20587384211065628 (2021)
84. B. Babakura, T. Nomhwange, A.E. Jean Baptiste, O. Dede, L. Taiwo, S. Abba, M. Soyemi, A.M. Idowu, M.T. Richard, F. Braka, et al., The challenges of insecurity on implementing vaccination campaign and its effect on measles elimination and control efforts: a case study of 2017/18 measles campaign in Borno State, Nigeria. Vaccine **39**, C66–C75 (2021)

85. D. Ali, A. Levin, M. Abdulkarim, U. Tijjani, B. Ahmed, F. Namalam, F. Oyewole, L. Dougherty, A cost-effectiveness analysis of traditional and geographic information system-supported microplanning approaches for routine immunization program management in northern Nigeria. Vaccine **38**(6), 1408–1415 (2020)
86. S. Shah, M. Goers, A. Zewde, B. Katz, I. Obaitan, O. Magbagbeola, K. Ssebambulidde, S. Hassany, A. Moussa, J. Mtengezo, et al., Hepatitis b awareness and understanding among healthcare workers in Africa, in *Hepatology*, vol. 68 (Wiley, Hoboken, 2018), p. 290A
87. H.O. Owie, P.A. Apanga, et al., Occupational health hazards prevailing among health-care workers in developing countries. J. AIDS Clin. Res. **7**(8) (2016). https://www.cabidigitallibrary.org/doi/pdf/10.5555/20163350994
88. O. O'Donnell, Access to health care in developing countries: breaking down demand side barriers. Cad. Saude Publica **23**, 2820–2834 (2007)
89. S.D. Torun, N. Bakırcı, Vaccination coverage and reasons for non-vaccination in a district of Istanbul. BMC Public Health **6**(1), 1–8 (2006)
90. A. Wendt, T.M. Santos, B.O Cata-Preta, L. Arroyave, D.R. Hogan, T. Mengistu, A.J.D. Barros, C.G. Victora, Exposure of zero-dose children to multiple deprivation: analyses of data from 80 low-and middle-income countries. Vaccines **10**(9), 1568 (2022)
91. C.E. Ozigbu, B. Olatosi, Z. Li, J.W. Hardin, N.L. Hair, Correlates of zero-dose vaccination status among children aged 12–59 months in sub-Saharan Africa: a multilevel analysis of individual and contextual factors. Vaccines **10**(7), 1052 (2022)
92. A. Majumdar, The primary education in developing countries and teacher's educational role, training and development. GPH-Int. J. Edu. Res. **3**(01), 01–15 (2020). https://gphjournal.org/index.php/er/article/view/265
93. M.E. Lockheed, A.M. Verspoor, et al., *Improving Primary Education in Developing Countries* (Oxford University Press for World Bank, Oxford, 1991)
94. BBC News, Italy bans unvaccinated children from school (2019). https://www.bbc.com/news/world-europe-47536981. Accessed 23 Jul 2023
95. N. Williams, H. Woodward, A. Majeed, S. Saxena, Primary care strategies to improve childhood immunisation uptake in developed countries: systematic review. JRSM Short Rep. **2**(10), 1–21 (2011)
96. Health.vic, Primary school immunisation requirements (2023). https://www.health.vic.gov.au/immunisation/primary-school-immunisation-requirements. Accessed 10 Aug 2023
97. NSW Government, Immunisation requirements (2023). https://www.nsw.gov.au/education-and-training/primary-and-high-school/starting-primary-school/enrolling-your-child/immunisation-requirements. Accessed 25 Aug 2023
98. M.M. Masadeh, K.H. Alzoubi, S.I. Al-Azzam, H.S. Al-Agedi, B.E. Abu Rashid, T.L. Mukattash, Public awareness regarding children vaccination in Jordan. Hum. Vaccines Immunother. **10**(6), 1762–1766 (2014)
99. J. Cassio De Moraes, M.C.C. Camargo, N.T. Rossetto Hidalgo, H. Aparecida Barbosa, V.L. Gattas, H. de G. Vasconcelos, C. Tavares Sacchi, I.M. Land Gral, B.A. Perkins, J.D. Wenger, et al., Protective efficacy of a serogroup b meningococcal vaccine in Sao Paulo, Brazil. Lancet **340**(8827), 1074–1078 (1992)
100. B.N. Tagbo, C.B. Eke, B.I. Omotowo, C.N. Onwuasigwe, E.B. Onyeka, U.O. Mildred, Vaccination coverage and its determinants in children aged 11-23 months in an urban district of Nigeria. World J. Vaccines **4**, 175–183 (2014). http://dx.doi.org/10.4236/wjv.2014.44020
101. F. Shahab, H. Hussain, H. Gul, Vaccination status and causes of under vaccination in paediatric patients admitted at Khyber teaching hospital Peshawar. J. Postgraduate Med. Inst. **27**(4), 439–444 (2013). https://www.jpmi.org.pk/index.php/jpmi/article/view/1447/1802
102. D. Kumar, A. Aggarwal, S. Gomber, Immunization status of children admitted to a tertiary-care hospital of north India: reasons for partial immunization or non-immunization. J. Health Popul. Nutr. **28**(3), 300 (2010)
103. S. Anand, T. Bärnighausen, Health workers and vaccination coverage in developing countries: an econometric analysis. Lancet **369**(9569), 1277–1285 (2007)

104. M. Ali, J.D. Clemens, J.-K. Park, L. Von Seidlein, V.D. Thiem, D.D. Trach, et al., The vaccine data link in Nha Trang, Vietnam: a progress report on the implementation of a database to detect adverse events related to vaccinations. Vaccine **21**(15), 1681–1686 (2003)
105. G. Babu, J. Olsen, S. Jana, S. Nandy, M. Farid, V.J. Sadhana, Evaluation of immunization cards and parental recall against gold standard for evaluating immunization coverage. Internet J. Epidemiol. **9** (2011)
106. N. Shrivastwa, B.W. Gillespie, G.E. Kolenic, J.M. Lepkowski, M.L. Boulton, Predictors of vaccination in India for children aged 12–36 months. Am. J. Prev. Med. **49**(6), S435–S444 (2015)
107. M.R. Francis, J.P. Nuorti, R.Z. Kompithra, H. Larson, V. Balraj, G. Kang, V.R. Mohan, Vaccination coverage and factors associated with routine childhood vaccination uptake in rural Vellore, Southern India, 2017. Vaccine **37**(23), 3078–3087 (2019)
108. C. Giambi, M. Del Manso, T. Dalla Zuanna, F. Riccardo, A. Bella, M.G. Caporali, A. Baka, N. Caks-Jager, T. Melillo, R. Mexia, et al., National immunization strategies targeting migrants in six European countries. Vaccine **37**(32), 4610–4617 (2019)
109. M. Miles, T.K. Ryman, V. Dietz, E. Zell, E.T. Luman, Validity of vaccination cards and parental recall to estimate vaccination coverage: a systematic review of the literature. Vaccine **31**(12), 1560–1568 (2013)
110. B.M. Craig, United states covid-19 vaccination preferences (CVP): 2020 hindsight. Patient **14**, 309–318 (2021)
111. A.L. Wagner, The use and significance of vaccination cards. Hum. Vaccines Immunother. **15**(12), 2844–2846 (2019)
112. M. Butt, R. Mohammed, E. Butt, S. Butt, J. Xiang, Why have immunization efforts in Pakistan failed to achieve global standards of vaccination uptake and infectious disease control? Risk Manag. Healthcare Policy **2020**, 111–124 (2020)
113. Centers for Disease Control and Prevention, Immunization information systems. https://www.cdc.gov/vaccines/programs/iis/index.html. Accessed 23 Jul 2023
114. UNICEF, Newborn health in humanitarian settings (2017). https://www.unicef.org/media/61561/file. Accessed 23 Jul 2023
115. World Health Organization, Who recommendations on newborn health: guidelines approved by the who guidelines review committee. Technical documents (2017)
116. Ö. Terzi, E.N. Gülen, C. Dündar, The causes of parental vaccine refusal: results of a survey from Giresun, Turkey. Turk. J. Pediatr. **63**(4), 618–625 (2021)
117. National Center for Immunization and Respiratory Diseases, Making the vaccine decision: Addressing common concerns (2023). https://www.cdc.gov/vaccines/parents/why-vaccinate/vaccine-decision.html. Accessed 4 Aug 2023
118. L. Selim, What is birth registration and why does it matter? (2019). https://www.unicef.org/stories/what-birth-registration-and-why-does-it-matter. Accessed 23 Jul 2023
119. C. Cappa, K. Gregson, T. Wardlaw, S. Bissell, Birth registration: a child's passport to protection. Lancet Glob. Health **2**(2), e67–e68 (2014)
120. C.H. Suppli, J.W. Dreier, M. Rasmussen, A.-M.N. Andersen, P. Valentiner-Branth, K. Mølbak, T.G. Krause, Sociodemographic predictors are associated with compliance to a vaccination-reminder in 9692 girls age 14, Denmark 2014–2015. Prev. Med. Rep. **10**, 93–99 (2018)
121. S.R. Newcomer, J. Graham, K. Irish, R.E. Freeman, C.S. Leary, B.K. Wehner, M.F. Daley, Identification of spatial clusters of undervaccination patterns among children aged< 24 months using immunization information system data, Montana, 2015–2019. Public Health Rep. **139**, 00333549231186603 (2023)
122. M.J. Uddin, M.S. Lily Horng, A. Labrique, L. Vasudevan, K. Zeller, M. Chowdhury, C.P. Larson, D. Bishai, N. Alam, Use of mobile phones for improving vaccination coverage among children living in rural hard-to-reach areas and urban streets of Bangladesh. Vaccine **34**(2), 276–283 (2016)

123. Public Health Agency of Sweden, National vaccination programme for children. https://www.folkhalsomyndigheten.se/the-public-health-agency-of-sweden/communicable-disease-control/vaccinations/. Accessed 23 Jul 2023
124. Canadian Paediatric Society, Impact: Canadian immunization monitoring program (2017). https://immunize.ca/resources/impact-canadian-immunization-monitoring-program-active. Accessed 23 Jul 2023
125. K. Dooling, M. Marin, M. Wallace, N. McClung, M. Chamberland, G.M. Lee, H.K. Talbot, J.R. Romero, B.P. Bell, S.E. Oliver, The advisory committee on immunization practices' updated interim recommendation for allocation of covid-19 vaccine—United States, December 2020. Morb. Mortal. Wkly. Rep. **69**(51–52), 1657 (2021)
126. K. Ferguson, A. Caplan, Love thy neighbour? Allocating vaccines in a world of competing obligations. J. Med. Ethics **47**(12), e20–e20 (2021)
127. L. Lataifeh, A. Al-Ani, I. Lataifeh, K. Ammar, A. AlOmary, F. Al-Hammouri, M. Al-Hussaini, Knowledge, attitudes, and practices of healthcare workers in Jordan towards the covid-19 vaccination. Vaccines **10**(2), 263 (2022)
128. I. Ceccato, A. Di Crosta, P. La Malva, L. Cannito, N. Mammarella, R. Palumbo, R. Palumbo, A. Di Domenico, Public opinion in vaccine allocation priority: who comes first? Psychol. Health **38**, 1194–1214 (2023)
129. S. Schumacher, J. Salmanton-García, O.A. Cornely, S.C. Mellinghoff, Increasing influenza vaccination coverage in healthcare workers: a review on campaign strategies and their effect. Infection **49**, 387–399 (2021)
130. S. Haviari, T. Bénet, M. Saadatian-Elahi, P. André, P. Loulergue, P. Vanhems, Vaccination of healthcare workers: a review. Hum. Vaccines Immunother. **11**(11), 2522–2537 (2015)
131. M. Hosseini, M. Ahmadi, B.E. Dixon, A service oriented architecture approach to achieve interoperability between immunization information systems in Iran, in *AMIA Annual Symposium Proceedings*, vol. 2014 (American Medical Informatics Association, Bethesda, 2014), p. 1797
132. D. Gray, Unvaccinated children banned from school during outbreaks (2019). https://www.healthline.com/health-news/unvaccinated-children-banned-from-schools-during-outbreaks. Accessed 24 Jul 2023
133. J.H. Tanne, US county bars unvaccinated children from public spaces amid measles emergency. Br. Med. J. (Online) **364** (2019)
134. L. Bever, Unvaccinated children banned from public spaces amid measles outbreak in New York suburb (2019). https://www.washingtonpost.com/health/2019/03/26/unvaccinated-children-banned-public-spaces-amid-measles-outbreak-new-york-suburb/. Accessed 20 Jul 2023
135. S. Long, NY county bans unvaccinated minors from public places. UWIRE Text (2019), pp. 1–1
136. L. Bever, New York county bans unvaccinated children from public spaces. Washingtonpost.com (2019)
137. N. Dudeja, T. Khan, D.T. Varughese, S.G. Abraham, M.M. Ninan, C.L. Prasad, R. Sarkar, G. Kang, Technologies for strengthening immunization coverage in India: a systematic review. Lancet Reg. Health Southeast Asia **23**, 100251 (2023)
138. A.M. Kazi, N. Ahsan, W. Mughis, S. Jamal, R. Allana, M. Raza, S. Muneer, M. Ayub Khan Mughal, H. Kaleemuddin, F. Sameen, et al., Usability and acceptability of a mobile APP for behavior change and to improve immunization coverage among children in Pakistan: a mixed-methods study. Int. J. Environ. Res. Public Health **18**(18), 9527 (2021)
139. K.M. Atkinson, J. Westeinde, R. Ducharme, S.E. Wilson, S.L. Deeks, N. Crowcroft, S. Hawken, K. Wilson, Can mobile technologies improve on-time vaccination? A study piloting maternal use of immunizeca, a pan-Canadian immunization APP. Hum. Vaccines Immunother. **12**(10), 2654–2661 (2016)

140. K. Wilson, K. Atkinson, M. Pluscauskas, C. Bell, A mobile-phone immunization record in Ontario: uptake and opportunities for improving public health. J. Telemed. Telecare **20**(8), 476–480 (2014)
141. K. Wilson, K.M. Atkinson, S.L. Deeks, N.S. Crowcroft, Improving vaccine registries through mobile technologies: a vision for mobile enhanced immunization information systems. J. Am. Med. Inform. Assoc. **23**(1), 207–211 (2016)
142. L.G. Scharf, R. Coyle, K. Adeniyi, J. Fath, L. Harris, S. Myerburg, M.B. Kurilo, E. Abbott, Current challenges and future possibilities for immunization information systems. Acad. Pediatr. **21**(4), S57–S64 (2021)
143. C. Magazzino, M. Mele, M. Coccia, A machine learning algorithm to analyse the effects of vaccination on covid-19 mortality. Epidemiol. Infect. **150**, e168 (2022)
144. C.Y. Lee, Y.-P.P. Chen, Machine learning on adverse drug reactions for pharmacovigilance. Drug Discov. Today **24**(7), 1332–1343 (2019)
145. K. Dick, A. Nordstrom, Identifying unvaccinated individuals in Canada: a predictive model (2016). arXiv preprint arXiv:1607.08656
146. C.A. Melton, O.A. Olusanya, N. Ammar, A. Shaban-Nejad, Public sentiment analysis and topic modeling regarding covid-19 vaccines on the Reddit social media platform: a call to action for strengthening vaccine confidence. J. Infect. Public Health **14**(10), 1505–1512 (2021)
147. A.R. Sanaullah, A. Das, A. Das, M.A. Kabir, K. Shu, Applications of machine learning for covid-19 misinformation: a systematic review. Soc. Netw. Anal. Min. **12**(1), 94 (2022)
148. A. Hussain, A. Tahir, Z. Hussain, Z. Sheikh, M. Gogate, K. Dashtipour, A. Ali, A. Sheikh, Artificial intelligence-enabled analysis of public attitudes on Facebook and twitter toward covid-19 vaccines in the United Kingdom and the united states: observational study. J. Med. Internet Res. **23**(4), e26627 (2021)
149. Y.-J. Hong, M. Piao, J. Kim, J.-H. Lee, Development and evaluation of a child vaccination chatbot real-time consultation messenger service during the covid-19 pandemic. Appl. Sci. **11**(24), 12142 (2021)
150. E. Jo, D.A. Epstein, H. Jung, Y.-H, Kim, Understanding the benefits and challenges of deploying conversational ai leveraging large language models for public health intervention, in *Proceedings of the 2023 CHI Conference on Human Factors in Computing Systems* (2023), pp. 1–16
151. A. Haleem, M. Javaid, R. Pratap Singh, R. Suman, Medical 4.0 technologies for healthcare: features, capabilities, and applications. Internet Things Cyber-Phys. Syst. **2**, 12–30 (2022)
152. G. Yang, Z. Pang, M. Jamal Deen, M. Dong, Y.-T. Zhang, N. Lovell, A.M. Rahmani, Homecare robotic systems for healthcare 4.0: visions and enabling technologies. IEEE J. Biomed. Health Inform. **24**(9), 2535–2549 (2020)
153. S.K.D. Houle, K. Atkinson, M. Paradis, K. Wilson, Canimmunize: a digital tool to help patients manage their immunizations. Can. Pharm. J./Revue des Pharmaciens du Canada **150**(4), 236–238 (2017)
154. A.M. Kazi, M. Ali, K. Ayub, H. Kalimuddin, K. Zubair, A. Nafey Kazi, A. Artani, S.A. Ali, Geo-spatial reporting for monitoring of household immunization coverage through mobile phones: findings from a feasibility study. Int. J. Med. Inform. **107**, 48–55 (2017)
155. M. Venkataraghavan, P. Rani, L. Ashok, C.R. Rao, V.C. Sekaran, T.K. Krishnapriya, "through their eyes, i can work"–rural physicians' perceptions about mobile phone use among community health workers–a qualitative analysis. Health Educ. **122**(2), 180–201 (2021)
156. K. Wilson, K.M. Atkinson, J. Westeinde, Apps for immunization: leveraging mobile devices to place the individual at the center of care. Hum. Vaccines Immunother. **11**(10), 2395–2399 (2015)
157. H. Anglada-Martinez, G. Riu-Viladoms, M. Martin-Conde, M. Rovira-Illamola, J.M. Sotoca-Momblona, C. Codina-Jane, Does mhealth increase adherence to medication? Results of a systematic review. Int. J. Clin. Pract. **69**(1), 9–32 (2015)

158. J. Adams, B. Bateman, F. Becker, T. Cresswell, D. Flynn, R. McNaughton, Y. Oluboyede, S. Robalino, L. Ternent, B.G. Sood, et al., Effectiveness and acceptability of parental financial incentives and quasi-mandatory schemes for increasing uptake of vaccinations in preschool children: systematic review, qualitative study and discrete choice experiment. Health Technol. Assess. **19**(94), 1–176 (2015)
159. J. Chen, X. Chen, C.-L. Chen, et al., A traceable blockchain-based vaccination record storage and sharing system. J. Healthcare Eng. **2022** (2022). https://doi.org/10.1155/2022/2211065
160. B. Yong, J. Shen, X. Liu, F. Li, H. Chen, Q. Zhou, An intelligent blockchain-based system for safe vaccine supply and supervision. Int. J. Inf. Manag. **52**, p. 7, 102024 (2020)

A Stacking Ensemble Approach for Robust Dengue Patient Detection from Complete Blood Count Data

Md. Sohanur Rahman, Imrat Jahan, Mohammad Kaosar Alam, Md. Nahiduzzaman, Abrar Shahriyar Hossain, Johayra Prithula, Shona Pedersen, and Muhammad E. H. Chowdhury

1 Introduction

Dengue fever is an arthropod-borne viral disease resulting from infection by the dengue virus (DENV) and is transmitted to humans primarily through the bites of infected Aedes aegypti mosquitoes. As delineated by Guzman et al. [1], DENV encompasses four distinct serotypes: DENV-1, DENV-2, DENV-3, and DENV-4, all predominantly vectored by Aedes aegypti. Jeffrey R. Powell [2] further elucidated that Aedes aegypti, a native African mosquito, is the primary vector for several arboviruses including Zika, yellow fever, dengue, and chikungunya. Moreover, it is postulated to be the principal vector for emerging viral diseases originating from Africa. The World Health Organization (WHO) [3] estimates that dengue poses a

M. S. Rahman · J. Prithula
Department of Electrical and Electronics Engineering, University of Dhaka, Dhaka, Bangladesh

I. Jahan
Department of Paediatric Dentistry, Bangabandhu Sheikh Mujib Medical University, Dhaka, Bangladesh

M. K. Alam · M. E. H. Chowdhury (✉)
Department of Electrical Engineering, Qatar University, Doha, Qatar
e-mail: mchowdhury@qu.edu.qa

M. Nahiduzzaman
Department of Electrical & Computer Engineering, Rajshahi University of Engineering & Technology, Rajshahi, Bangladesh
e-mail: nahiduzzaman@ece.ruet.ac.bd

A. S. Hossain
Department of Computer Science and Engineering, Qatar University, Doha, Qatar

S. Pedersen
Department of Basic Medical Sciences, College of Medicine, Qatar University, Doha, Qatar
e-mail: spedersen@qu.edu.qa

M. E. H. Chowdhury, S. Kiranyaz (eds.), *Surveillance, Prevention, and Control of Infectious Diseases*, https://doi.org/10.1007/978-3-031-59967-5_7

risk to nearly 50% of the global populace, with an annual incidence ranging between 100 to 400 million cases. While the majority of DENV infections might manifest as asymptomatic or mild clinical presentations, severe and occasionally fatal outcomes can arise from DENV infections.

The global distribution of Ae. aegypti is significantly influenced by climatic conditions. Temperatures below 10 °C hinder both larval development and adult survivability as noted by Slosek 1986 [4] and Hopp and Foley 2001 [5]. Beserra et al. [6] identified the optimal temperature bracket for growth, reproductive efficacy, and lifespan to be between 22 and 32 °C. Within this thermal range, elevated temperatures expedite the oviposition process in Ae. aegypti, leading to an augmented egg-laying frequency [7]. These climatic conditions, combined with dense urban settlements, render the subtropical regions and the Indian subcontinent particularly conducive for Ae. aegypti proliferation.

Dengue manifests in two primary clinical forms: dengue fever and severe dengue. Dengue fever, as characterized by Simmons et al. [8], typically presents with symptoms like high fever, rashes, myalgia, arthralgia, and cephalalgia. Severe dengue, often referred to as dengue hemorrhagic fever or dengue shock syndrome, exhibits clinical features such as plasma leakage, fluid accumulation, respiratory distress, pronounced hemorrhaging, and potential organ impairment. Such severe cases possess a fatality risk. Annually, the WHO approximates a staggering 50 million dengue infections globally. The expanded footprint of dengue and its vectors can be attributed to factors like urban sprawl, demographic expansion, augmented global mobility, lackluster vector control strategies, among others. Presently, over half of the global population resides in regions predisposed to dengue transmission [9].

The life cycle of the Aedes mosquito encompasses four distinct phases: egg, larva, pupa, and adult. Research by Christophers (1960) revealed that female mosquitoes deposit their eggs on damp substrates near stagnant water sources. Remarkably, these eggs can endure desiccation for extended periods, maintaining their viability. When submerged, typically within a day, the eggs hatch into larvae [10]. These larvae then feed on organic detritus and microorganisms present in the water. As outlined by Judson (1960), the larval phase persists for approximately 6–8 days, succeeded by the pupal phase which spans 2–3 days [11]. Subsequent to this metamorphosis, the adult mosquito emerges. It's noteworthy that while females necessitate a blood meal for egg production, males do not bite for sustenance but feed primarily on nectar.

Prompt diagnosis of dengue is pivotal as it facilitates immediate therapeutic interventions, thereby enhancing patient prognosis. A study conducted by Lee et al. [12] indicated that patients diagnosed and treated within the initial 72 hours of symptom onset experienced reduced hospitalization durations and exhibited a diminished mortality rate in comparison to those with belated diagnoses. Early administration of intravenous rehydration notably mitigates the complications of severe dengue, such as plasma leakage, shock, and hemorrhage. Moreover, it fosters the precise management and vigilant monitoring of critical indicators.

NS1, also known as Non-structural protein, is a glycoprotein found in the dengue virus. It is highly conserved and weights around 40-46KDa. This protein is believed to be held responsible in some degree reproducing the virus [13]. The enzyme-linked immunoassay (ELISA) test has confirmed the presence of elevated levels of dengue NS1 antigen in the blood and furthermore infected individuals has shown 10 ng/ml of soluble hexameric NS1 in their blood sample [14]. NS1 test are conducted through Enzyme immunoassays (EIAs) or immunochromatographic (ICT) techniques; these assays are specific to various flaviviruses. A rigorous investigation unveils that the combined sensitivity and specificity of single enzyme immunoassay (EIA) based NS1 tests were 67% and 99% respectively, whereas for immunochromatographic based NS1 tests, they were 71% and 99% respectively [15]. One of the main drawbacks of the NS1 detection approach is its failure to identify the infection in samples taken during the latter stages of dengue. The drawback can be explained as the scarcity of NS1 antigen and the presence of the particular antibody in the bloodstream. Hence, a considerable precaution is maintained when diagnosing NS1 in patients who have been unwell for at least 5 days or in cases of secondary dengue [15]. Machine learning algorithms can learn patterns from different blood count information related to the patients and deliver possible outcome for the infected person which saves the trouble to go through various NS1 tests.

Machine learning-based algorithms do a phenomenal job in assisting different disease conditions which ultimately separates a sick person from a healthy person with minimum effort. Hence, various machine learning architectures and work pipelines has been developed over the years to attribute in providing optimum condition in health care facilities. A certain study [16] utilized Xray images to train transfer learning algorithm to detect pneumonia using chest radiographs. Chowdhury et al. [17] proposed an architecture which utilizes photoplethysmography (PPG) signal to develop a machine learning model which introduces a cuffless blood pressure (BP) measurement system to assist with Hypertension. A early detection system was proposed which was crucial in detecting patients with precarious situation with mortality risk in Covid19 pandemic time [18]. Another machine learning implementation incorporated in during the outbreak of Covid19 included a prognostic model using blood biomarkers to for severity forecasting of patients [19]. Shuzan et al. [20] proposed an architecture to predict respiration rate and blood oxygen saturation rate using ppg signal which made use of machine learning models.

Dengue ranks among the top 10 global health threats, as per WHO's classification, and its rapid proliferation means an outbreak can potentially afflict thousands. Contemporary research points towards the potential of machine learning in formulating predictive models that harness clinical and laboratory data for early and accurate dengue diagnosis. For instance, in their endeavor to predict dengue outbreaks in Malaysia, Majeed et al. [21] devised and juxtaposed six distinct long short-term memory (LSTM) architectures: LSTM, Stacked LSTM (S-LSTM),

LSTM with temporal attention (TA-LSTM), S-LSTM with temporal attention (STA-LSTM), LSTM with spatial attention (SA-LSTM), and S-LSTM with spatial attention (SSA-LSTM). These models were trained and assessed utilizing a dataset chronicling monthly dengue incidences in Malaysia from 2010 to 2016, with prediction variables encompassing climatic, topographical, demographic, and land-use metrics. Among these, the SSA-LSTM emerged as the most proficient in predicting dengue outbreaks.

In a related study, Rocha & Giesbrecht [22] embarked on constructing machine learning frameworks using data sourced from São Luís do Maranhão, a municipality located in Brazil's Maranhão state. Given the regional specificity of this study, which inherently limited the volume of data, oversampling techniques such as synthetic minority over-sampling technique (SMOTE), adaptive synthetic sampling approach (ADASYN), and density-based synthetic minority oversampling technique (DBSMOTE) were deployed to synthesize additional data. The models ingested input variables like neighborhood-specific dengue case data spanning 2014–2020, as well as associated climatic, geographical, and environmental variables. The Random Forest model, refined with the DBSMOTE technique, showcased superior performance metrics with an area under the curve (AUC) of 75.1%, a sensitivity rate of 75.43%, and a specificity of 60.53%.

Though early detection and appropriate medical intervention can significantly reduce the mortality rates associated with severe dengue, a specific treatment remains elusive. In light of this, machine learning is emerging as a valuable tool in the battle against dengue. Manoharan et al. [23] introduced a Hybrid convolutional neural network with tanh long and short term memory (CNN-TLSTM) model, enhanced by ATLBO, which incorporated symptoms and external factors for swift and accurate dengue diagnosis. This model demonstrated commendable performance metrics, achieving an accuracy of 96.9%, precision of 95.7%, and recall of 96.8%. By incorporating a system that synergizes IoT, fog-cloud computing, and advanced deep learning, this work addressed challenges like underreporting and misdiagnoses. When tested in real-time settings, this model outperformed existing methodologies, enabling identification of high-risk regions and facilitating instantaneous reporting to health authorities. Similarly, Mayrose et al. [24] proposed the application of AI in scrutinizing peripheral blood smear (PBS) images to assist clinicians in dengue diagnosis. Their tool detected dengue-associated platelet variations and thrombocytopenia using blob detection techniques. Employing machine learning, they extracted pivotal features from lymphocyte nuclei, enhancing the SVM classifier's accuracy to 95.74% through feature selection and other methodologies. A distinct research initiative [25] used a dataset collated from Chittagong Medical College Hospital and Dhaka Medical College Hospital in Bangladesh, applying decision tree (DT) and random forest (RF) machine learning methodologies for categorization. The decision tree model demonstrated superiority, achieving a 79% accuracy. Gomes et al. [26] leveraged Support Vector Machines

(SVM) for classifying dengue fever patients into two categories: Dengue Fever (DF) and Dengue Hemorrhagic Fever (DHF). By analyzing gene expression patterns, their model achieved an impressive 96% accuracy. Another study [27] emphasized early detection of severe dengue in children. By analyzing data from 742 Colombian children with dengue, the authors found the SVM with a Gaussian kernel to have the best diagnostic capability, with an receiver operating characteristic - area under the curve (ROC AUC) of 0.75. Mello-Román et al. [28] contrasted artificial neural networks (ANN) and SVMs in diagnosing early dengue. The ANN multilayer perceptron emerged as the most efficacious model, attaining an average accuracy of 96%. Chakraborty et al. [29] put forth a hybrid of autoregressive integrated moving average and neural network autoregressive (ARIMA-NNAR) model, which amalgamated the linear modeling prowess of ARIMA with the nonlinear capabilities of NNAR. This model outperformed standalone models in forecasting dengue outbreaks. Another investigation [28] applied IBM SPSS Modeler to evaluate categorization models, with the artificial neural network and Multilayer Perceptron (ANN-MLP) classifier achieving a sensitivity of 96%. K. Ming et al. [30], in their Vietnamese study, employed gradient boosting to differentiate dengue from other acute febrile illnesses, securing a median AUROC of 0.86. Overall, the study showed promise for supervised learning to support healthcare systems through passive surveillance for dengue in endemic regions.

The primary objective of this work is to construct a machine learning pipeline incorporating established state-of-the-art algorithms, with the aim of producing accurate classification outcomes for distinguishing between dengue positive and negative individuals. The main aim of this pipeline is to effectively discriminate individuals who are undergoing a dengue test and later on deliver the appropriate clinical prescription. In an effort to achieve the previously stated goal, sophisticated machine learning techniques were employed to construct a resilient classifier. This project employed suitable feature predictors for the aim of classification. The aforementioned key attributes, when paired with the most optimal classification model, were applied in the formulation of a nomogram founded on logistic regression with multiple variables. Afterwards, the nomogram conducted a procedure of validation to gauge its prognostic characteristics.

The subsequent sections of the chapter are structured in the following manner: Sect. 2 delves into the methodologies employed in this study, encompassing a comprehensive elucidation of the datasets utilized in this article, as well as an intricate exposition of the intricacies involved in the pre-processing phases of data for machine learning classifiers and the stacking machine learning algorithm and validation using nomogram as well. Section 3 provides an analysis of the outcomes derived from the classification models, as well as an examination of the stacking machine learning model and nomogram. The chapter ultimately ended in Sect. 4 with concluding remarks.

2 Methodology

In this study, we adopted a specific methodology to scrutinize clinical datasets associated with dengue patients. These datasets were subsequently harnessed to cultivate a proficient model aimed at discerning dengue-positive and dengue-negative individuals. By devising this model, the intention was to alleviate the administrative burden in clinical settings, thus facilitating an enhanced focus on delivering apt care and services to the visiting patients. Three discrete datasets, all pertaining to individuals diagnosed with dengue, were engaged in this research. These datasets were subjected to meticulous cleaning and transformation to ensure uniformity. This was followed by crucial preprocessing steps. Post data preparation, optimal features were delineated via various feature ranking techniques. Multiple traditional machine learning models were then trained using these selected features. Throughout the training phase, Shapley values were leveraged to discern the influential attributes for each classification. To optimize the final outcomes, we incorporated a stacking-based meta-classifier developed in-house to derive improved results. A schematic representation of the methodological stages was incorporated in Fig. 1, providing a sound understanding of the whole process.

2.1 Dataset Description

In the context of the dengue project, complete blood counts (CBC) and demographic data were collected from data from two hospitals of Bangladesh. These databases

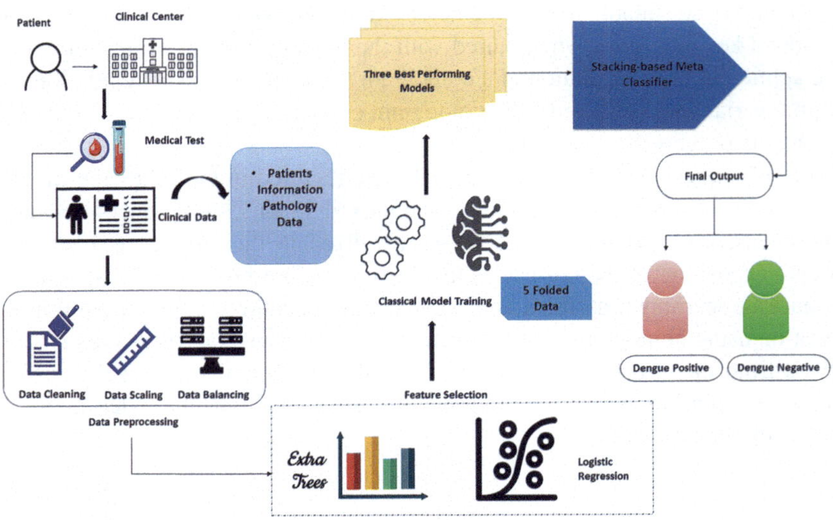

Fig. 1 Methodological overview of dengue classification study

capture a range of patient conditions, with data both from healthy individuals and those confirmed to have dengue. The datasets used in this research were collected from Bangladesh, specifically during a dengue outbreak that emerged in the summer season. The study was approved by the local ethical committee and written informed consent was taken from the subjects.

The dengue-related data comprises three distinct subsets as they are collected from three different hospitals.

- **Dengue Positive Patient Dataset:** The dataset encompasses a total of 248 samples with 22 distinct CBC and demographic features, alongside some additional columns of miscellaneous nature (additional tests and patient status data).
- **Dengue Negative Dataset:** The dataset is structured in a clinical format and encapsulates details pertaining to dengue negative outcomes patients, comprises 252 data entries distributed across 26 columns, each representing distinct attributes.

2.2 *Data Preprocessing*

Prior to incorporating the final dataset into the model training pipeline, several preprocessing steps were considered. The emphasis during this phase was on data cleaning, consolidating datasets into a unified format, imputing any absent values, and refining the dataset for optimal usability. After ensuring the dataset was in its most conducive state, it was subjected to a folding operation, marking the culmination of the preprocessing phase for this dataset. Subsequent to these preparatory tasks, the focus transitioned to the model training segment.

2.2.1 Data Cleaning

The dataset comprising diagnosed dengue fever cases, approximately 60% of the total entries have missing values across several columns. In order to mitigate the presence of highly synthetic data, it was decided to eliminate these columns. The dataset in question has three columns that are non-predictive in nature: serial number, patient id, and the specific type of dengue virus the patient was exposed to. As these columns offer no predictive value, they were deemed extraneous to the model's training and were subsequently removed. Additionally, the dataset, barring the subset concerning diagnosed dengue cases, does not include the Erythrocyte Sedimentation Rate (ESR) column. This column was also discarded to maintain uniformity for potential dataset merging in the future. Gender classification presented discrepancies between the dengue positive and negative datasets. Hence, steps were taken to ensure they were represented uniformly. Similarly, the platelets and white blood cell counts in the dengue dataset varied in their scaling. While the majority of the data points were scaled on a centennial metric, some deviated significantly, indicating that they were scaled correctly prior to inclusion. To rectify this, abnormally high values were rescaled to align with the majority. Given the precision of the dengue dataset regarding confirmed positive cases, it was essential to acknowledge that mixing data from healthy and dengue-positive patients might compromise the discriminatory power of the model. In terms of generating the ground truth label, the dengue-diagnosed dataset served as the positive class, denoting dengue positivity. Conversely, Dengue Negative Dataset cases from the respective dataset represented the negative class, signifying Dengue Negative class.

2.2.2 Missing Data Imputation

It is a pivotal step in machine learning projects, as it deals with the challenge of addressing missing values within a dataset. Typically, machine learning models are trained on numerical data. Absent instances, however, can introduce non-numerical anomalies during the training phase. Addressing this challenge can either involve the removal of data points or the adoption of a mathematical imputation strategy that leverages existing values within a column to fill the voids. Opting for the latter is the advocated approach in this context, since discarding data might result in significant information loss, which could prove vital in subsequent phases of the project [31].

The Multivariate Imputation by Chained Equations (MICE) approach was employed to address the presence of missing values in the clinical biomarkers of the patients. The aforementioned approach is often utilized in clinical machine learning endeavors [32].

Figure 2 illustrates the cases that are absent within the dataset. Every feature within the dataset displays some degree of missing values. Among the evaluated variables MPV(fL) exhibits the most pronounced occurrence of missing values.

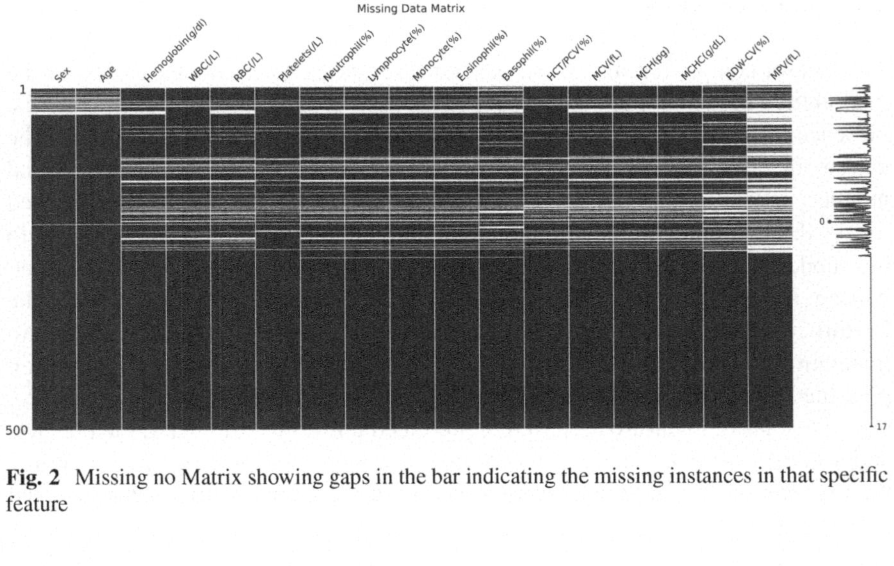

Fig. 2 Missing no Matrix showing gaps in the bar indicating the missing instances in that specific feature

On the other end of the spectrum, the gender and age of the patients' columns demonstrate the fewest missing values, both lacking an identical number of samples. The remaining columns consistently indicate a uniform number of missing values. The gaps within this dataset were addressed using the MICE algorithm, which employs methods such as averaging and regression relation based on available data to fill the void.

2.3 *Statistical Analysis*

A proper statistical analysis is imperative to learn statistical association between a target feature and a predictor feature which ultimately indicates the significance of that predictor feature with respect to the target feature. For such a scenario, p-value comes into play. It's a factor which provides measurement of likelihood of an outcome when null hypothesis is irrelevant [33]. Mean and standard deviation (std) is responsible for providing central tendency of a feature and how the data points deviate from that central value.

When a predictor feature followed normal distribution, t-test was utilized for test statistic. The t-test is an often-employed statistical method for evaluating hypotheses relating to population means. It is a necessary tool to observe whether the mean of a sample deviates significantly from a hypothesized mean. It may generate genuine distinction when the differences in observation may be attributed to random sampling. The p-value of such testing acts as a prime indicator of the level of support against the null hypothesis. Therefore, p-values are very unlikely to have risen due to random chance, whereas a high p-value indicates that the observed difference could plausibly be attributed to random variability [34]. The Wilcoxon Rank-sum technique is employed in our work to conduct statistical analysis when a predictor feature was not normally distributed. The proposed methodology efficiently calculates test statistics by considering the sample sizes and the sum of rankings corresponding to each attribute which ultimately generates p-value [35].

2.4 *Data Scaling*

It is a common practice in order to obtain optimal results by representing the data in a generalized style. Consequently, scaling the data during the pre-processing phase before model training can substantially reduce potential biases arising from differing feature distributions. This ensures an equitable contribution from each feature. Various research has provided evidence of enhanced performance in machine learning models through the utilization of normalization approaches [36]. Utilizing the Z-score data scaling approach effectively mitigates any inadvertent bias that may arise from the presence of varied features through a specific mathematical computation.

$$z_f = \frac{x_f - \mu_f}{\sigma_f} \tag{1}$$

In this context, z_f, x_f, μ_f, and σ_f represent the scaled value, original value, mean of the feature variable, and standard deviation of that specific feature, respectively in the Eq. 1. This scaling method alters the feature values to conform to a Gaussian normal distribution. However, a limitation of this scaling strategy is its susceptibility to outlier values within the variable.

2.5 *Data Balancing*

Class level data imbalance can skew the training of a model, potentially leading to biased results. Given this circumstance, achieving a more favorable outcome may be possible by addressing and rectifying the existing imbalance. In light of this, the Synthetic Minority Oversampling Technique (SMOTE) was implemented to balance the Dengue Positive class. SMOTE is one of the state of the arts algorithms to resolve predicaments such as imbalance [37]. It is important to note that since the dengue-positive cases are 248 and dengue-negative cases are 252, the dataset is mostly balanced.

An investigation was conducted to examine the association among the attributes. Figure 3 displays a heatmap that showcases the correlation scores of all the features. The correlation matrix reveals that within the upper triangle, two features have an absolute correlation value exceeding 0.80. The strongest correlation is typically observed between neutrophil and lymphocyte levels, indicating that, in dengue cases, a decrease in lymphocyte proportion accompanied by an increase in neutrophil count. There exists a pronounced positive correlation of 0.84 between hematocrit and hemoglobin levels. This correlation has clinical significance because hematocrit quantifies the volume of red blood cells, which are the carriers of hemoglobin. Consequently, such a robust association is both expected and justifiable. Even though these variables might not be selected for intensive training from a purely mathematical perspective, their clinical importance in relation to dengue cannot be undermined. The initial inclination to eliminate features with strong intercorrelations was reconsidered. To provide a thorough understanding of the data distribution across features, a pair-plot is shown in Fig. 4.

As elucidated in the aforementioned paragraph, the pair plot reveals a negative correlation between the Neutrophil (%) and Lymphocyte (%) variables and a strong positive correlation between Hematocrit and Hemoglobin variable.

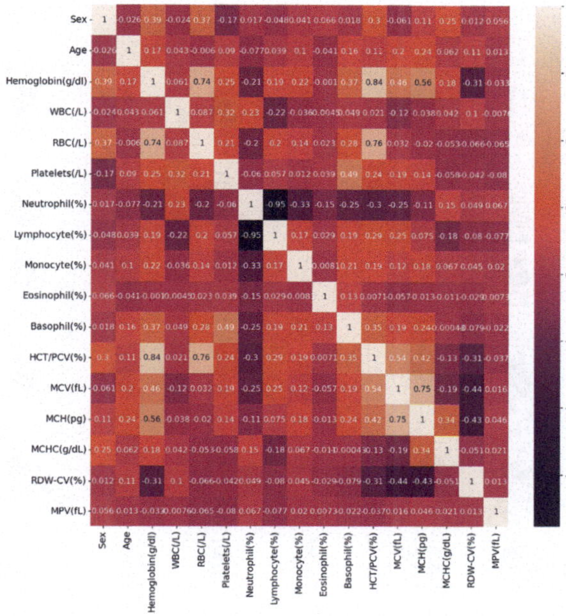

Fig. 3 Correlation Matrix displaying correlations among features

2.6 *Feature Ranking and Selection*

In this study, we utilized four different feature ranking techniques: XGBoost, Random Forest, Extra trees, and genetic feature extractor. After evaluating the results obtained from these algorithms, Extra tree emerged as a preferred technique. This choice was driven by the observation that Extra tree yielded a more balanced distribution across the features compared to its counterparts.

The Extra Trees Classifier is a type of ensemble learning technique that combines the predictions of multiple independent decision trees organized in a collection known as a "forest" to generate its classification output. Fundamentally, it exhibits a very strong resemblance to the Random Forest Classifier, it predominantly deviates based on its strength in building decision tree within the forest.

In the context of the Extra Trees Forest, it is worth noting that each Decision Tree is constructed using the original training dataset. During the creation of each tree, at each decision node, a subset of k features is randomly chosen from the complete collection of features. Within this particular subset, each decision tree operates autonomously to identify the optimal feature for dividing the data, relying on a distinct mathematical criterion, commonly referred to as the Gini Index. The utilization of a randomly selected subset of features leads to the generation of several decision trees that are not correlated with each other.

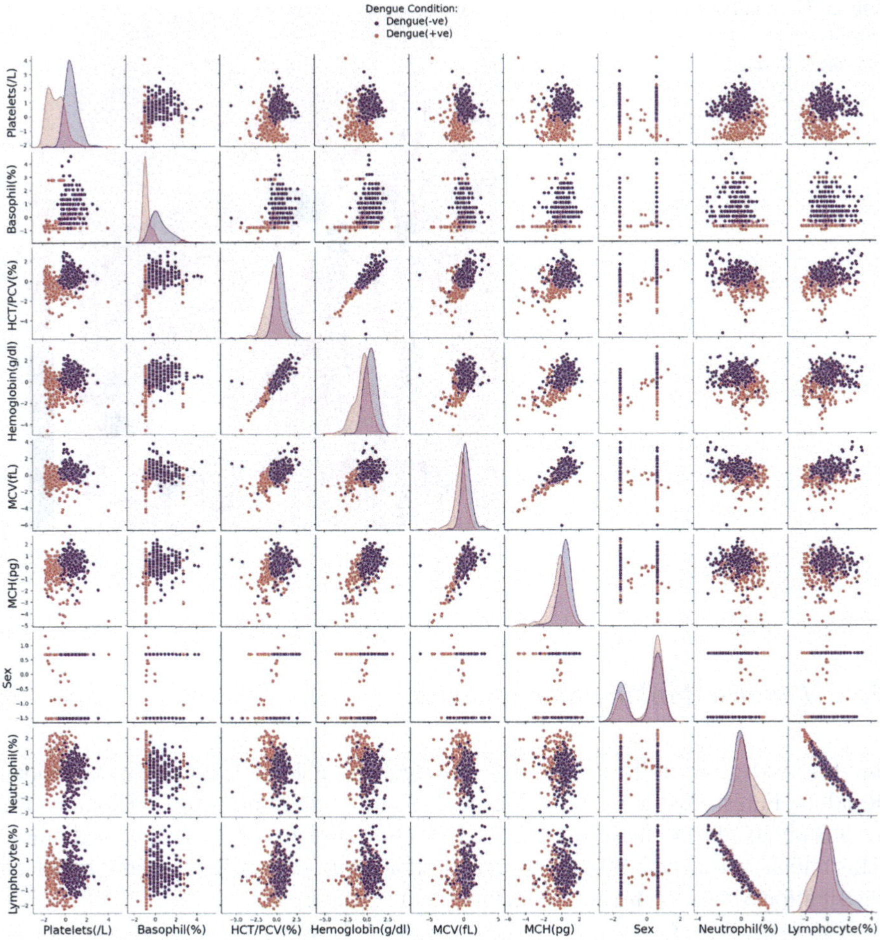

Fig. 4 Pair-plot showing relationship between features

Following the process of feature ranking, logistic regression is employed to efficiently select the essential number of features for training the models. Consider our dataset as a set in the type where x represents the input characteristics and y represents the target feature consisting of binary values of 0 and 1. If we denote p as the expected probability of individual recordings, we can create a formula represented by an equation.

$$y = \ln\left(\frac{p}{1-p}\right) = \beta x \tag{2}$$

In Eq. 2, β represents the hyperparameters of the model. The relationship between the target feature and input feature can be represented linearly. Based on the aforementioned relationship, we prioritize the highest outcome exhibited by the amount of features and proceed to train the model. Based on this knowledge, 10 features were selected to start the model training process.

2.7 *Stacking-Based Meta-Classifier for Model Training*

In this study, we devised a Stacking Algorithm framework to realize the end goal of model training. This design amalgamates several top-tier traditional machine learning models, seamlessly integrating the attributes of the dataset with their respective ground truth output. A total of 13 classical machine learning was subjected to traning in this study, which are Multilayer perceptron (MLP) [38], Linear Discriminant Analysis (LDA) [39], Extreme Gradient Boosting (XGB) [40], Logistic Regression (LR) [41], Support Vector Machine (SVM) [42], Extreme Randomized Tree (ExtraTree) [43], Adaptive Boosting (Adaboost) [44], K-nearest neighbors (KNN) [45], Gradient Boosting [46], Categorical Boosting (Catboost) [47], Light Gradient Boosting Machine (LGBM), Elastic Net, Random Forest (RF) [48].

The aforementioned models were trained on the dataset. Subsequently, the prediction probabilities obtained from this initial training served as input for the stacking meta classifier. Detailed refinements and an accompanying block diagram elucidating the stacking procedure will be presented in subsequent sections.

In Fig. 5, the variable p represents the quantity of samples, while the variable q denotes the number of trained features. The aforementioned features were derived from the feature selection scheme that was previously discussed. Utilizing folded data with selected features, classical machine learning models were trained which expose prediction probabilities for each sample. Based on three best performing models, prediction probabilities for each sample were used as input and hence a meta-classifier was constructed which considers the leading score of probability score for a specific sample and the final result was assimilated.

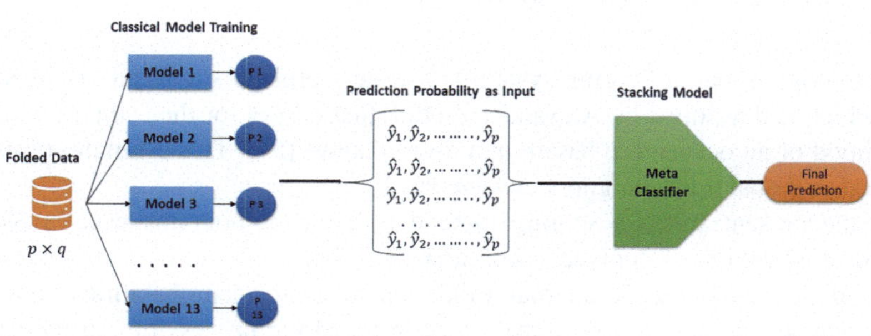

Fig. 5 Stacking Machine Learning algorithm framework

2.8 Model Interpretability

The analysis of the fundamental logic behind a model that has generated an outcome is frequently essential, considering its significance and usefulness in many real-world scenarios and association with human understanding. Nevertheless, professionals still face significant challenges when it comes to interpreting complex models like ensemble or deep learning models, despite their impressive capacity to achieve high accuracy on contemporary and extensive datasets. This scenario presents a dilemma where the desire for accuracy conflicts with the ability to elucidate the underlying reasoning behind the model's results. Several algorithms have been recently developed to aid users in interpreting the outcomes of intricate models, with the aim of addressing this issue. Nevertheless, there remains a dearth of lucidity concerning the interrelationships between these methods and the particular circumstances in which one approach has to be given precedence over another.

The SHAP framework, often referred to as SHapley Additive exPlanations, is a comprehensive framework and set of methodologies utilized to enhance the interpretability of models, particularly in the field of machine learning and predictive modelling. The primary aim of the SHAP (SHapley Additive exPlanations) architecture is to facilitate users in understanding how the input properties of a model contribute to its predictions. The primary objective of the SHAP architecture is to offer insights into individual predictions generated by a machine learning model. Instead of providing a general summary of the model's behavior, this particular interpretable architecture leverages game theory to achieve its objective by incorporating Shapley values into the study. The Shapley values represent a technique used to assign a measure of importance to each individual information within a projected outcome. This allows for the quantification of the degree to which each feature has influenced the total prediction. The aforementioned values are derived from the idea of equity in the allocation of credit for a prediction across multiple qualities [49, 50].

2.9 Nomogram-Based Scoring System

The Nomogram-based Scoring system is a widely utilized statistical visualization tool which is developed by Alexander Zlotnik that allows for the estimation of the likelihood of an occurrence based on a given dataset [51]. This estimation follows prediction probabilities ranging between 0 to 1.

In the present study, a scoring method utilizing nomograms was developed by the application of logistic regression. The approach utilized in this study involved the utilization of internal validation to estimate probabilities based on fundamental biomarkers. Additionally, we initiated the process of calibrating the internal validation by aligning it with the ground truth labels and the prediction likelihood of the occurrences. A threshold by every feature was visually displayed using Decision Curve Analysis (DCA). All these operations were done using Stata 15 software.

2.10 Performance Measures

In order to evaluate the results demonstrated by the models, many performance testing measures were employed, including the ROC (Receiver Operating Characteristic) curve, AUC (Area Under the Curve), as well as Accuracy, Precision, Recall, Specificity, and F1-score. The dataset underwent a 5-fold cross-validation process, where the data was divided into training and testing sets using an 80–20 ratio.

The mathematical description of the performance measures is depicted in Eqs. 3, 4, 5, 6, and 7:

$$Accuracy_{class\_x} = \frac{TP_{class\_x} + TN_{class\_x}}{TP_{class\_x} + TN_{class\_x} + FP_{class\_x} + FN_{class\_x}} \tag{3}$$

$$Precsion_{class\_x} = \frac{TP_{class\_x}}{TP_{class\_x} + FP_{class\_x}} \tag{4}$$

$$Recall_{class\_x} = \frac{TP_{class\_x}}{TP_{class\_x} + FN_{class\_x}} \tag{5}$$

$$Spcificity_{class\_x} = \frac{TN_{class\_x}}{TN_{class\_x} + FP_{class\_x}} \tag{6}$$

$$F1 - Score_{class\_x} = \frac{2 \times Precsion_{class\_x} \times Recall_{class\_x}}{Precsion_{class\_x} + Recall_{class\_x}} \tag{7}$$

where class_x = Dengue positive and Dengue negative

Here TP, TN, FP, FN is the abbreviated form of True Positive, True Negative, False Positive, False Negative respectively.

AUC score is the redeeming factor for a classifier to provide adequate classification report indicating whether the binary classification result is properly identifying positive class as positive class and negative class as negative class.

3 Results and Discussion

3.1 Statistical Analysis

A detailed statistical analysis was conducted on the dataset. The dataset utilized for this study has distinct features, with the age of patients being interpreted as a continuous variable. Additionally, clinical biomarkers were statistically analyzed for both Dengue positive and Dengue negative cases. Based on the features present in the training set, most of the features followed normal distribution except for platelets, eosinophil, mpv and age. Hence, t-test was implemented for normally distributed biomarkers and rank-sum for the exceptions to extract p-value. With the exception of eosinophil, all the biomarkers had association with the ground truth label as shown by p-value less than 0.05. Demographically, the dataset predominantly consists of male patients, accounting for approximately 69.3%, while females constitute the remaining 30.7% of the non-missing samples.

Table 1 provides a comprehensive statistical analysis of the biomarkers from inception to conclusion. There appears to be a strong positive association between platelet counts and the dengue diagnostic tests. Typically, healthy individuals have platelet counts around 281 ± 65.1, whereas those diagnosed with an ailment showed reduced platelet counts averaging 117 ± 89.9. This trend aligns with clinical observations, as dengue-affected individuals often manifest decreased platelet counts compared to their healthy counterparts. The White Blood Cell counted was 6.5 ± 2.03 (10^9/L) on average in dengue-negative patients and 5.7 ± 3.34 (10^9/L) in dengue-positive patients. The packed volume test revealed that the hematocrit levels of healthy individuals were 48.0 ± 6.10 (%) and those of sick patients were 40.1 ± 6.78 (%), respectively. The Red Blood Cell Count (RBC) exhibited an average of 5.36 ± 0.506 (10^12/L) for dengue-negative individuals and 4.90 ± 0.79 (10^12/L) for dengue-positive patients in the sample under consideration. Collectively, these statistical insights highlight the discernible differences in clinical test values between dengue-positive and dengue-negative patients.

3.2 Best Feature Combination

As outlines in the preceding sections, we employed four distinct feature ranking algorithms. Of these, logistic regression was used to ascertain the optimal combination of characteristics required for training the model. The Extra tree technique provided the highest ranking for the features, with a set of 8 features emerging as the most effective.

When utilizing Extra trees for feature ranking, the significance score of each feature is observed. The algorithm accumulates the magnitudes of relevance across all trees. The aggregated scores are calculated based on the statistical mean and are employed to evaluate the attributes within the dataset. Subsequently, these scores are harnessed to rank the features in a descending hierarchy, positioning the most influential features at the top. Figure 6 depicts the outcome of the feature ranking process executed using the Extra tree algorithm. For the distinction between the dengue positive and dengue negative classes, the chosen variables comprised Platelets count, Basophil percentage, Hemoglobin, Gender, Mean Corpuscular Volume, Neutrophil percentage, Hematocrit percentage, Red Blood Cell count, Mean Corpuscular Hemoglobin, Mean Corpuscular Hemoglobin Concentration.

The conventional machine learning models were trained using the optimal combination of findings. Three models with the highest performance were selected

Table 1 Statistical Analysis

Features	Acronym	Unit	Missing Rate (%)	Dengue(−ve) [Mean ± std]	Dengue(+ve) [Mean ± std]	Overall [Mean ± std]	P-value
Hemoglobin (HGB)	HGB	g/dL	9	15.7 ± 1.57	13.3 ± 2.26	14.7 ± 2.25	<0.001
White Blood Cell (WBC)	WBC	$\times 10^9$/L	8	6.5 ± 2.03	5.7 ± 3.34	6.1 ± 2.73	<0.001
Red Blood Cell (RBC)	RBC	$\times 10^{12}$/L	10	5.36 ± 0.506	4.90 ± 0.79	5.16 ± 0.684	<0.001
Platelets (PLT)	PLT	$\times 10^9$/L	6	281 ± 65.1	117 ± 89.9	205 ± 113	<0.001 (ranksum)
Neutrophil (NEUT)	NEUT	(%)	10	47.3 ± 14.0	57.9 ± 16.3	51.9 ± 15.9	<0.001
Lymphocyte (LYM)	LYM	(%)	10	42.7 ± 13.6	33.6 ± 14.9	38.7 ± 14.9	<0.001
Monocyte (MONO)	MONO	(%)	10	7 ± 2.65	5.8 ± 3.40	6.4 ± 3.06	<0.001
Eosinophil (EO)	EO	(%)	10	2.3 ± 2.04	2.2 ± 2.24	2.2 ± 2.13	0.56
Basophil (BASO)	BASO	(%)	12	0.40 ± 0.257	0.037 ± 0.19	0.25 ± 0.292	<0.001
Hematocrit (Packed Cell Volume Test) (HCT/PCV)	HCT/PCV	(%)	8	48.0 ± 6.10	40.1 ± 6.78	44.4 ± 7.52	<0.001
Mean Corpuscular Volume (MCV)	MCV	fL	11	90.1 ± 7.49	81.7 ± 8.64	86.4 ± 9.02	<0.001
Mean Corpuscular Hemoglobin (MCH)	MCH	pg	11	29.4 ± 2.00	27.2 ± 3.16	28.4 ± 2.79	<0.001
Mean Corpuscular Hemoglobin Concentration (MCHC)	MCHC	g/dL	11	32.6 ± 2.23	33.0 ± 2.76	32.8 ± 2.48	0.057
Red Cell Distribution Width- Coefficient of Variation (RDW-CV)	RDW-CV	(%)	14	12.9 ± 1.08	13.5 ± 1.71	13.1 ± 1.40	<0.001
Mean Platelet Volume (MPV)	MPV	fL	25	9.92 ± 1.10	10.7 ± 7.74	10.2 ± 4.52	<0.001
Age	N/A	Year	4	36.7 ± 12.1	30.7 ± 15.4	33.8 ± 14.0	<0.001

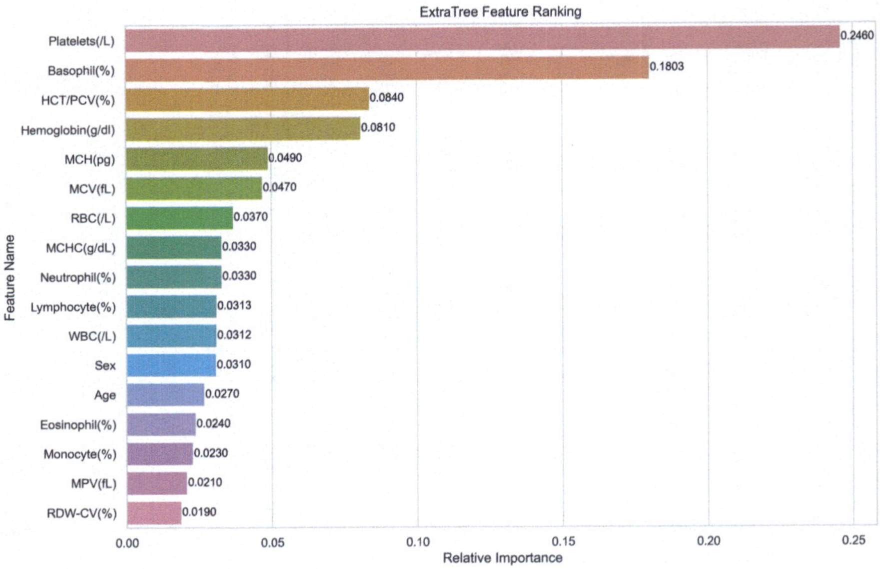

Fig. 6 Bar plot featuring feature importance posed variables for Extra Tree algorithm

for the Stacking Classifier, and the best result was retrieved from these models. The results for both conditions are presented in the table.

3.3 Classification Using Classical ML and Stacking Model

Among the conventional models, the Extra Tree classifier, Adaboost classifier, and CatBoost Classifier demonstrated superior performance. Subsequently, the metaclassifier was constructed using these three models as the basis for its prediction probability. On that note, the metaclassifier underwent further training using the models. The XGBoost classifier demonstrated the highest performance among all other classifiers, achieving an accuracy of 97.8%, precision score of 97.82%, recall of 97.8%, specificity of 97.82%, and an F1-score of 97.80%. This outcome surpassed all previous results. The implementation of a metaclassifier resulted in a notable enhancement in the overall performance of all models, with the exception of AdaBoost and Catboost. The outcome did not exhibit any enhancement in result ensuing to the implementation of stacking. The outcomes of these approaches can be observed in the provided Table 2.

Stacking based algorithm developed improved the performance of XGBoost classifier by around 6% compared to its prior result as shown in the confusion matrix of Fig. 7.

Table 2 Classical and Stacking machine learning classification result

	Classical Result					Stacking Based Meta Classifier Result				
Models	Accuracy	Precision	Recall	Specificity	F1-Score	Accuracy	Precision	Recall	Specificity	F1-Score
MLP Classifier	95.6	95.60	95.6	95.61	95.60	96.8	96.81	96.8	96.81	96.80
LDA	94.2	94.32	94.2	94.16	94.20	97.0	97.00	97.00	97.01	97.00
XGBoost	91.8	91.80	91.8	91.79	91.80	**97.8**	**97.82**	**97.8**	**97.82**	**97.80**
LR	95.6	95.60	95.6	95.59	95.60	96.8	96.81	96.8	96.81	96.80
SVM	95.2	95.21	95.2	95.21	95.20	96.8	96.81	96.8	96.81	96.80
Extra Tree	**97.2**	**97.22**	**97.2**	**97.22**	**97.20**	97.4	97.40	97.4	97.41	97.40
AdaBoost	**97.6**	**97.63**	**97.6**	**97.62**	**97.60**	97.0	97.00	97.0	97.01	97.00
KNN	93.8	94.25	93.8	93.88	93.79	96.0	96.01	96.0	96.01	96.00
GradientBoost	93.4	93.44	93.4	93.42	93.40	97.0	97.00	97.0	97.01	97.00
CatBoost	**97.2**	**97.20**	**97.2**	**97.21**	**97.20**	97.2	97.20	97.2	97.21	97.20
LGBM	94.2	94.20	94.2	94.19	94.20	96.8	96.80	96.8	96.80	96.80
ElasticNet	95.2	95.20	95.2	95.20	95.20	96.8	96.81	96.8	96.81	96.80
RandomForest	97.0	97.00	97.0	97.01	97.00	96.8	96.80	96.8	96.81	96.8

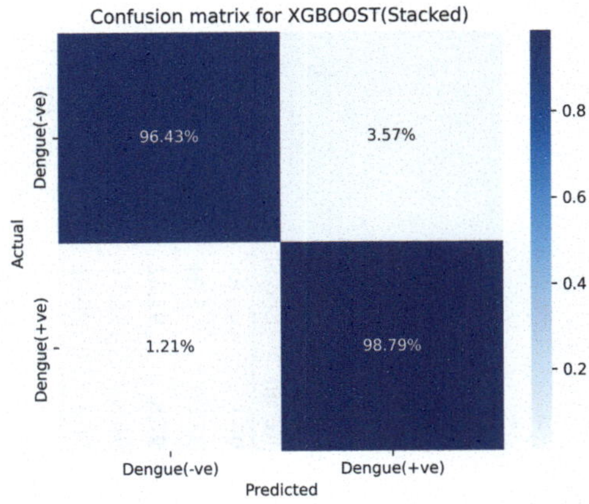

Fig. 7 Confusion Matrix for Stacking-Based XGBoost model

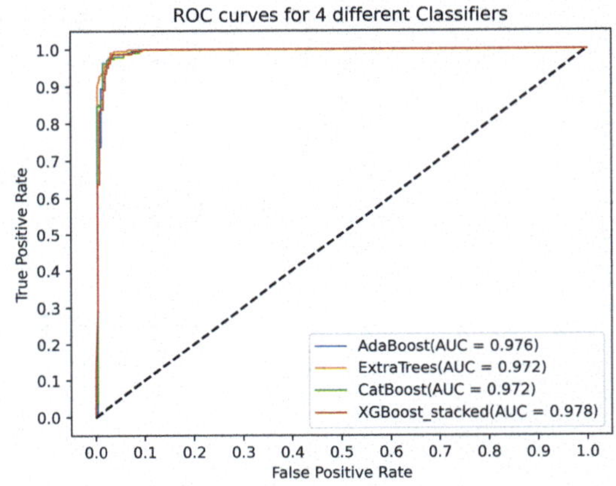

Fig. 8 ROC for classical models and the best stacking model

The above result exemplified a considerable robustness and authenticity as both classes were classified consecutively conveyed 96.43% and 98.79% for both dengue positive and dengue negative class as shown in Fig. 7. So, no class wise bias was evident in the outcome.

Region of convergence (ROC) diagram is presented in Fig. 8 for best performing classical models which is showing AUC score of 0.976 for AdaBoost, 0.972 for Extra Tree and 0.972 as well for CatBoost. XGBoost meta-classifier shows 0.978 as AUC score. As this score indicates the quality of distinguishing the two classes, it is safe enough to assume XGBoost stacked would be able to recognize best in classifying individual classes specifically.

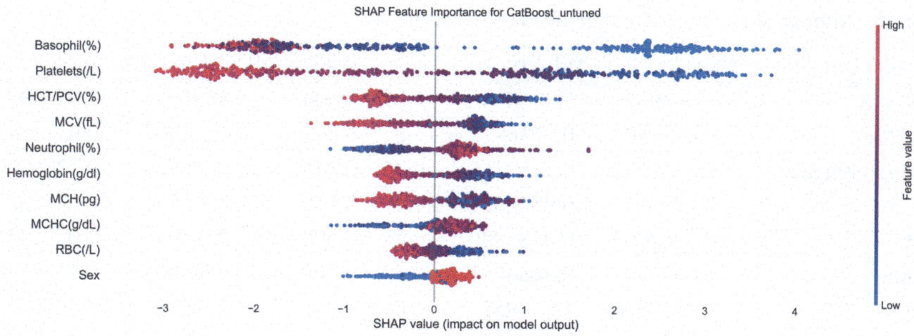

Fig. 9 SHAP summary plot depicting all trained biomarkers' contribution on XGBoost classifier

3.4 *Model Interpretability*

The SHAP analysis is depicted in Fig. 9 for best performing the classical machine learning models. It reveals a significant negative contribution from Platelet counts and Basophil percentage in accurately identifying the dengue condition.

The SHAP summary plot reveals that high platelet counts and basophil counts are associated with a higher feature value in the context of dengue classification. This suggests that an increase in platelet counts, and basophil percentage contributes to the dengue negative class. Conversely, a decrease in platelet and basophil feature values is strongly associated with the dengue positive class. This finding aligns with clinical observations, as individuals infected with dengue typically exhibit a low platelet count. This implies that Platelets and Basophil play a significant role in distinguishing instances that do not have the dengue virus and vice versa as the distribution is broader in the summary plot which exhibits contribution on model outcome. Ibtehaz et al. [52] made use of SHAP to interpret contribution of each spectrum on the prediction on their proposed RamanNet, which has motivated us to use in this work.

3.5 *Nomogram-Based Result Analysis*

The study entailed developing a predictive analysis represented through a nomogram. This algorithm simplified the intricate computations of the characteristics and generated projected probabilities of outcomes using the training features, hence facilitating comprehension of the model's outputs in a linear manner. To facilitate comprehension of the visual representation, a nomogram analysis has been shown in Table 3. The features name has been represented as abbreviated form which was used in the dataset.

Table 3 Nomogram analysis for dengue classification

Dengue Condition	Coef.	Std. Err.	z	P > |z|	[95% Conf. Interval]	
basophil	−4.968942	0.976636	−5.09	0.000	−6.883187	−3.054697
plateletsl	−0.0289805	0.0036818	−7.87	0.000	−0.0361967	−0.0217644
hemoglobingdl	−0.6838781	0.7167472	−0.95	0.340	−2.088677	−0.7209207
hctpcv	−0.079611	0.0566052	−1.41	0.160	−0.1905551	0.031333
mcvfl	−0.1561695	0.0384826	−4.06	0.000	−0.231594	−0.080745
mchpg	0.0932294	0.3684881	0.25	0.800	−0.628994	0.8154528
rbcl	0.1259263	1.971952	0.06	0.949	−3.739029	3.990881
neutrophil	0.0481766	0.019558	2.46	0.014	0.0098437	0.0865096
rdwcv	0.2423517	0.2302528	1.05	0.293	−0.2089354	0.6936388
monocyte	−0.1334566	0.106867	−1.25	0.212	−0.3429121	0.0759989
_cons	26.33161	10.76026	2.45	0.014	5.241882	47.42134

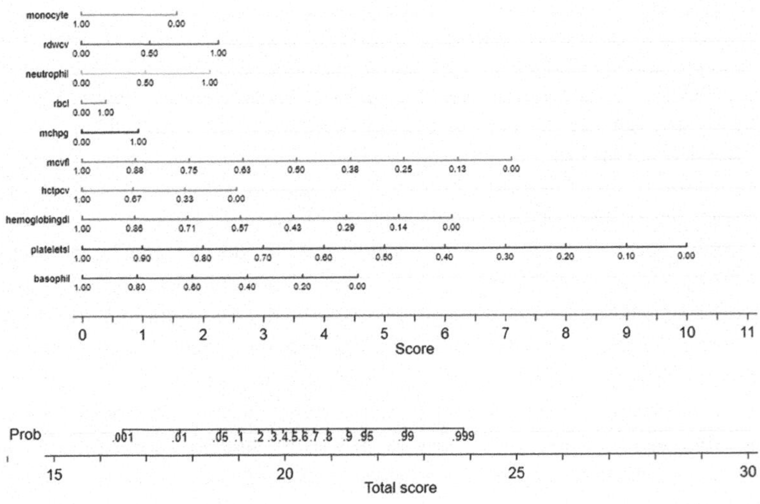

Fig. 10 Nomogram for predicting probability of outcome from dengue test

The z-value is a widely utilized metric that determines the placement of an outcome inside the nomogram. As the number of z-value movements increases in favor of a higher score, the significance of the related independent feature becomes increasingly apparent. The nomogram depicted in Fig. 10 illustrates that platelet count exhibits the most extensive dispersion, consistent with the elevated score indicated in the table and reflected in the nomogram. Some features contributed faintly compared to the score shown in feature ranking bar-plot in Fig. 4, where it ranked quite high. The difference in contribution to both of methods is due to the different procedure followed. Nomogram regression analysis employed z-value, which yielded low contribution to those features like mchpg, rbcl whereas extratrees utilized accuracy to individual trees in its algorithm.

This projects nomogram is shaped based on existing features on the dataset and outcome of each event and computed the probabilistic result in the bottom scale. This probabilistic value represents a certain scoring result for each outcome. As the prediction probabilities in the nomogram mainly marks the probabilities of an outcome being a dengue positive class. Hence, probability greater than 0.5 marks the outcome as dengue positive and less than 0.5 contributes toward dengue negative class. As it becomes excessively difficult to discern an outcome between positive and negative class, safer option is fixing a cut-score of 0.4 probability score to distinguish between the classes. Total score scale beneath the probability values introduces a scoring scheme to assist the health-care providers to promptly separate between dengue positive and dengue negatively class through the nomogram. Dengue negative class yields a value approximately between 16.5 and 20 and nomogram score between 20 and 24 justifies a patient's being diagnosed with dengue. Health-care providers can make use of this score to swiftly provide reports of a patient, most of the probability distribution is marked around 80–99.9% and 0.1–20% meaning proper binary classification. A small portion of the scaling is between them indicating the samples have mixed probabilistic value for the classes.

This study showcases the utilization of internal validation to establish a calibration method for evaluating and assessing the predictive accuracy of logistic regression's probability estimates illustrated in Fig. 11. A notable proportion of the calibration belt is situated along the diagonal bisector, exhibiting a uniform distribution between the regions above and below it. Consequently, logistic regression has a slight bias towards the overfitting zone. However, calibration still maintains a close relationship with the ideal calibration. Figure 12 depicts an illustration of the overall benefits that each all the predictors utilized in the study brings to the table during the decision-making process for the model in classifying between two dengue classes.

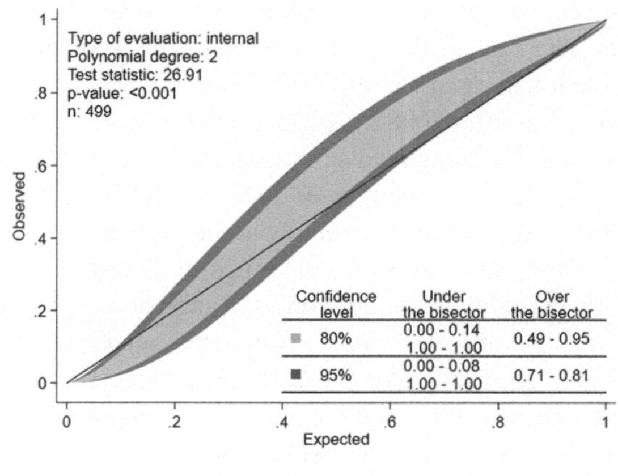

Fig. 11 Calibration using internal validation for dengue classification

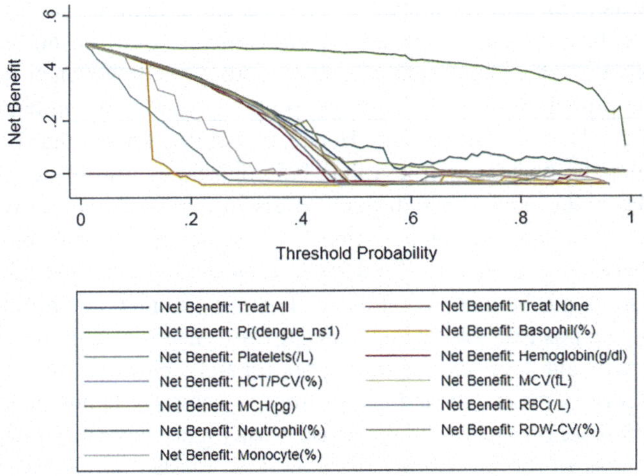

Fig. 12 Decision Curve Analysis (DCA) for analyzing different features and probability predictions of dengue classification

3.6 *Discussion*

Dengue is the most widespread and swiftly proliferating viral illness transmitted by mosquitoes. A comprehensive investigation was conducted to examine the occurrences of dengue cases worldwide over the period from 1990 to 2019, yielding prompt insights on the fatality rates observed among patients across various age groups. In the 1990s, a significant proportion of dengue-related mortality were observed in patients who were below the age of 5. The aforementioned situation underwent substantial transformation over the course of time, as evidenced by the fact that in the year 2019, a majority of the casualties were experienced by individuals aged 15–49 [53]. Bhouwmik et al. [54] conducted a study in Bangladesh spanning from 2008 to 2022, which revealed a significant increase in mortality rates attributed to dengue fever. Specifically, the study found that the proportion of deaths solely caused by dengue in 2022 was 32.14%. The statement implies a potentially dire future scenario arising from the prevalence of dengue.

This study can contribute much in distinguishing between dengue infected individuals and healthy individuals. Bangladesh has faced its most extensive and severe dengue outbreak to date, surpassing all previous records since the government started recording cases in 2000 [55]. Hence, clinical centers were overloaded with patients. Our proposed methodology may provide potential outcome based on blood counts from blood test, which can act as a early warning mechanism for infected person and take medical care accordingly before the situation becomes dire. The research employed basic preprocessing methods as described in the methodology section, which encompassed formatting of numerical values in uniform condition and standardization of data. According to the Extra tree feature ranking method, the variables that were most significant in differentiating between individuals classified as dengue positive and dengue negative were identified. The training stages for model classification consisted of the following variables: platelet count, basophil percentage, hemoglobin levels, gender, mean corpuscular volume, neutrophil percentage, hematocrit percentage, red blood cell count, mean corpuscular hemoglobin, and mean corpuscular hemoglobin concentration. After conducting an initial analysis, it was shown that the features identified by the Extra tree model demonstrated higher effectiveness compared to other attributes based on feature selection. In our classification challenge, a total of thirteen machine learning models were evaluated. Among these models, Catboost, Adaboost, and Extra tree demonstrated the highest performance. The final stacking model was constructed by utilizing three models, namely the XGBoost model. This stacking model demonstrated an overall accuracy of 97.8%, a precision score of 97.82%, a recall of 97.8%, a specificity of 97.82%, and an F1-score of 97.80%. Rahman et al. [56] was able to improve overall performance using stacking which achieved superior performance, with weighted precision, sensitivity, specificity, total accuracy, and F1-score of 91.44%, 91.44%, 91.44%, 91.45%, and 91.45% respectively. The performance of the model in accurately categorizing patients with dengue illness was satisfactory. The XGBoost algorithm demonstrated superior performance with an AUC score of 0.978, suggesting its exceptional ability to effectively distinguish between binary classifications.

The study primarily consisted of a demographic of younger patients who were infected, in comparison to the demographic of uninfected patients. Sick individuals exhibited reduced platelet counts due to the direct impact of the dengue virus on platelet function within the human body. As a result, there was a decrease observed in the white blood count, red blood count, and hemoglobin levels, while there appeared to be an increase in the percentage of neutrophils. Leukopenia, also known as a low white blood cell count, is characterized by a decrease in the number of white blood cells. This disorder is mostly caused by viral invasion of the bone marrow and subsequent suppression of the immune system. A reduction in red blood cell (RBC) count and hemoglobin levels can occur as a result of various factors, including heightened vascular permeability, hemorrhaging, and, in more severe instances, shock. Neutrophils assume a critical part in the body's immunological response to infections. Elevated neutrophil levels are a component of the innate immune response to combat the dengue virus. The observed elevation in neutrophil count frequently coincides with a concomitant reduction in lymphocyte count, a characteristic finding in individuals afflicted with an infection. Therefore, trained predictor variables are significant from clinical prospect as well.

Table 4 presents a comparative analysis. In their study, Sarma et al. [25] conducted an implementation of the Decision Tree and Random Forest algorithms. The results indicated that the Decision Tree algorithm exhibited superior performance compared to the Random Forest algorithm, reaching an accuracy rate of 79%. T.-S. Ho et al. [57] utilized 4 biomarkers to train 3 models: DNN, DT, LR which achieved an accuracy between 83.75% to 85.87%. In their study, Mello-Román et al. [28] conducted 3 stage operation to impute the missing values. The study

Table 4 Results comparison among similar literatures

Authors	Approach	Evaluation
Sarma et al. [25]	Median imputation, Decision Tree, Random Forest	Decision Tree: 79% Accuracy
T.-S. Ho et al. [57]	Four key variables: Age, body temperature, white blood cells and platelet counts. Models: Deep neural network (DNN), decision tree (DT), logistic regression (LR)	DT, DNN and LR achieved an AUC of 84.60% ± 0.03%, 85.87% ± 0.54%, 83.75% ± 0.17% respectively.
Mello-Román et al. [28]	Mean imputation, data split: 90:10 ratio. Models: ANN, SVM	ANN: 96% Accuracy, 96% Sensitivity, 97% Specificity
This Work	**MICE Imputation, Extra tree feature selection, 13 Classical Machine Learning Model, Stacking-Based Meta XGBoost Classifier**	**Accuracy of 97.8%, a precision score of 97.82%, a recall of 97.8%, a specificity of 97.82%, and an F1-score of 97.80%, AUC 0.978.**

revealed to be excluding the features with 20% of samples missing and getting rid of the features which have more than 80% of samples to be missing values, which marks the first 2 stages. In the last stage of operation, features missing values in between the percentiles were filled using the mean of the feature's relevant values and testing on 10% of splitted data, their proposed methodology were able to achieved a high level of accuracy (96%), sensitivity (97%), and specificity (97%) using an Artificial Neural Network (ANN). Our proposed pipline followed a more robust procedure from preprocessing to model training. Instead of imputing based on statistical mean value, our work employed state-of-the-arts imputation algorithm MICE. Then we sorted out the best number and combination of features using extratree feature selection to provide optimum number of relevant features to train the model on. Mello-Román et al. [28] tested the performance of the model on only 10% of unseen data. Our methodology followed standard 80:20 ratio and 5-fold cross validation which justifies the model being tested on entire dataset instead of only a portion of the dataset. The results of this study demonstrated a high level of performance, achieving an accuracy of 97.8%. Additionally, precision was measured at 97.82%, recall at 97.8%, specificity at 97.82%, and the F1-score at 97.80% achieved through stacking-based XGBoost metaclassifier. The area under the curve (AUC) was calculated to be 0.978, surpassing the findings reported in the compared literature. Stacking ensemble model outperformed ANN in terms of evalution metrics. Stacking algorithms is a state-of-the-arts machine learning algorithms which takes advantage of multiple base level learner to create a robust model. Rather than learning patterns from the dataset from the scratch, this algorithms exploits predicted probabilistic values from multiple models to train a robust model, whereas ANN has to learn patterns from the dataset from the scratch. As a result, ANN fall behind in terms of performance to stacking ensemble model.

This work elucidates interesting possibilities for further investigation and progression. The dataset exploited in this study is of limited size, and the presence of disparities between classes is negligible. However, in intricate events, this may not hold true, as the numerical discrepancy between two separate cases of dengue symptoms might possess significant consequences on the decision of classification. A promising approach for future study involves integrating data from many clinical facilities throughout different regions of Bangladesh. This approach aims to develop a broader framework that can yield a very robust classification tool for effectively managing Dengue outbreaks in any geographical area within Bangladesh. In addition, it would be beneficial to do an external validation of this model applying a dengue dataset from geographically diverse places for future research pursuits.

4 Conclusion

This study demonstrates the potential of using machine learning techniques in addressing the urgent challenge of fast and accurate diagnosis of dengue patients. Given the serious clinical repercussions and high mortality rates associated with Dengue, there is an imperative need for swift and precise diagnosis. Our study not only highlights this critical need but also presents a comprehensive solution. Using meticulous methodology, we assimilated data from diverse sources, including dengue tests, and routine blood tests. SMOTE, Stacking-Based Meta-Classifier, and Nomogram-Based Scoring System improve the classification accuracy of Dengue patients. XGBoost classifier emerged as the most effective model with an accuracy of 97.8%, underscoring its proficiency. This study sheds light on the prospects of achieving accurate dengue patient classification, providing insights into the pivotal attributes influencing the decisions of the model, thereby facilitating clinical interpretation. The culmination of this endeavor holds significant ramifications for the medical realm, enabling timely interventions and judicious resource deployment. By harnessing the capabilities of machine learning, we set the stage for enhanced disease management, aiming to diminish the impact of Dengue on global health systems.

Code and Data Availability Statement Code for data cleaning and analysis is provided as part of the replication package and is available at https://github.com/Sohan2087/A-Stacking-Ensemble-Approach-for-Robust-Dengue-Patient-Detection-from-Complete-Blood-Count-Data.

Conflicts of Interest Authors have no conflict of interest to declare.

References

1. M.G. Guzman et al., Dengue: A continuing global threat. Nat. Rev. Microbiol. **8**(12), S7–S16 (2010). https://doi.org/10.1038/nrmicro2460
2. J.R. Powell, Mosquito-borne human viral diseases: Why Aedes aegypti?, (in eng). Am. J. Trop. Med. Hygi. **98**(6), 1563–1565 (2018). https://doi.org/10.4269/ajtmh.17-0866
3. W. H. O. Who, Dengue and severe dengue, (in English), *World Health Organization: WHO* (2023). [Online]. Available: https://www.who.int/news-room/fact-sheets/detail/dengue-and-severe-dengue
4. J. Slosek, Aedes aegypti mosquitoes in the Americas: A review of their interactions with the human population, (in eng). Soc. Sci. Med. **23**(3), 249–257 (1986). https://doi.org/10.1016/0277-9536(86)90345-x
5. M.J. Hopp, J.A. Foley, Global-scale relationships between climate and the dengue fever vector, Aedes Aegypti. Clim. Chang. **48**(2), 441–463 (2001). https://doi.org/10.1023/A:1010717502442
6. E.B. Beserra, C.R.M. Fernandes, S.A.D.O. Silva, L.A.D. Silva, J.W.D. Santos, Efeitos da temperatura no ciclo de vida, exigências térmicas e estimativas do número de gerações anuais de Aedes aegypti (Diptera, Culicidae). Iheringia. Série Zoologia **99**, 142–148 (2009)
7. E.A.P.D.A. Costa, E.M.D.M. Santos, J.C. Correia, C.M.R.D. Albuquerque, Impact of small variations in temperature and humidity on the reproductive activity and survival of Aedes aegypti (Diptera, Culicidae). Revista Brasileira de Entomologia **54**, 488–493 (2010)
8. C.P. Simmons, J.J. Farrar, N. van Vinh Chau, B. Wills, Dengue. N. Engl. J. Med. **366**(15), 1423–1432 (2012). https://doi.org/10.1056/NEJMra1110265
9. A. Wilder-Smith, D.J. Gubler, Geographic expansion of dengue: The impact of international travel. Med. Clin. North Am. **92**(6), 1377–1390 (2008). https://doi.org/10.1016/j.mcna.2008.07.002
10. H.A. Karam, J.C.B. da Silva, A.J.P. Filho, J.L.F. Rojas, Dynamic modelling of dengue epidemics in function of available enthalpy and rainfall (in English). Open J. Epidemiol **6**(1), 50–79 (2015). https://doi.org/10.4236/ojepi.2016.61007
11. B. Byttebier, M.S. De Majo, S. Fischer, Hatching response of Aedes aegypti (Diptera: Culicidae) eggs at low temperatures: Effects of hatching media and storage conditions. J. Med. Entomol. **51**(1), 97–103 (2014). https://doi.org/10.1603/me13066
12. V.J. Lee, D.C.B. Lye, Y. Sun, G. Fernandez, A. Ong, Y.S. Leo, Predictive value of simple clinical and laboratory variables for dengue hemorrhagic fever in adults. J. Clin. Virol. **42**(1), 34–39 (2008). https://doi.org/10.1016/j.jcv.2007.12.017
13. D. Muller, P. Young, *Molecular Virology and Control of Flaviviruses* (Caister Academic Press, 2012)
14. B. Shenoy, A. Menon, S. Biradar, Diagnostic utility of dengue NS1 antigen. Pediatr. Infect. Dis. **6**(3), 110–113 (2014)
15. H. Zhang et al., NS1-based tests with diagnostic utility for confirming dengue infection: A meta-analysis. Int. J. Infect. Dis. **26**, 57–66 (2014)
16. T. Rahman et al., Transfer learning with deep convolutional neural network (CNN) for pneumonia detection using chest X-ray. Appl. Sci. **10**(9), 3233 (2020) [Online]. Available: https://www.mdpi.com/2076-3417/10/9/3233
17. M.H. Chowdhury et al., Estimating blood pressure from the Photoplethysmogram signal and demographic features using machine learning techniques. Sensors **20**(11), 3127 (2020) [Online]. Available: https://www.mdpi.com/1424-8220/20/11/3127
18. M.E.H. Chowdhury et al., An early warning tool for predicting mortality risk of COVID-19 patients using machine learning. Cogn. Comput. (2021). https://doi.org/10.1007/s12559-020-09812-7
19. T. Rahman et al., Mortality prediction utilizing blood biomarkers to predict the severity of COVID-19 using machine learning technique, (in eng). Diagnostics (Basel, Switzerland) **11**(9) (2021). https://doi.org/10.3390/diagnostics11091582

20. M.N.I. Shuzan et al., Machine learning-based respiration rate and blood oxygen saturation estimation using Photoplethysmogram signals, (in eng). Bioengineering (Basel, Switzerland) **10**(2) (2023). https://doi.org/10.3390/bioengineering10020167
21. M.A. Majeed, H.Z.M. Shafri, Z. Zulkafli, A. Wayayok, A deep learning approach for dengue fever prediction in Malaysia using LSTM with spatial attention. Int. J. Environ. Res. Public Health **20**(5), 4130 (2023) [Online]. Available: https://www.mdpi.com/1660-4601/20/5/4130
22. F.P. Rocha, M. Giesbrecht, Machine learning algorithms for dengue risk assessment: A case study for São Luís do Maranhão. Comput. Appl. Math. **41**(8), 393 (2022). https://doi.org/10.1007/s40314-022-02101-z
23. S.N. Manoharan, K.M.V.M. Kumar, N. Vadivelan, A novel CNN-TLSTM approach for dengue disease identification and prevention using IoT-fog cloud architecture. Neural. Process. Lett. **55**(2), 1951–1973 (2023). https://doi.org/10.1007/s11063-022-10971-x
24. H. Mayrose, G.M. Bairy, N. Sampathila, S. Belurkar, K. Saravu, Machine learning-based detection of dengue from blood smear images utilizing platelet and lymphocyte characteristics. Diagnostics **13**(2), 220 (2023) [Online]. Available: https://www.mdpi.com/2075-4418/13/2/220
25. D. Sarma, S. Hossain, T. Mittra, M.A.M. Bhuiya, I. Saha, R. Chakma, Dengue prediction using machine learning algorithms, in *2020 IEEE 8th R10 Humanitarian Technology Conference (R10-HTC)*, (2020), p. 1–6. https://doi.org/10.1109/R10-HTC49770.2020.9357035
26. A.L.V. Gomes et al., Classification of dengue fever patients based on gene expression data using support vector machines. PLoS One **5**(6), e11267 (2010). https://doi.org/10.1371/journal.pone.0011267
27. W. Caicedo-Torres, Á. Paternina, H. Pinzón, Machine learning models for early dengue severity prediction, in *Advances in Artificial Intelligence - IBERAMIA 2016*, ed. by M.M. Cham, G.H.J. Escalante, A. Segura, J.D.D. Murillo, (Springer International Publishing, 2016), pp. 247–258
28. J.D. Mello-Román, J.C. Mello-Román, S. Gómez-Guerrero, M. García-Torres, Predictive models for the medical diagnosis of dengue: A case study in Paraguay, (in eng). Comput. Math. Methods Med. **2019**, 7307803 (2019). https://doi.org/10.1155/2019/7307803
29. T. Chakraborty, S. Chattopadhyay, I. Ghosh, Forecasting dengue epidemics using a hybrid methodology. Phys. A Statist. Mech. Appl. **527**, 121266 (2019). https://doi.org/10.1016/j.physa.2019.121266
30. D.K. Ming et al., The diagnosis of dengue in patients presenting with acute febrile illness using supervised machine learning and impact of seasonality, (in English). Front. Digit. Health, Original Research **4** (2022). https://doi.org/10.3389/fdgth.2022.849641
31. H. Hegde, N. Shimpi, A. Panny, I. Glurich, P. Christie, A. Acharya, MICE vs PPCA: Missing data imputation in healthcare. Inform. Med. Unlock. **17**, 100275 (2019). https://doi.org/10.1016/j.imu.2019.100275
32. J.R. Stevens, A. Suyundikov, M.L. Slattery, Accounting for missing data in clinical research, (in eng). JAMA **315**(5), 517–518 (2016). https://doi.org/10.1001/jama.2015.16461
33. T. Dahiru, P - value, a true test of statistical significance? A cautionary note, (in eng). Ann. Ibadan Postgrad. Med. **6**(1), 21–26 (2008). https://doi.org/10.4314/aipm.v6i1.64038
34. T.K. Kim, T test as a parametric statistic. kja **68**(6), 540–546 (2015). https://doi.org/10.4097/kjae.2015.68.6.540
35. J. Cuzick, A Wilcoxon-type test for trend, (in eng). Stat. Med. **4**(1), 87–90 (1985). https://doi.org/10.1002/sim.4780040112
36. D. Singh, B. Singh, Investigating the impact of data normalization on classification performance. Appl. Soft Comput. **97**, 105524 (2020). https://doi.org/10.1016/j.asoc.2019.105524
37. N.V. Chawla, K.W. Bowyer, L.O. Hall, W.P. Kegelmeyer, SMOTE: Synthetic minority oversampling technique. J. Artif. Intell. Res. **16**, 321–357 (2002)
38. S.S.S.J. Surendiran, N. Yuvaraj, M. Ramkumar, C.N. Ravi, R.G. Vidhya, Classification of diabetes using multilayer perceptron, in *2022 IEEE International Conference on Distributed Computing and Electrical Circuits and Electronics (ICDCECE), 23–24 April 2022*, (2022), pp. 1–5. https://doi.org/10.1109/ICDCECE53908.2022.9793085

39. D.K. Choubey, M. Kumar, V. Shukla, S. Tripathi, V.K. Dhandhania, Comparative analysis of classification methods with PCA and LDA for diabetes. Curr. Diabetes Rev. **16**(8), 833–850 (2020)
40. M.A.A. Faisal et al., An investigation to study the effects of Tai Chi on human gait dynamics using classical machine learning. Comput. Biol. Med. **142**, 105184 (2022)
41. F. Haque et al., A machine learning-based severity prediction tool for the Michigan neuropathy screening instrument. Diagnostics **13**(2), 264 (2023)
42. S.S. Keerthi, S.K. Shevade, C. Bhattacharyya, K.R.K. Murthy, Improvements to Platt's SMO algorithm for SVM classifier design. Neural Comput. **13**(3), 637–649 (2001). https://doi.org/10.1162/089976601300014493
43. A. Sharaff, H. Gupta, Extra-tree classifier with metaheuristics approach for email classification, in *Advances in Computer Communication and Computational Sciences: Proceedings of IC4S 2018*, (Springer, 2019), pp. 189–197
44. A. Khandakar et al., A machine learning model for early detection of diabetic foot using thermogram images. Comput. Biol. Med. **137**, 104838 (2021). https://doi.org/10.1016/j.compbiomed.2021.104838
45. G. Guo, H. Wang, D. Bell, Y. Bi, K. Greer, KNN model-based approach in classification, in *On the Move to Meaningful Internet Systems 2003: CoopIS, DOA, and ODBASE*, ed. by R. Meersman, Z. Tari, D.C. Schmidt, (Springer, Berlin, Heidelberg, 2003), pp. 986–996
46. A. Natekin, A. Knoll, Gradient boosting machines, a tutorial. Front. Neurorobot. **7**, 21 (2013)
47. M. Al-Sarem, F. Saeed, W. Boulila, A.H. Emara, M. Al-Mohaimeed, M. Errais, Feature selection and classification using CatBoost method for improving the performance of predicting Parkinson's disease, in *Advances on Smart and Soft Computing: Proceedings of ICACIn 2020*, (Springer, 2021), pp. 189–199
48. M. Pal, Random forest classifier for remote sensing classification. Int. J. Remote Sens. **26**(1), 217–222 (2005). https://doi.org/10.1080/01431160412331269698
49. S.M. Lundberg, S.-I. Lee, A unified approach to interpreting model predictions, in *NIPS'17: Proceedings of the 31st International Conference on Neural Information Processing Systems*, (Curran Associates Inc., Red Hook, 2017), pp. 4768–4777
50. An introduction to explainable AI with Shapley values — SHAP latest documentation, ed (2023)
51. A. Zlotnik, V. Abraira, A general-purpose nomogram generator for predictive logistic regression models. Stata J. **15**(2), 537–546 (2015) [Online]. Available: https://econpapers.repec.org/article/tsjstataj/v_3a15_3ay_3a2015_3ai_3a2_3ap_3a537-546.htm
52. N. Ibtehaz, M.E.H. Chowdhury, A. Khandakar, S. Kiranyaz, M.S. Rahman, S.M. Zughaier, RamanNet: A generalized neural network architecture for Raman spectrum analysis. Neural Comput. & Applic. **35**(25), 18719–18735 (2023). https://doi.org/10.1007/s00521-023-08700-z
53. X. Yang, M.B. Quam, T. Zhang, S. Sang, Global burden for dengue and the evolving pattern in the past 30 years. J. Travel Med. **28**(8), taab146 (2021)
54. K.K. Bhowmik, J. Ferdous, P.K. Baral, M.S. Islam, Recent outbreak of dengue in Bangladesh: A threat to public health, (in eng). Health Sci. Rep. **6**(4), e1210 (2023). https://doi.org/10.1002/hsr2.1210
55. ACAPS Briefing note - Bangladesh 2023 Dengue Outbreak (26 September 2023) - Bangladesh, ed (2023)
56. T. Rahman et al., QCovSML: A reliable COVID-19 detection system using CBC biomarkers by a stacking machine learning model. Comput. Biol. Med. **143**, 105284 (2022). https://doi.org/10.1016/j.compbiomed.2022.105284
57. T.-S. Ho et al., Comparing machine learning with case-control models to identify confirmed dengue cases. PLoS Negl. Trop. Dis. **14**(11), e0008843 (2020). https://doi.org/10.1371/journal.pntd.0008843

Interpretable Deep Learning Model for Tuberculosis Detection Using X-Ray Images

Md. Faysal Ahamed, Md. Nahiduzzaman, Md. Rabiul Islam, Tawsifur Rahman, Khandaker Reajul Islam, Ahmed Balla Abdalla Altyeb, and Muhammad E. H. Chowdhury

1 Introduction

Tuberculosis (TB) remains a primary global health concern, causing many deaths as one of the leading infectious diseases. In the year 2021, an estimated worldwide population of 10.6 million individuals suffered the effects of TB. The responsibility was allocated among a population consisting of 6 million males, 3.4 million

M. F. Ahamed
Department of Electrical & Computer Engineering, Rajshahi University of Engineering & Technology, Rajshahi, Bangladesh

M. Nahiduzzaman
Department of Electrical & Computer Engineering, Rajshahi University of Engineering & Technology, Rajshahi, Bangladesh
e-mail: nahiduzzaman@ece.ruet.ac.bd

M. R. Islam
Department of Computer Science & Engineering, Rajshahi University of Engineering & Technology, Rajshahi, Bangladesh

T. Rahman
Department of Biomedical Engineering, Johns Hopkins University, Baltimore, MD, USA

K. R. Islam
Department of Physiology, Faculty of Medicine, University Kebangsaan Malaysia, Kuala Lumpur, Malaysia
e-mail: p111445@siswa.ukm.edu.my

A. B. A. Altyeb
Department of Urology, Hamad Medical Corporation, Doha, Qatar
e-mail: aaltyeb@hamad.qa

M. E. H. Chowdhury (✉)
Department of Electrical Engineering, Qatar University, Doha, Qatar
e-mail: mchowdhury@qu.edu.qa

M. E. H. Chowdhury, S. Kiranyaz (eds.), *Surveillance, Prevention, and Control of Infectious Diseases*, https://doi.org/10.1007/978-3-031-59967-5_8

females, and 1.2 million individuals in the younger age group, including many nations and age ranges [1]. Early diagnosis and proper treatment are a must for a successful cure. Although Chest X-rays (CXRs) are commonly used to detect and screen for pulmonary TB, depending on expert interpretation may introduce subjectivity and inefficiencies, ultimately leading to misdiagnosis and poor patient outcomes [2]. While antimicrobial drugs effectively treat this bacterial disease caused by Mycobacterium tuberculosis [3–6]. It is crucial to continue improving the accuracy of TB detection and diagnosis to enhance patient care and effectively manage the disease. The need for more skilled radiologists in low-income and remote regions is a cause for concern. This makes it crucial to utilize computer-assisted diagnostic (CAD) systems for broad pulmonary tuberculosis screening by carefully examining CXR images. Combining deep convolutional neural network (CNN) models and easily accessible large datasets has led to the widespread use of computer vision techniques. The scarcity of trained radiologists is even more pronounced in resource-limited areas, especially in underserved regions and rural settings. The healthcare sector is a priority area for people seeking quality care and services. However, healthcare struggles with a gap between public expectations and service delivery, which comes with significant budget allocation. An essential aspect of this environment is the subjectivity and differences in medical data evaluation, made more complex by the image quality and exhaustion experienced by medical professionals. The application of machine learning in healthcare has garnered growing attention, as its potential for transformative impact has emerged as a prominent topic in the ongoing medical diagnosis sector [7].

CNNs have proven to be effective in detecting various abnormalities in chest X-ray samples, including but not limited to tuberculosis, pneumonia, cancer, COVID, and other diseases [8–26]. Several researchers have utilized conventional machine learning techniques to distinguish between tuberculosis (TB) and healthy lung conditions or non-TB pulmonary infections by analyzing chest X-ray (CXR) images [27–32].

Singh et al. [32] conducted a study introducing a novel approach for detecting tuberculosis (TB) in chest X-rays. This approach consisted of three main stages: separating the lung image from the X-ray, generating a set of texture and shape features from the segmented data, and combining these features into a vector that feeds a robust machine learning algorithm called a support vector machine (SVM). The study's results were remarkable, with an AUC of 0.98 and 0.96 for the MC and CHN datasets, respectively, indicating high accuracy. Additionally, the algorithm exhibited a specificity of 100%, meaning that it was exceptionally proficient in identifying healthy X-rays.

A study by Hernandez et al. [33] used a various CNN models to automatically categorize tuberculosis (TB) patients based on chest X-ray (CXR) images, achieving a commendable accuracy rate of 86%. In another approach, Lopes et al. [34] utilized pre-trained CNN models derived from the ImageNet dataset to distinguish patients with TB from those without, using CXR images. Ahsan et al. [35] introduced modifications to an existing CNN model for TB identification, yielding accuracy rates of 81.25% and 80% with and without image augmentation techniques, respectively. Pre-trained CNN models were also explored and exhibited an impressive TB detection accuracy of 94.89%, as demonstrated by Yadav et al. [36]. To improve it more, Abbas et al. [37] proposed a novel CNN architecture via a class decomposition approach. However, it is worth noting that training pre-trained CNN models using TB culture test images could potentially introduce uncertainty when compared to classification based on widely accessible CXRs. Finally, Chang et al. [38] employed a transfer learning strategy on TB culture images and achieved notable outcomes, achieving a sensitivity of 98% and a precision of 99% in categorizing TB cases. Pasa et al. [39] conducted a study using support vector machines (SVMs) and CNNs. They developed a simplified CNN model that prioritizes efficiency without sacrificing accuracy. Additionally, the potential of CNNs for visualization has yet to be fully explored. They assessed the usefulness of saliency maps and grad-CAMs as visualization techniques for TB, providing a radiological viewpoint on their relevance and usefulness.

In their study, Nguyen et al. [40] looked into how transfer learning could be used in medical imaging for TB detection. They presented an enhanced technique for transfer learning that outperformed the custom of using only ImageNet weights. Low-level features obtained using ImageNet weights were also ineffective for imaging tasks involving modalities such as X-rays. The scientists devised a unique plan to train models inside a multiclass multilabel framework to gather low-level characteristics. Classifying TB performed better using this method than training from randomly initialized conditions. They presented a more successful training paradigm, especially pertinent in contexts with limited data, like the healthcare industry. With the help of transfer learning from various pre-trained CNN models, Tahir et al. [18] achieved incredible performance in identifying different coronavirus families (SARS, MERS, and COVID-19) from CXR images. Their method achieved sensitivities higher than 90%, significantly improving the discrimination between these virus families. Ismael et al. [16] utilized a dataset of CXR images in their study, focusing on the potential of deep learning methods to identify COVID-19 through image analysis. Their findings showed that the ResNet50 model's features achieved an impressive accuracy rate of 94.7% when classified using the support vector model (SVM) with a linear kernel. This study demonstrates the effectiveness of advanced techniques in detecting COVID-19 through CXR image analysis.

This research was motivated by the studies above and aimed to employ a novel lightweight CNN to differentiate CXR images. The study also aims to categorize TB patients into groups using explainable AI with SHAP for early diagnosis and treatment. The notable contributions of the study are outlined below:

- By merging a TB benchmark dataset named NIAID with another set comprising cases of non-TB conditions (bacterial and viral pneumonia), we have carefully curated a dataset comprising 7700 CXR images. This collection includes 3500 Normal (healthy) cases, 3500 non-TB cases (bacterial and viral pneumonia), and 700 TB cases.
- Using this distinct dataset, a novel Lightweight Parallel CNN (LP-CNN) framework was proposed for TB classification. Our framework establishes a new

performance benchmark on this dataset, achieving the highest levels of accuracy observed in diagnosing and assessing TB using CXR images alone.

- We conduct a comprehensive analysis, delving into various aspects such as parameters, convolutional layers, and compactness, and draw comparisons with other advanced transfer learning (TL) models.
- In addition, we leverage the SHAP visualization technique to offer insights into the model's decision-making process as it classifies CXR images in real-time.

2 Methodology

2.1 Proposed Framework

Initially, we gathered the dataset from reputable sources and created a custom set by examining each CXR sample in the class category. After performing image pre-processing (resizing, Contrast-Limited Adaptive Histogram Equalization (CLAHE), normalization), the samples were separated into training, validation, and testing sets. The proposed LP-CNN model was evaluated on this dataset by extracting the most prominent features simultaneously. Explainable artificial intelligence (XAI) with SHAP was used for black-box model comprehension. Figure 1 provides a comprehensive overview of the proposed structure.

2.2 Dataset Collection

To conduct the research, we manually collected data sets from various sources. The study focused solely on CXR samples captured from the posterior-to-anterior or anterior-to-posterior viewpoints, which radiologists commonly use. The dataset includes images of non-tuberculosis (non-TB) pneumonia, including both bacterial

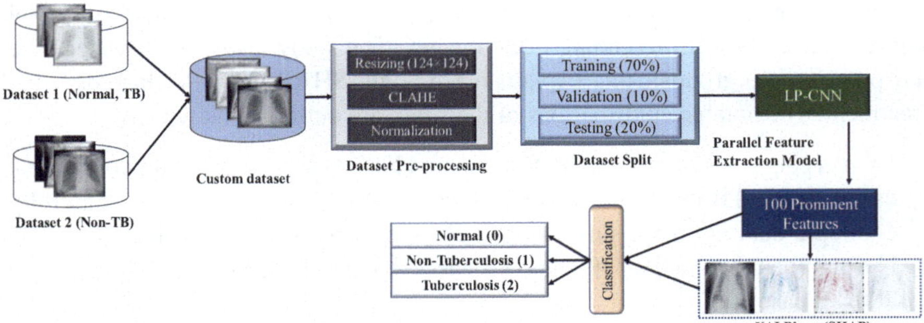

Fig. 1 Proposed framework for multiclass classification from CXR images

Table 1 The number of samples in each class

Disease Class	Training set	Validation set	Testing set
Normal (0)	2520	280	700
Non-TB (1)	2520	280	700
TB (2)	2520	280	700
Total	7560	840	2100

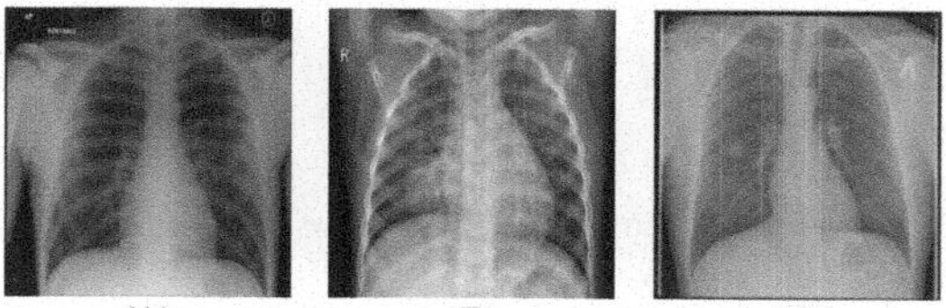

Fig. 2 Samples of CXR images which contain (**a**) normal (healthy), (**b**) non-TB (Bacterial and viral pneumonia) and (**c**) Tuberculosis (TB)

and viral variants and tuberculosis (TB) cases. TB and normal CXR images (dataset 1) were sourced from the National Institute of Allergy and Infectious Diseases (NIAID) [41]. The NIAID TB gateway program dataset comprises approximately 3037 chest X-ray images showing indications of tuberculosis from nearly 3087 distinct cases. The dataset 2 included 5863 X-ray images captured in JPEG format, categorized as either pneumonia or normal [42]. The images were extracted from historical cohorts of pediatric patients, specifically anterior-posterior chest X-ray images. Before the chest X-ray analysis, a preliminary screening process was conducted to exclude scans that were of poor quality or unreadable, ensuring the quality of the dataset. In order to address the possible consequences arising from diagnostic inconsistencies, a third expert conducted a thorough examination of the evaluation set. The selected samples for the investigation are specified in Table 1, which includes the number of combined balanced datasets. The categorization process involves the allocation of samples into separate sets for training (70%), validation (10%), and testing (20%). Figure 2 exhibits normal, non-TB, and TB CXRs samples.

2.3 Pre-processing

A sequence of transformations (CLAHE, resizing, and normalization) was applied to optimize image quality to prepare CXR images for analysis (Fig. 3). This was crucial to ensure the images were suitable for utilization within the LP-CNN model for TB classification. The first step involved Contrast Limited Adaptive Histogram Equalization (CLAHE), which dynamically adjusted pixel intensities to improve the visibility of anatomical structures and subtle features [43]. Normalization helped standardize pixel intensities, stabilizing the neural network's training and promoting consistent convergence. This was crucial to ensure the images were suitable for utilization within the LP-CNN model for TB classification. In addition, resizing the images to a uniform size of 124×124 pixels helped streamline batch processing

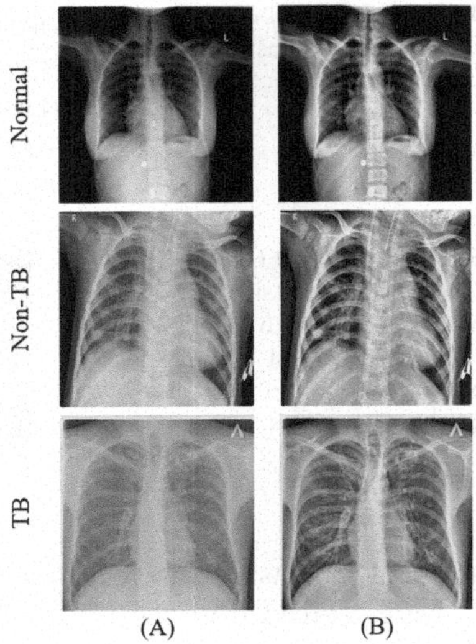

Fig. 3 Samples of CXR images which contain (**a**) before and (**b**) after pre-process

and feature extraction by the CNN models while maintaining critical information's integrity and optimizing computational efficiency. The preprocessing pipeline was designed to enhance image quality, ensure uniformity, and enable precise and robust classification performance.

2.4 Lightweight Parallel Convolutional Neural Network (LP-CNN)

The extraction of notable features from a CNN model has emerged as particularly challenging due to computational complexity and the number of layers. In practical, real-world situations, an optimal design reduces the number of parameters and computational complexity to ensure efficient implementation. Additionally, fewer parameters and layers can extract sufficient discriminant features. In contrast, a larger number of parameters increases the risk of overfitting and the computational time requirement to process patient samples. The architecture of the lightweight parallel CNN is illustrated in Fig. 4.

The CNN model is structured with eight convolutional layers (CLs), divided into two distinct components: a functional segment and a sequential segment. The functional segment consists of four interconnected CLs that operate parallelly; this strategic design was chosen to improve the model's computational efficiency. These specific CLs were meticulously selected through trial and error, resulting in optimized performance. The idea of utilizing parallel CLs was initially introduced by Szegedy et al. [44]. Sequential processing of the four CLs consumes more time than parallel execution, presenting a notable advantage in rapidly reducing the time

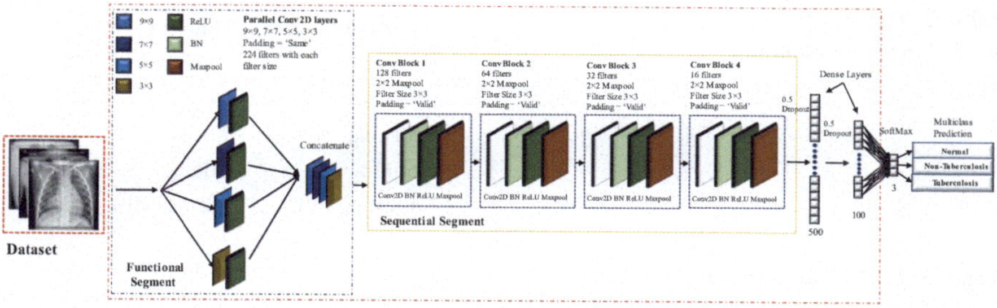

Fig. 4 Proposed LPNCNN architecture for feature extraction

demands [45, 46]. Each CL had a dimension of 32, while the kernels were sized as follows: 3 × 3 for the first, 5 × 5 for the second, 7 × 7 for the third, and 9 × 9 for the fourth, respectively. Krizhervsky et al.'s research architecture was followed, which recommended larger kernel sizes and the connections between them to improve classification performance, affecting kernel size preference [45, 47]. Diverse kernels were considered to extract relevant features, as distinct kernels generate distinct feature maps, aiming for optimal classification performance. Ultimately, these kernels were seamlessly concatenated to achieve a comprehensive and effective feature representation. Such a configuration ensured the efficient capture of essential features, accommodating their diverse sizes without compromise. In the first six CLs, a 'SAME' padding size was kept so that important information could be taken from the edges of the CXR images. This method extracted the image's features, even at the edges. Subsequently, the cumulative CL outputs were combined and moved into the sequential segment. This section implemented batch normalization (BN) and max pooling with a 2 × 2 kernel size to establish a connection for every CL. Four consecutive CLs were used at the sequential segment as filter sizes 128, 64, 32, and 16, while keeping "valid" padding sizes and with a 3 × 3 kernel. The four CLs used the rectified linear unit (ReLU) activation function. Two fully connected (FC) layers were added to handle feature extraction, with the final FC layer as the final layer. In order to reduce overfitting and accelerate training, 50% of nodes were randomly deactivated. Two drops (one after the first FC layer and one after the final CL) were applied with a probability of 0.5 each. Half of the nodes were randomly deactivated to prevent overfitting and speed up the training process. Two dropouts were implemented with a probability of 0.5 each, one after the first fully connected layer and one after the final convolutional layer. Table 2 provides an in-depth glance at the hyperparameters. A selection of 100 features was derived from the final fully connected (FC) layer through an iterative process of experimentation and improvement. The summary of the model with its parameters is shown in Table 3. Following the trial-and-error method, we chose 100 epochs to allow the model to converge effectively while avoiding overfitting. We also chose a batch size of 64 to make sure efficient training while making the most of the available computing resources.

Table 2 Hyperparameters utilized in model training

Hyperparameters	Values/Types
Epoch	100
Batch size	64
Learning rate	0.001
Optimizer	Adam
Loss function	Sparse cross entropy

Table 3 LP-CNN model summary

Layer type	Output shape	Params
Functional	(None, 124, 124, 1024)	126976
conv2d_211 (Conv2D)	(None, 122, 122, 128)	1179776
batch_normalization_207	(None, 122, 122, 128)	512
activation_203 (Activation)	(None, 122, 122, 128)	0
max_pooling2d_4	(None, 61, 61, 128)	0
conv2d_212 (Conv2D)	(None, 59, 59, 64)	73792
batch_normalization_208	(None, 59, 59, 64)	256
activation_204	(None, 59, 59, 64)	0
max_pooling2d_5	(None, 29, 29, 64)	0
conv2d_213	(None, 27, 27, 32)	18464
batch_normalization_209	(None, 27, 27, 32)	128
activation_205	(None, 27, 27, 32)	0
max_pooling2d_6	(None, 13, 13, 32)	0
lastconv	(None, 11, 11, 16)	4624
batch_normalization_210	(None, 11, 11, 16)	64
activation_206	(None, 11, 11, 16)	0
max_pooling2d_7	(None, 5, 5, 16)	0
dropout	(None, 5, 5, 16)	0
flatten_6	(None, 400)	0
dense_6	(None, 500)	200500
batch_normalization_211	(None, 500)	2000
dropout_1	(None, 500)	0
DenseLastTB	(None, 100)	50100
batch_normalization_212	(None, 100)	400
dropout_2	(None, 100)	0
dense_7	(None, 3)	303
Total parameters:	1,657,895	
Trainable parameters:	1,656,215	
Non-trainable parameters:	1680	

2.5 *Transfer Learning Models*

In tuberculosis classification, we rely on various transfer learning models, including DenseNet169 [48], DenseNet201 [49], InceptionResNetV2 [50], VGG19 [51], and

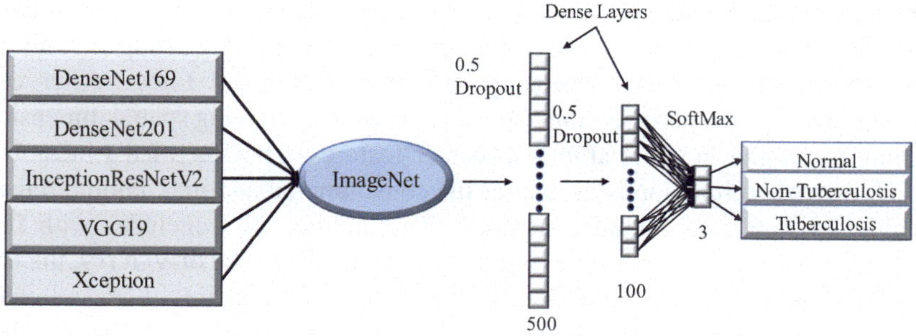

Fig. 5 Multiclass classification using TL models

Xception [52]. These models effectively categorize TB cases into normal, non-TB, and TB. They can extract meaningful image features by leveraging pre-existing knowledge from extensive datasets. Through fine-tuning, they can capture complex patterns and subtle nuances in CXR images, utilizing a limited amount of data tailored to our target task. These pre-existing models have undergone rigorous training on over 14 million image classifications encompassing a diverse range of 1000 categories within the ImageNet database. Our primary objective is to evaluate these models' classification performance and resource utilization thoroughly. This will involve thoroughly analyzing performance metrics, model parameters, and layer sizes for training and testing. Once the models are initialized, we boost the precision of class identification by incorporating two FC layers consisting of 500 and 100 nodes. Figure 5 provides an illustrative depiction of these TL models.

The DenseNet169 architecture assures each layer receives inputs from all antecedent layers, facilitating comprehensive information exchange. These layers, which are organized into dense units, facilitate the integration of features from different dimensions. Transition layers maintain essential data while managing dimensions. Multiclass classification is enabled by FC layers concluding in a SoftMax activation function. The interplay of dense connections, transitions, and FC layers in DenseNet169 improves feature extraction, allowing accurate and efficient image classification. DenseNet201 is organized into dense blocks, where sequential layers collaborate to extract and combine features at different scales. Transition layers, strategically inserted between dense blocks, manage feature map dimensions while preserving crucial information. These layers employ pooling and convolutional operations to control computational complexity. DenseNet201 employs fully connected (FC) layers for classification tasks, culminating in a SoftMax activation function. The InceptionResNetV2 uses residual connections boosted by ResNet architecture to make the training process more efficient and effective. These connections help to prevent the vanishing gradient problem and allow information to flow smoothly between layers. This means the network can be deeper without sacrificing its ability to learn and represent complex features. During classification, the InceptionResNetV2 uses fully connected (FC) layers, which end with a SoftMax activation function. This function allows for precise and accurate multi-class categorization. The VGG19 is a convolutional neural network architecture renowned for its deep and structured design, consisting of multiple convolutional layers (CL) comprising several convolutional filters. After each convolutional layer, a max-pooling (MP) layer is added, reducing spatial dimensions and improving the model's ability to detect features. The Rectified Linear Unit (ReLU) activation function is used after the convolutional and max-pooling layers, allowing for nonlinear feature extraction. The architecture concludes with fully connected (FC) layers responsible for classification. In the case of VGG19, the final FC layer employs the SoftMax activation function and contains three individual FC layers, enabling the model to represent intricate features and classify them effectively. Xception is an advanced CNN architecture that reconceives depth-wise separable convolutions for feature extraction. Xception employs a series of deep-separable convolutions at its core, augmenting its ability to recognize complex image patterns. This innovative design reduces the number of parameters substantially, resulting in streamlined computation without forsaking precision. The architecture of Xception is similar to Inception's, utilizing parallel branches to capture information at multiple dimensions. This contributes to the model's robust image analysis capabilities by effectively identifying local and global features. In the classification phase of Xception, fully connected (FC) layers culminate in a SoftMax activation function, enabling precise multi-class categorization.

2.6 Classification Metrics and Loss Function

To assess and compare the performance of various classifiers, we analyzed ROC curves and calculated the area under the curve (AUC) and precision, recall, F1 score, and accuracy. AUC was selected as the benchmark for evaluation. When assessing classification models, it is important to consider key metrics like precision, recall, F1 score, and accuracy. Precision measures the ratio of correctly predicted positive instances to total predicted positives, helping to reduce false positives. Meanwhile, recall (also known as sensitivity or true positive rate) evaluates the ratio of correctly predicted positive instances to total actual positives, aiming to minimize false negatives. The F1 score is especially useful for imbalanced datasets as it balances precision and recall, considering false positives and negatives. Finally, accuracy determines the proportion of correctly predicted instances, providing an overall measure of model correctness. Sparse cross entropy loss function measures the difference between predicted class probabilities and actual class labels, with a focus on scenarios where classes are imbalanced or sparsely distributed. The formula of the corresponding classification metrics is:

$$precision = \frac{True\_Positive}{True\_Positive + False\_Positive} \tag{1}$$

$$recall = \frac{True\_Positive}{True\_Positive + False\_Negative} \tag{2}$$

$$accuracy = \frac{True\_Positive + True\_Negative}{True\_Positive + True\_Negative + False\_Positive + False\_Negative} \tag{3}$$

$$F1\_Score = 2 \times \frac{precision \times recall}{precision + recall} \tag{4}$$

$$Loss_{SCE} = -\sum_{i=1}^{n} truth\_label_i \times \log\left(soft\max\_probability_i\right) \tag{5}$$

3 Experiment Set-Up and Analysis

Table 4 provides a comprehensive overview of the training setup implemented in the proposed framework.

The following section entails a comprehensive evaluation of the test set data, where we constructed both the ROC-AUC curve and confusion matrix to determine the total accuracy and weighted evaluation metrics.

3.1 Results of Proposed LP-CNN Model

Initially, we thoroughly evaluated CXR images to classify them as normal (0), non-TB (1), or TB (2). Our primary focus was on the novel LP-CNN model, and we

Table 4 Experimental set-up

Name	Parameters
Programming language	Python
Environment	PyCharm Community Edition (2021.2.3)
Backend	Keras with TensorFlow
Processor	Intel(R) Core (TM) i9-11900K
Installed RAM	32 GB
GPU	NVIDIA GeForce, RTX 3090 Ti 24 GB
Operating system	Windows 10 Pro
Input	Chest X-ray images
Input size	124 × 124

Table 5 Class-wise classification performances on LP-CNN model

Classes	Precision	Recall	F1-score	Accuracy (%)	AUC (%)
Normal (0)	0.99	1.00	0.99	99.43	99.95
Non-TB (1)	0.99	1.00	1.00	99.76	100
TB (2)	0.99	0.98	0.99	99.19	99.85
Average (μ) ± SD (σ) (%)	99 ± 1.36E-16	98.33 ± 0.0115	99.33 ± 0.0057	99.46	99.93

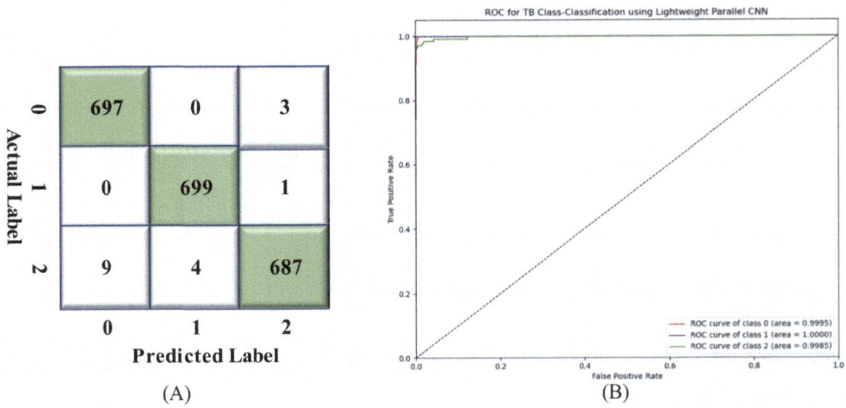

Fig. 6 (**a**) Confusion metrics for LP-CNN model and (**b**) class-wise ROCs for multiclass classifications

established a range of performance metrics to gauge its efficacy. These metrics comprised precision, recall, f1, accuracy, and AUC. Table 5 provides a summary of the performance scores for each category. The model proposed in this study showed exceptional performance in multiclass classification, especially in detecting specific classes. It demonstrated high average precision (99 ± 1.36E-16%), recall (98.33 ± 0.0115%), F1 score (99.33 ± 0.0057%), accuracy (99.46%), and AUC (99.93%). The LP-CNN achieved perfect detection scores of 100% in recall and F1 for non-TB CXR classification. Across all metrics, the average scores were above 98%, indicating the model's satisfactory performance evaluation. The average AUC score was an impressive 99.93%. The corresponding confusion metrics (CM) for the three classes, illustrated in Fig. 6a, showcase the model's outstanding detection capabilities. The class-wise ROC curves in Fig. 6b show complete area coverage of 100% in the non-TB class, while TB and normal CXR images achieved commendable scores of 99.95% and 99.85%, respectively.

3.2 Performances Comparisons among SOTA TL Models

In this study, the implementation of TL models to improve the classification of Chest X-ray (CXR) images was investigated, with a focus on three major categories: Normal, Non-Tuberculous (Non-TB) diseases, and Tuberculosis (TB). TL presents a promising method for improving the classification of CXR images, which is essential for early disease detection. Utilizing pre-trained CNN architectures on large-scale image datasets, we fine-tuned these models using our selected CXR dataset. Transfer learning substantially improved the accuracy, precision, recall, f1, and AUC of disease classification across all three classes, according to the findings of our study. These models exhibited a remarkable capacity to generalize novel and unobserved cases, a crucial aspect of their clinical deployment. In addition, we conducted exhaustive analyses of model comprehension, shedding light on the features driving the classification decisions.

The CMs of the DenseNet169, DenseNet201, InceptionResnetV2, VGG19, and Xception models are shown in Fig. 7. The performance analysis by class is displayed in Table 6. VGG19 attained the highest average precision, recall, F1, accuracy and AUC compared to other models, 98.67 $\pm$ 0.0115%, 98.67 $\pm$ 0.0115%, 98.67 $\pm$ 0.0115%, 98.48%, and 99.92%, respectively. DensNet1201 attained the second highest f1 and accuracy of 98.33 $\pm$ 0.0002% and 98.19%, respectively, improving 0.345% and 0.294% over the second-best VGG19 model. Moreover, DenseNet169, DenseNet201, and VGG19 have a 100% detection rate for non-TB CXR classification. According to our evaluation of various models, DenseNet201 had the second-best performance score for identifying normal chest X-ray (CXR) images, with precision, recall, and f1 scores. VGG19 achieved a maximum area score of 99.92%. However, identifying tuberculosis (TB) can be challenging as it can coexist with other pulmonary diseases and exhibit various manifestations,

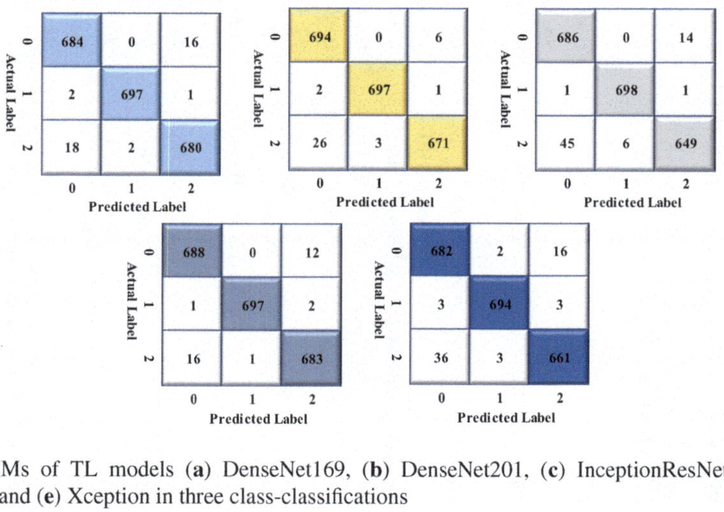

Fig. 7 CMs of TL models (**a**) DenseNet169, (**b**) DenseNet201, (**c**) InceptionResNetV2, (**d**) VGG19, and (**e**) Xception in three class-classifications

Table 6 Performance comparison on SOTA TL models

Model name	Diseases class	Precision	Recall	F1-score	Accuracy (%)	AUC (%)
DenseNet169	Normal (0)	0.97	0.98	0.97	–	99.84
	Non-TB (1)	1.00	1.00	1.00	–	100
	TB (2)	0.98	0.97	0.97	–	99.82
	Average (%)	98.33 ± 0.0002	98.33 ± 0.0002	98 ± 0.0173	98.14	99.88
DensNet1201	Normal (0)	0.96	0.99	0.98	–	99.88
	Non-TB (1)	1.00	1.00	1.00	–	99.98
	TB (2)	0.99	0.96	0.97	–	99.82
	Average (%)	98.33 ± 0.0004	98.33 ± 0.0004	98.33 ± 0.0002	98.19	99.89
InceptionResNetV2	Normal (0)	0.94	0.98	0.96	–	99.42
	Non-TB (1)	0.99	1.00	0.99	–	99.97
	TB (2)	0.98	0.93	0.95	–	99.15
	Average (%)	97 ± 0.0264	97 ± 0.036	96.67 ± 0.0208	96.81	99.51
VGG19	Normal (0)	0.98	0.98	0.98	–	99.89
	Non-TB (1)	1.00	1.00	1.00	–	100
	TB (2)	0.98	0.98	0.98	–	99.87
	Average (%)	**98.67 ± 0.0115**	**98.67 ± 0.0115**	**98.67 ± 0.0115**	**98.48**	**99.92**
Xception	Normal (0)	0.95	0.97	0.96	–	99.54
	Non-TB (1)	0.99	0.99	0.99	–	99.98
	TB (2)	0.97	0.94	0.96	–	99.47
	Average (%)	97 ± 0.02	96.67 ± 0.025	97 ± 0.017	97	99.66

[a]Bold values indicate best results

including extrapulmonary TB. Overall, the TB classification result was satisfactory. Regarding performance, VGG19 had the highest AUC score of 99.92%, which was 0.03% better than the second-best score of 99.89% achieved by DenseNet201. For the Normal CXR Class, VGG19 achieved the top AUC score of 99.89%. The DenseNet169 and VGG19 models had a perfect 100% AUC score for the non-TB class. Figure 8 shows the class-wise ROC-AUC curves for all TL models.

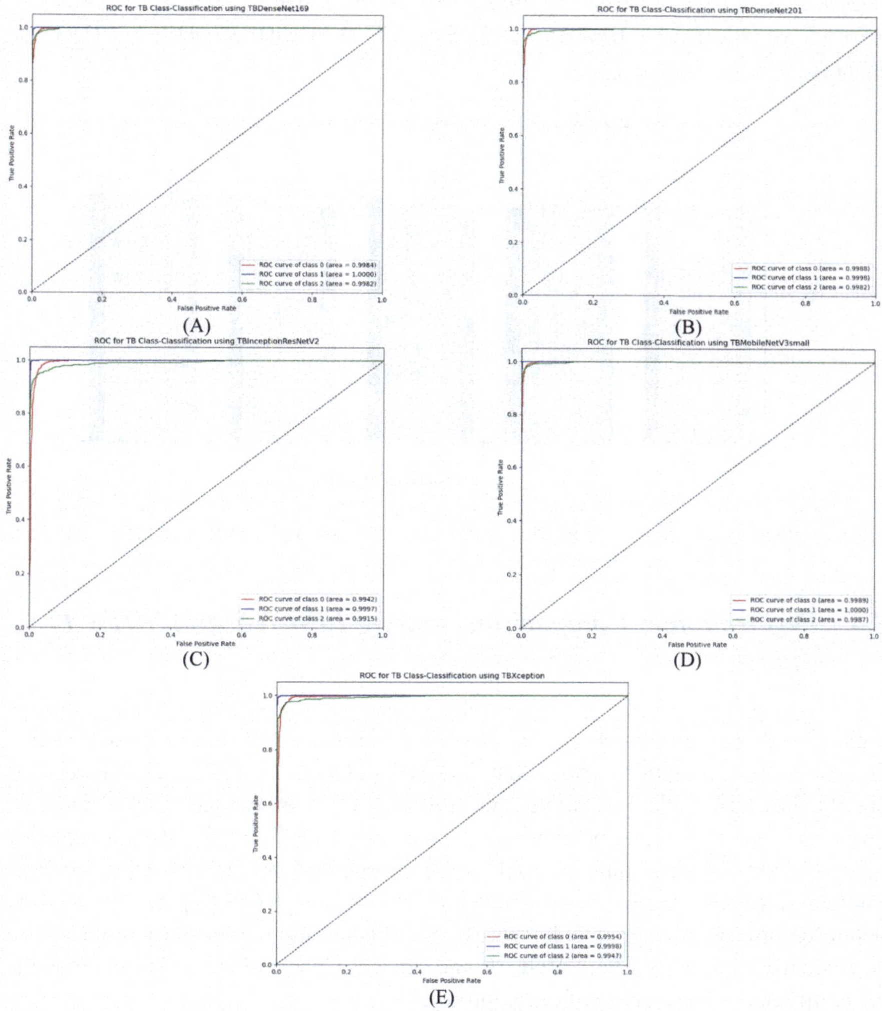

Fig. 8 Class-wise ROC of TL models (**a**) DenseNet169, (**b**) DenseNet201, (**c**) InceptionResNetV2, (**d**) VGG19, and (**e**) Xception in three class-classifications

Table 7 Performance comparison among the LP-CNN and SOTA TL models, where 'm' denotes average

Model name	mP (%)	mR (%)	mF1 (%)	Acc (%)	AUC (%)
DenseNet169	98.33 ± 0.0002	98.33 ± 0.0002	98 ± 0.0173	98.14	99.88
DenseNet1201	98.33 ± 0.0004	98.33 ± 0.0004	98.33 ± 0.0002	98.19	99.89
InceptionResNetV2	97 ± 0.0264	97 ± 0.036	96.67 ± 0.0208	96.81	99.51
VGG19	98.67 ± 0.0115	**98.67 ± 0.0115**	98.67 ± 0.0115	98.48	99.92
Xception	97 ± 0.02	96.67 ± 0.025	97 ± 0.017	97	99.66
LP-CNN (proposed)	**99 ± 1.36E-16**	98.33 ± 0.0115	**99.33 ± 0.0057**	**99.46**	**99.93**

[a]Bold values indicate best results

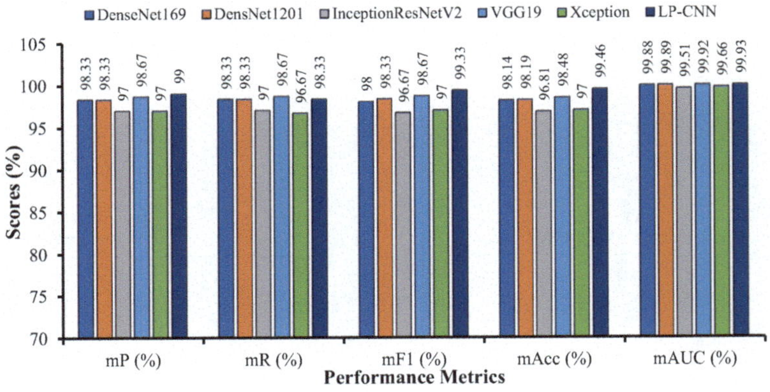

Fig. 9 Comparative performance metrics scores among proposed LP-CNN and SOTA TL models

3.3 *Performances Comparisons among LP-CNN and SOTA TL Models*

Table 7 provides a detailed comparison of TL models with the proposed model. Our previous evaluations show that VGG19 outperforms other TL models, as clearly shown in Table 6. However, our novel LP-CNN model has made significant progress, with an average precision rate exceeding VGG19 by 0.33%, an accuracy rate of 0.99% higher, and an AUC subtly improved by 0.01%. Despite these impressive results, there are some nuances to consider. VGG19 performs slightly better regarding average recall scores, but interestingly, the F1 score remains consistently high across both VGG19 and our LP-CNN model. This indicates the reliability and effectiveness of our approach.

To better understand these findings, we have included Fig. 9, which visually represents the performance metrics of all models. This graph reinforces our proposed model's advantages in classifying CXR diseases. In conclusion, after assessing various models for CXR disease classification, it is evident that each has individual abilities and strengths. However, our LP-CNN model outshines the rest with its exceptional performance across multiple evaluation metrics.

Table 8 Computational resources comparison among the proposed LP-CNN and TL models

Performance criteria	LP-CNN (proposed)	DenseNet169	DenseNet201	Inception ResNetV2	VGG19	Xception
Total parameters (million)	**1.658**	14.14	20.05	54.95	20.485	24.139
Trainable parameters (million)	**1.656**	1.498	1.728	0.614	0.461	3.277
Number of layers (CL)	**8**	598	710	783	25	135
Size (megabytes)	**19.1**	66.9	91.4	216	81.7	117

[a]Bold values indicate the best results

3.4 Computational Resource Comparison

Comparing computational resources for CXR classification is essential to optimize the efficacy and efficiency of diagnostic procedures. By evaluating the computational requirements of various models, healthcare institutions can make informed decisions regarding resource allocation, hardware infrastructure, and model selection. This analysis contributes to developing real-time applications, scalability for large-scale inspections, and energy-efficient deployments. In addition, it enables the identification of models that strike the optimal balance between accuracy and interpretability, fostering diagnostic outcomes in clinical settings that are reliable and well-explained. Table 8 provides a comprehensive comparison of various deep learning models, with an emphasis on the LP-CNN model. Due to its efficient resource utilization and compact design, LP-CNN emerges as a compelling alternative. LP-CNN has fewer parameters than models such as DenseNet169 (14.14 million), DenseNet201 (20.05 million), InceptionResNetV2 (54.95 million), VGG19 (20.485), and Xception (24.139 million). The efficiency of the LP-CNN model is accentuated by its trainable parameters, which total 1.656 million. LP-CNN balances model complexity and performance compared to DenseNet169 (1.498 million) and DenseNet201 (1.728 million). In addition, the modest depth of LP-CNN, as indicated by its eight CL, contrasts with the complexity of architectures such as DenseNet169 (598 CL), DenseNet201 (710 CL), InceptionResNetV2 (783 CL), VGG19 (25 CL), and Xception (135 CL). LP-CNN has a model size of only 19.1 megabytes, an advantage due to its efficient resource utilization. Compared to other models like DenseNet169 (66.9 MB), DenseNet201 (91.4 MB), InceptionResNetV2 (216 MB), VGG19 (81.7 MB), and Xception (117 MB), LP-CNN stands out because of its smaller size. In conclusion, the LP-CNN model provides an efficient and effective method for classifying CXRs. Its compact architecture, an optimal number of parameters, and resource-conscious design position it as a promising solution for accurate and expeditious medical image analysis, demonstrating its potential for implementation and deployment in real-world healthcare settings. Figure 10 illustrates a bar chart of computational resources.

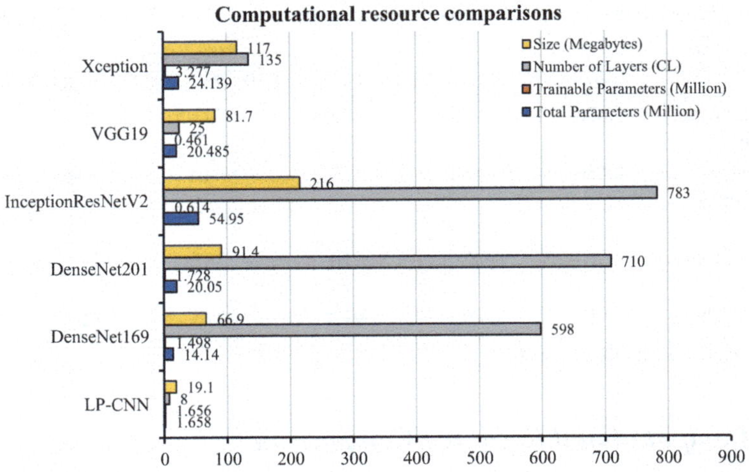

Fig. 10 Computational resource comparison among proposed LP-CNN and others

3.5 *Comparative Analysis with Others Work*

The LP-CNN (three-class classification) approach outshines all other models examined in detecting tuberculosis (see Table 9). SVM, CNN, and transfer learning methods were investigated, but the evaluation scores differed from the LP-CNN model. The LP-CNN model accurately identified classes with exceptional precision with a mean Precision (mP) of 99%. Its mean Recall (mR) of 98.33% effectively captures instances of true positivity. The model's mean F1-score (mF1) of 99.33% demonstrates an exceptional balance of precision and recall for accurate diagnosis. The LP-CNN model's mean Accuracy (mAcc) of 99.46% is outstanding, proving its predictions are consistently accurate.

Furthermore, the LP-CNN model's AUC rises to an exceptional 99.93%, which is a testament to its ability to differentiate between normal, non-TB, and TB cases. In contrast, other state-of-the-art models had AUC values ranging from 66 to 98.18%. The LP-CNN model's performance is indisputably dominant, and its extraordinary evaluation scores conclusively establish its superiority. It sets a new standard for tuberculosis classification in chest X-ray images.

4 Model Interpretability with SHAP

The use of SHAP (Shapley Additive Explanations) in combination with the LP-CNN model for tuberculosis (TB) classification is significant in enhancing the model and improving medical diagnosis. The model categorizes cases into Normal, non-TB, and TB, and the integration of SHAP provides a deeper understanding

Table 9 Comparative analysis with proposed model with others work

References	Dataset	CXR samples	Methodology	Evaluation scores
Singh et al. [32]	CHN, MC	805	Support vector machine (SVM)	Specificity- 100% and AUC- 96%
Pasa et al. [39]	MC, Belarus, and CHN	1111	CNN	AUC- 90% (CNH), 92.5% (combined), and 81.1% (MC)
Nguyen et al. [40]	CHN, MC	805	Fine-tuned DenseNet	AUC- 82% (MC) and 94% (CHN)
Hernández et al. [33]	CHN, MC	805	Three TL models	Accuracy- 86%
Ahsan et al. [35]	CHN, MC	805	VGG19	Accuracy- 81.25% (augmented) and 80% (w/o augmented)
Jaeger et al. [53]	Private dataset	135	CNN (binary class with TB)	AUC- 66%
Meraj et al. [54]	CHN, MC	805	CNN	AUC- 85%
Bhosale et al. [55]	NIH	10,800	CNN (nine class with TB)	AUC-98.18%
Yang et al. [56]	NIAD TB	2233	ML classifier	Accuracy- 72%
Our	**NIAID and CELL**	**10,500**	**LP-CNN (three class classification)**	**mP- 99%, mR- 98.33%, mF1- 98.33%, mAcc- 99.46%, and AUC- 99.93%**

[a]Bold values indicate the best results

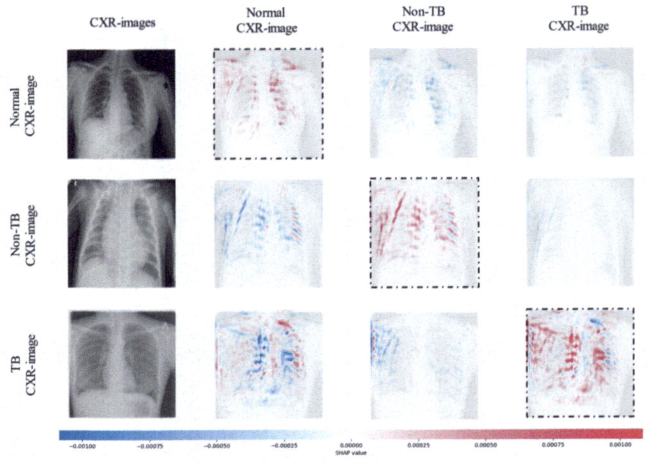

Fig. 11 Model insight visibility on prediction using SHAP

of the model's predictive outcomes. This transparency fosters trust in its decision-making process within the medical domain. In deep learning and medical diagnosis, the model must be interpretable. SHAP addresses complex models' "black box" nature by attributing individual feature contributions to the model's predictions. This transparency enables healthcare practitioners and experts to comprehend the rationale behind each prediction, allowing for better insights. It is crucial to build confidence in the model's performance and integrate it into the clinical workflow. The interpretation of SHAP values through red and blue points further enhances the model's interpretability. The red points represent features that push the model's prediction toward the particular class, highlighting the diagnostically relevant areas of the image. On the other hand, blue points indicate features contributing to the model's prediction to the other classes. This visual representation helps medical professionals identify the specific regions within a chest X-ray that influence the model's classification, aiding them in validating the model's findings. We can connect advanced deep-learning techniques with valuable medical insights by integrating SHAP with the LP-CNN model.

Figure 11 illustrates the process of gaining insights from CXR images. In the top row, the highest concentration of red pixels in the initial column signifies images falling into the normal category. The second row reveals the maximum red points clustered in the second column, corresponding to the non-TB class. An image in the third row displays a red point in the first and third columns. However, the predominant number of red points in the third column is attributed to being categorized as TB. TB image classification risks misclassification due to multiple sections with red points, a challenge overcome by our LP-CNN model's accurate discernment. It empowers healthcare practitioners to leverage the model's predictive capabilities and gain a clearer understanding of the image features that drive those predictions. This synergy between machine learning and medical expertise can improve diagnostic accuracy, streamline clinical decision-making, and enhance patient care in tuberculosis classification and beyond.

5 Conclusion

This study introduces a new LP-CNN (Lightweight Parallel CNN) method for detecting tuberculosis in Chest X-ray images. LP-CNN is designed to have fewer parameters and layers, making it simpler than other models. The process involves two main steps: identifying TB-infected images from Healthy and non-TB (Bacterial and viral pneumonia) cases and enhancing model interpretability using SHAP in the context of CXR images. LP-CNN performs better than other pre-trained deep learning models, achieving an impressive accuracy of 99.46% with CLAHE pre-processing. The study also introduces a novel stacking strategy, which results in exceptional scores of 99% precision, 98.33% recall, 98.33% F1-score, and 99.93% AUC. This sets a new benchmark in the field of TB detection. By incorporating SHAP, the LP-CNN model gains enhanced interpretability, providing insight into the reasoning behind its predictions and establishing its role as a reliable diagnostic tool. This innovative TB detection framework can speed up timely detection, especially without medical experts. This rapid and accurate diagnostic tool may save countless lives by preventing incorrect or delayed diagnoses.

References

1. Tuberculosis, (n.d.). https://www.who.int/news-room/fact-sheets/detail/tuberculosis. Accessed 14 Aug 2023
2. S.K. Sharma, A. Mohan, Tuberculosis: From an incurable scourge to a curable disease-journey over a millennium. Indian J. Med. Res. **137**, 455 (2013)
3. C. Silverman, An appraisal of the contribution of mass radiography in the discovery of pulmonary tuberculosis. Am. Rev. Tuberc. **60**, 466–482 (1949)
4. A.H. van't Hoog, H.K. Meme, K.F. Laserson, J.A. Agaya, B.G. Muchiri, W.A. Githui, L.O. Odeny, B.J. Marston, M.W. Borgdorff, Screening strategies for tuberculosis prevalence surveys: The value of chest radiography and symptoms. PLoS One **7**, e38691 (2012)
5. A.P. Brady, Error and discrepancy in radiology: Inevitable or avoidable? Insights Imaging **8**, 171–182 (2017)
6. A.J. Degnan, E.H. Ghobadi, P. Hardy, E. Krupinski, E.P. Scali, L. Stratchko, A. Ulano, E. Walker, A.P. Wasnik, W.F. Auffermann, Perceptual and interpretive error in diagnostic radiology—Causes and potential solutions. Acad. Radiol. **26**, 833–845 (2019)
7. H. Greenspan, B. Van Ginneken, R.M. Summers, Guest editorial deep learning in medical imaging: Overview and future promise of an exciting new technique. IEEE Trans. Med. Imaging **35**, 1153–1159 (2016)
8. V. Acharya, G. Dhiman, K. Prakasha, P. Bahadur, A. Choraria, M. Sushobhitha, J. Sowjanya, S. Prabhu, K. Chadaga, W. Viriyasitavat, S. Kautish, AI-assisted tuberculosis detection and classification from chest X-rays using a deep learning normalization-free network model. Comput. Intell. Neurosci. **2022**, 2399428 (2022). https://doi.org/10.1155/2022/2399428
9. M.E.H. Chowdhury, T. Rahman, A. Khandakar, S. Al-Madeed, S.M. Zughaier, S.A.R. Doi, H. Hassen, M.T. Islam, An early warning tool for predicting mortality risk of COVID-19 patients using machine learning. Cogn. Comput. (2021). https://doi.org/10.1007/s12559-020-09812-7

10. A. Iqbal, M. Usman, Z. Ahmed, An efficient deep learning-based framework for tuberculosis detection using chest X-ray images. Tuberculosis **136**, 102234 (2022). https://doi.org/10.1016/j.tube.2022.102234
11. M.E.H. Chowdhury, T. Rahman, A. Khandakar, R. Mazhar, M.A. Kadir, Z.B. Mahbub, K.R. Islam, M.S. Khan, A. Iqbal, N.A. Emadi, M.B.I. Reaz, M.T. Islam, Can AI help in screening viral and COVID-19 pneumonia? IEEE Access **8**, 132665–132676 (2020). https://doi.org/10.1109/ACCESS.2020.3010287
12. M. Nahiduzzaman, M.R. Islam, R. Hassan, ChestX-Ray6: Prediction of multiple diseases including COVID-19 from chest X-ray images using convolutional neural network. Expert Syst. Appl. **211**, 118576 (2023). https://doi.org/10.1016/j.eswa.2022.118576
13. M.R. Islam, M. Nahiduzzaman, Complex features extraction with deep learning model for the detection of COVID19 from CT scan images using ensemble based machine learning approach. Expert Syst. Appl. **195**, 116554 (2022). https://doi.org/10.1016/j.eswa.2022.116554
14. M. Yamaç, M. Ahishali, A. Degerli, S. Kiranyaz, M.E.H. Chowdhury, M. Gabbouj, Convolutional sparse support estimator-based COVID-19 recognition from X-ray images. IEEE Trans. Neural Netw. Learn. Syst. **32**, 1810–1820 (2021). https://doi.org/10.1109/TNNLS.2021.3070467
15. A.M. Tahir, M.E.H. Chowdhury, A. Khandakar, T. Rahman, Y. Qiblawey, U. Khurshid, S. Kiranyaz, N. Ibtehaz, M.S. Rahman, S. Al-Maadeed, S. Mahmud, M. Ezeddin, K. Hameed, T. Hamid, COVID-19 infection localization and severity grading from chest X-ray images. Comput. Biol. Med. **139**, 105002 (2021). https://doi.org/10.1016/j.compbiomed.2021.105002
16. A.M. Ismael, A. Şengür, Deep learning approaches for COVID-19 detection based on chest X-ray images. Expert Syst. Appl. **164**, 114054 (2021). https://doi.org/10.1016/J.ESWA.2020.114054
17. S. Kazemzadeh, J. Yu, S. Jamshy, R. Pilgrim, Z. Nabulsi, C. Chen, N. Beladia, C. Lau, S.M. McKinney, T. Hughes, A.P. Kiraly, S.R. Kalidindi, M. Muyoyeta, J. Malemela, T. Shih, G.S. Corrado, L. Peng, K. Chou, P.-H.C. Chen, Y. Liu, K. Eswaran, D. Tse, S. Shetty, S. Prabhakara, Deep learning detection of active pulmonary tuberculosis at chest radiography matched the clinical performance of radiologists. Radiology **306**, 124–137 (2022). https://doi.org/10.1148/radiol.212213
18. A.M. Tahir, Y. Qiblawey, A. Khandakar, T. Rahman, U. Khurshid, F. Musharavati, M.T. Islam, S. Kiranyaz, S. Al-Maadeed, M.E.H. Chowdhury, Deep learning for reliable classification of COVID-19, MERS, and SARS from chest X-ray images. Cogn. Comput., 1–21 (2022)
19. Y. Qiblawey, A. Tahir, M.E.H. Chowdhury, A. Khandakar, S. Kiranyaz, T. Rahman, N. Ibtehaz, S. Mahmud, S.A. Maadeed, F. Musharavati, M.A. Ayari, Detection and severity classification of COVID-19 in CT images using deep learning. Diagnostics **11** (2021). https://doi.org/10.3390/diagnostics11050893
20. M. Nahiduzzaman, M.O. Faruq Goni, M. Robiul Islam, A. Sayeed, M. Shamim Anower, M. Ahsan, J. Haider, M. Kowalski, Detection of various lung diseases including COVID-19 using extreme learning machine algorithm based on the features extracted from a lightweight CNN architecture. Biocybern. Biomed. Eng. **43**, 528–550 (2023). https://doi.org/10.1016/j.bbe.2023.06.003
21. T. Rahman, A. Khandakar, Y. Qiblawey, A. Tahir, S. Kiranyaz, S. Bin Abul Kashem, M.T. Islam, S. Al Maadeed, S.M. Zughaier, M.S. Khan, M.E.H. Chowdhury, Exploring the effect of image enhancement techniques on COVID-19 detection using chest X-ray images. Comput. Biol. Med. **132**, 104319 (2021). https://doi.org/10.1016/j.compbiomed.2021.104319
22. S. Hansun, A. Argha, S.-T. Liaw, B.G. Celler, G.B. Marks, Machine and deep learning for tuberculosis detection on chest X-rays: Systematic literature review. J. Med. Internet Res. **25**, e43154 (2023). https://doi.org/10.2196/43154
23. O. Sarkar, M.R. Islam, M.K. Syfullah, M.T. Islam, M.F. Ahamed, M. Ahsan, J. Haider, Multi-scale CNN: An explainable AI-integrated unique deep learning framework for lung-affected disease classification. Technologies **11** (2023). https://doi.org/10.3390/technologies11050134
24. T. Rahman, A. Khandakar, M.A. Kadir, K.R. Islam, K.F. Islam, R. Mazhar, T. Hamid, M.T. Islam, S. Kashem, Z.B. Mahbub, M.A. Ayari, M.E.H. Chowdhury, Reliable tuberculosis

detection using chest X-ray with deep learning, segmentation and visualization. IEEE Access **8**, 191586–191601 (2020). https://doi.org/10.1109/ACCESS.2020.3031384
25. T. Rahman, M.E.H. Chowdhury, A. Khandakar, K.R. Islam, K.F. Islam, Z.B. Mahbub, M.A. Kadir, S. Kashem, Transfer learning with deep convolutional neural network (CNN) for pneumonia detection using chest X-ray. Appl. Sci. **10** (2020). https://doi.org/10.3390/app10093233
26. S.I. Nafisah, G. Muhammad, Tuberculosis detection in chest radiograph using convolutional neural network architecture and explainable artificial intelligence. Neural Comput. & Applic. (2022). https://doi.org/10.1007/s00521-022-07258-6
27. J. Melendez, B. Van Ginneken, P. Maduskar, R.H.H.M. Philipsen, K. Reither, M. Breuninger, I.M.O. Adetifa, R. Maane, H. Ayles, C.I. Sánchez, A novel multiple-instance learning-based approach to computer-aided detection of tuberculosis on chest X-rays. IEEE Trans. Med. Imaging **34**, 179–192 (2014)
28. S. Jaeger, A. Karargyris, S. Antani, G. Thoma, Detecting tuberculosis in radiographs using combined lung masks, in *2012 Annual International Conference of the IEEE Engineering in Medicine and Biology Society*, (2012), pp. 4978–4981
29. B. Van Ginneken, S. Katsuragawa, B.M. ter Haar Romeny, K. Doi, M.A. Viergever, Automatic detection of abnormalities in chest radiographs using local texture analysis. IEEE Trans. Med. Imaging **21**, 139–149 (2002)
30. H. Das, A. Nath, An efficient detection of tuberculosis from chest X-rays. Int. J. Adv. Res. Comput. Sci. Manag. Stud. **3**, 149–154 (2015)
31. T. Nishtar, S. Burki, F.S. Ahmad, T. Ahmad, Diagnostic accuracy of computer aided reading of chest x-ray in screening for pulmonary tuberculosis in comparison with Gene-Xpert. Pakistan J. Med. Sci. **38**, 62–68 (2022). https://doi.org/10.12669/pjms.38.1.4531
32. N. Singh, S. Hamde, Tuberculosis detection using shape and texture features of chest X-rays, in *Innovations in Electronics and Communication Engineering Proceedings 7th ICIECE 2018*, (2019), pp. 43–50
33. A. Hernández, Á. Panizo, D. Camacho, An ensemble algorithm based on deep learning for tuberculosis classification, in *Intelligent Data Engineering and Automated Learning—IDEAL 2019, 20th International Conference, Manchester, UK, November 14–16, 2019, Proceedings, Part I 20*, (2019), pp. 145–154
34. U.K. Lopes, J.F. Valiati, Pre-trained convolutional neural networks as feature extractors for tuberculosis detection. Comput. Biol. Med. **89**, 135–143 (2017)
35. M. Ahsan, R. Gomes, A. Denton, Application of a convolutional neural network using transfer learning for tuberculosis detection, in *2019 IEEE International Conference on Electro Information Technology (EIT)*, (2019), pp. 427–433
36. O. Yadav, K. Passi, C.K. Jain, Using deep learning to classify X-ray images of potential tuberculosis patients, in *2018 IEEE International Conference on Bioinformatics and Biomedicine (BIBM)*, (2018), pp. 2368–2375
37. A. Abbas, M.M. Abdelsamea, M.M. Gaber, Detrac: Transfer learning of class decomposed medical images in convolutional neural networks. IEEE Access **8**, 74901–74913 (2020)
38. R.-I. Chang, Y.-H. Chiu, J.-W. Lin, Two-stage classification of tuberculosis culture diagnosis using convolutional neural network with transfer learning. J. Supercomput. **76**, 8641–8656 (2020)
39. F. Pasa, V. Golkov, F. Pfeiffer, D. Cremers, D. Pfeiffer, Efficient deep network architectures for fast chest X-ray tuberculosis screening and visualization. Sci. Rep. **9**, 6268 (2019)
40. Q.H. Nguyen, B.P. Nguyen, S.D. Dao, B. Unnikrishnan, R. Dhingra, S.R. Ravichandran, S. Satpathy, P.N. Raja, M.C.H. Chua, Deep learning models for tuberculosis detection from chest X-ray images, in *2019 26th International Conference on Telecommunications (ICT)*, (2019), pp. 381–385
41. A. Rosenthal, A. Gabrielian, E. Engle, D.E. Hurt, S. Alexandru, V. Crudu, E. Sergueev, V. Kirichenko, V. Lapitskii, E. Snezhko, V. Kovalev, A. Astrovko, A. Skrahina, J. Taaffe, M. Harris, A. Long, K. Wollenberg, I. Akhundova, S. Ismayilova, A. Skrahin, E. Mammadbayov, H. Gadirova, R. Abuzarov, M. Seyfaddinova, Z. Avaliani, I. Strambu, D. Zaharia, A. Muntean,

E. Ghita, M. Bogdan, R. Mindru, V. Spinu, A. Sora, C. Ene, S. Vashakidze, N. Shubladze, U. Nanava, A. Tuzikov, M. Tartakovsky, The TB portals: An open-access, web-based platform for global drug-resistant- tuberculosis data sharing and analysis. J. Clin. Microbiol. **55**, 3267–3282 (2017). https://doi.org/10.1128/JCM.01013-17

42. D.S. Kermany, M. Goldbaum, W. Cai, C.C.S. Valentim, H. Liang, S.L. Baxter, A. McKeown, G. Yang, X. Wu, F. Yan, J. Dong, M.K. Prasadha, J. Pei, M. Ting, J. Zhu, C. Li, S. Hewett, J. Dong, I. Ziyar, A. Shi, R. Zhang, L. Zheng, R. Hou, W. Shi, X. Fu, Y. Duan, V.A.N. Huu, C. Wen, E.D. Zhang, C.L. Zhang, O. Li, X. Wang, M.A. Singer, X. Sun, J. Xu, A. Tafreshi, M.A. Lewis, H. Xia, K. Zhang, Identifying medical diagnoses and treatable diseases by image-based deep learning. Cell **172**, 1122–1131.e9 (2018). https://doi.org/10.1016/j.cell.2018.02.010
43. K. Koonsanit, S. Thongvigitmanee, N. Pongnapang, P. Thajchayapong, Image enhancement on digital x-ray images using N-CLAHE, in *2017 10th Biomedical Engineering International Conference (BMEiCON)*, (2017), pp. 1–4. https://doi.org/10.1109/BMEiCON.2017.8229130
44. C. Szegedy, W. Liu, Y. Jia, P. Sermanet, S. Reed, D. Anguelov, D. Erhan, V. Vanhoucke, A. Rabinovich, Going deeper with convolutions, in *Proceedings of the 2015 IEEE Conference on Computer Vision and Pattern Recognition (CVPR)*, (2015), pp. 1–9
45. M. Nahiduzzaman, M. Robiul Islam, M. Omaer Faruq Goni, M. Shamim Anower, M. Ahsan, J. Haider, M. Kowalski, Diabetic retinopathy identification using parallel convolutional neural network based feature extractor and ELM classifier. Expert Syst. Appl. **217**, 119557 (2023). https://doi.org/10.1016/j.eswa.2023.119557
46. M. Nahiduzzaman, M.O.F. Goni, R. Hassan, M.R. Islam, M.K. Syfullah, S.M. Shahriar, M.S. Anower, M. Ahsan, J. Haider, M. Kowalski, Parallel CNN-ELM: A multiclass classification of chest X-ray images to identify seventeen lung diseases including COVID-19. Expert Syst. Appl. **229**, 120528 (2023). https://doi.org/10.1016/j.eswa.2023.120528
47. A. Krizhevsky, I. Sutskever, G.E. Hinton, ImageNet classification with deep convolutional neural networks. Commun. ACM **60**, 84–90 (2017). https://doi.org/10.1145/3065386
48. R. Tri Wahyuningrum, A. Kusumaningsih, W. Putra Rajeb, I.K. Eddy Purnama, Classification of corn leaf disease using the optimized DenseNet-169 model, in *Proceedings of the 2021 the 9th International Conference on Information Technology: IoT and Smart City*, (2021), pp. 67–73
49. C. Zhao, R. Shuai, L. Ma, W. Liu, D. Hu, M. Wu, Dermoscopy image classification based on StyleGAN and DenseNet201. IEEE Access **9**, 8659–8679 (2021)
50. Y. Bhatia, A. Bajpayee, D. Raghuvanshi, H. Mittal, Image captioning using Google's inception-resnet-v2 and recurrent neural network, in *2019 Twelfth International Conference on Contemporary Computing (IC3)*, (2019), pp. 1–6
51. T.R.G.V. Sudha, A convolutional neural network classifier VGG-19 architecture for lesion detection and grading in diabetic retinopathy based on deep learning. Comput. Mater. Contin. **66**, 827–842 (2021). https://doi.org/10.32604/cmc.2020.012008
52. F. Chollet, Xception: Deep learning with depthwise separable convolutions, in *Proceedings of the IEEE Conference on Computer Vision and Pattern Recognition (CVPR)*, (Institute of Electrical and Electronics Engineers Inc, 2017), pp. 1251–1258. https://doi.org/10.1109/CVPR.2017.195
53. S. Jaeger, O.H. Juarez-Espinosa, S. Candemir, M. Poostchi, F. Yang, L. Kim, M. Ding, L.R. Folio, S. Antani, A. Gabrielian, Others, detecting drug-resistant tuberculosis in chest radiographs. Int. J. Comput. Assist. Radiol. Surg. **13**, 1915–1925 (2018)
54. S.S. Meraj, R. Yaakob, A. Azman, S. Rum, A. Shahrel, A. Nazri, N.F. Zakaria, Detection of pulmonary tuberculosis manifestation in chest X-rays using different convolutional neural network (CNN) models. Int. J. Eng. Adv. Technol. (IJEAT) **9**, 2270–2275 (2019)
55. Y.H. Bhosale, K.S. Patnaik, IoT deployable lightweight deep learning application for COVID-19 detection with lung diseases using RaspberryPi, in *2022 International Conference on IoT and Blockchain Technology (ICIBT)*, (2022), pp. 1–6
56. F. Yang, H. Yu, K. Kantipudi, M. Karki, Y.M. Kassim, A. Rosenthal, D.E. Hurt, Z. Yaniv, S. Jaeger, Differentiating between drug-sensitive and drug-resistant tuberculosis with machine learning for clinical and radiological features. Quant. Imaging Med. Surg. **12**, 675–687 (2022). https://doi.org/10.21037/qims-21-290

Continuous Physiological Signal Monitoring Using Wearables for the Early Detection of Infectious Diseases: A Review

S. K. Somasundaram, S. Sridevi, Murugappan Murugappan, and B. Vinoth Kumar

1 Introduction

Infectious diseases (ID) are one of the most important types of diseases which affect nearly 17 million people in the world per year. According to a recent report from the World Health Organization, 14% of deaths are due to ID [1]. There are several types of ID, such as Pneumonia, AIDS/HIV, Malaria, Tuberculosis, diarrhea, Chickenpox, Hepatitis B, Measles, Mumps, and others. Among the different types of ID, Tuberculosis, HIV/AIDS, and Malaria are the top three infectious diseases that have caused a greater number of casualties over the years in the World [2]. Pathogen detection is one of the most important steps in designing a diagnosis and developing a control management strategy to reduce the infection spread and save human/plant lives. Wearables may provide useful information for ID surveillance and early detection mechanisms, but they cannot replace conventional medical

S. K. Somasundaram · S. Sridevi
Department of Information Security, School of Computer Science and Engineering, Vellore Institute of Technology, Vellore, Tamil Nadu, India

M. Murugappan (✉)
Intelligent Signal Processing (ISP) Research Lab, Department of Electronics and Communication Engineering, Kuwait College of Science and Technology, Doha, Kuwait

Department of Electronics and Communication Engineering, School of Engineering, Vels Institute of Sciences, Technology, and Advanced Studies, Chennai, India

Center of Excellence for Unmanned Aerial Systems (CoEUAS), Universiti Malaysia Perlis, Perlis, Malaysia
e-mail: m.murugappan@kcst.edu.kw

B. Vinoth Kumar
Department of Information Technology, PSG College of Technology, Coimbatore, Tamil Nadu, India
e-mail: bvk.it@psgtech.ac.in

M. E. H. Chowdhury, S. Kiranyaz (eds.), *Surveillance, Prevention, and Control of Infectious Diseases*, https://doi.org/10.1007/978-3-031-59967-5_9

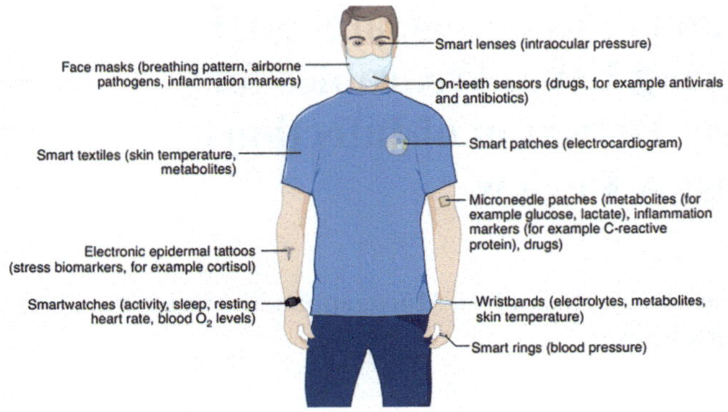

Fig. 1 Wearable sensors used for ID detection [6]

diagnosis or testing. The conventional testing methods are based on the samples of blood, urine, and other human products to detect ID. Whenever wearable data shows odd patterns, a medical examination and testing should be performed to confirm whether an infectious illness exists. However, lab testing-based pathogen detection takes a longer time compared to a faster diagnosis result through wearable sensors and AI tools. In addition, when collecting medical data using wearable sensors, the user's permission and privacy are crucial considerations. In terms of the diagnosis of ID, wearable sensors, artificial intelligence (AI) tools based on text inputs, and non-contact sensors are also widely used to detect ID. As a part of public health surveillance and early disease identification, wearable sensor devices play an important role in tracking and observing infectious diseases.

Some of the major advantages of using wearable sensors to predict ID are: (i) wearable sensors are completely non-invasive and non-intrusive (ii) they can provide a continuous monitoring of physiological activity (iii) cost cost-effective and portable and smaller in size, and (iv) provide more reliable and accurate information about human physiological activity. In recent years, researchers have developed a non-invasive wearable sensor to predict the ID such as H1N1 and rhinovirus due to viral infection 24 hours before onset with a maximum detection rate of 90% using random forest (RF) models [3]. Detecting abnormal heart rate variability (HRV), skin temperature (ST), galvanic skin response (GSR), and resting heart rate (HR) through wearable sensors could be used to predict the ID before its onset (Fig. 1) [3]. Similarly, the most recent study has also predicted influenza A (H3N2) using a wearable sensor and AI before 23 hours of onset [4]. A detailed review of different biomedical wearable sensor-based infectious disease detection and the use of AI have been documented in [5]. Some of the most common physiological parameters that could be used to detect the ID are given below:

- Body Temperature [7]: Infectious disorders can be categorized and tracked using body temperature, although it is often used as one of many signs rather than a reliable diagnostic tool. However, it is important to remember that body temperature alone cannot diagnose a particular infectious condition. A diagnosis can only be made based on additional indicators, clinical evaluations, test results (e.g. PCR or serological tests), and medical history. In addition to assessing temperature data for disease prediction, other factors like specific variations in temperature and non-transmission factors that cause fever should also be considered.

- Heart rate variability (HRV) [8]: Symptoms of infection and illness can be detected by variations in heart rate variability (HRV) parameters. The difference between a person's normal HRV and a disease's normal range can be an indication that the disease is on its way. Infectious diseases are often monitored and classified using HRV and heart rate (HR). Additionally, other clinical data, including symptoms, results of testing, and past medical records, must be analyzed together with HRV data. These factors, however, should not be used as stand-alone diagnostic instruments since they are merely part of an in-depth assessment of a patient's illness. Further, individual variances in HRV should be considered when interpreting the results, as well as variables like activity level and stress.
- Respiratory Rate (RR) [9]: Many wearable devices have features that can track breathing rates. According to studies, respiratory illnesses may cause changes in breathing rate. It is important to evaluate breathing data analysis in the context of other clinical information. Physical examination results, laboratory test results (such as lung function tests or chest X-rays), and health history are also considered. The measurements should be used as part of a complete assessment, not as a diagnostic tool on their own. Furthermore, these data may be affected by individual variations in respiration rate (or) stress (or) physical exertion.
- Blood Oxygen Saturation (SpO2) [10]: Monitoring the blood oxygen level plays a crucial role in monitoring the respiratory system's health. This is called blood oxygen saturation (SpO2). A sudden decline in SpO2 could be a sign of respiratory problems, including infections. Even though SpO2 measurements are useful, they should also be compared with other clinical data, such as physiological signs, physical examination results, laboratory results (like blood gas analyses and chest X-rays), and past medical history. As a result, SpO2 measurements should not be used as a standalone diagnostic tool since they are just one component of surveillance to predict infectious diseases. A SpO2 reading may be used by patients and medical professionals to assess the condition of their respiratory system in depth.
- Cough Detection [11]: In the near future, advanced wearable sensors may be able to recognize coughing patterns using microphones and artificial intelligence (AI) techniques. Some infections can cause coughing more frequently. Methods for predicting and monitoring coughs can differ based on the amount of data and the level of accuracy they provide.
- Geolocation and Contact Tracing [12, 13]: Global Positioning System or Bluetooth technology may be used in wearables to monitor behaviors and interactions with others. In the event of an outbreak of an illness, this kind of data may

be useful for locating contacts. A GPS and contact monitoring program's effectiveness in predicting infectious infections depends on the accuracy of the data, prompt recognition, and public compliance.

In recent years, ChatGPT [14] has also been used to diagnose the ID through text/speech/image inputs. Compared to the conventional methods of testing in labs for pathogens using chemicals, disease detection through wearable sensors and AI tools is costlier. Current research attempts to adopt a multidisciplinary approach for both the identification of underlying pathogenic agents and the control of infectious diseases. In AI, Machine Learning algorithms (MLA) are most widely used to detect ID. According to a recent report, the majority of the work has focused on bacteria-based ID detection followed by viruses, tuberculosis, and other pathogens [15]. Indeed, disease detection is mostly considered by researchers through different modality-based inputs followed by prediction, early prediction, prognosis, and others. In [16], the authors have developed a wearable sensor that is placed on a suprasternal notch to extract the data on cardio-respiratory function, physical activity, and cough sounds over a short period to detect COVID-19. The proposed system has been tested with a limited number of COVID-19 and normal controls (14 subjects) and achieved a maximum Area Under Curve (AUC) of 94% using a logistic regression classifier. They also reported that the heart rate, respiration rate, and other physiological parameters of a COVID-19 patient are completely different from normal controls. In a recent study, the researchers used wearable sensors in smartwatches to monitor heart rate signals and steps to detect SARS-CoV-19 at an early stage. The experimental results have proved that real-time algorithms can detect COVID-19 at an early stage using AI algorithms [17].

The major physiological indicators and the type of wearable sensors used to collect the physiological responses to detect the ID are given in Table 1. It also shows the optimal range of the physiological parameters and the risk stratification methods. From the table, it is highly evident that physiological responses such as HR, HRV, ST, and GSR are most preferably used for predicting or diagnosing ID using wearable sensors.

1.1 Objective and Collection of Articles

In this review, we have collected several articles related to Infectious Diseases (ID) detection using conventional (lab-based) and wearable sensors from different sources. Later, we removed the papers which are not relevant to this review such as the papers that are related to conventional methods-based ID detection, non-wearable sensor-based ID detection, and the literature review articles relevant to ID and non-infectious disease (NID) detection. Figure 2 shows the overview of collecting the paper for this review.

Table 1 Wearable devices and physiological indicators to detect the Infectious Disease

Physiological Parameters	Device used	Normal range	Symptom Identification	Pattern Recognition	Risk stratification	Disease Diagnosis
Body Temperature [7]	Smartwatches, Wearable Thermometer Patches, smart rings, and clothing	98.6 °F or 37 °C	Warm or cold, sweating, or shivering	Early morning—lowest temperatures Late afternoon or early evening—the highest temperature	High	Influenza (Flu), COVID-19, Malaria, Tuberculosis (TB), gastroenteritis, cellulitis, and viral hepatitis
Heart Rate (HR) and Heart Rate Variability (HRV) [8]	Smartwatches, Fitness Trackers, Chest Straps, Wearable ECG Monitors and Wearable HRV Monitors	Heart rate—60 to 100 beats per minute (bpm). High HRV—50 to 200 ms Low HRV—below 50 ms	Fatigue, stress, anxiety, or changes in heart rate,	Depends on person's activities such as resting, exercise, and so forth.	High	Tachycardia, Sepsis, Viral Myocarditis, Respiratory Infections
Respiratory Rate [9]	Smartwatches, Fitness Trackers, Chest Straps, Smart Clothing, Dedicated Respiratory Rate Monitors	Adults: 12–20 breaths per minute Infants (1–12 months): 25–40 breaths per minute Young children (1–5 years): 20–30 breaths per minute Older children (6–12 years): 12–20 breaths per minute Adolescents (13–17 years): 12–16 breaths per minute	Rapid Breathing (Tachypnoea), Shallow Breathing, Cyanosis, Nasal Flaring, Chest Pain	Count the Respiratory Rate, Observe the Rhythm, Assess the Depth, Listen for Abnormal Sounds	High	Tachypnoea, Bradypnea, Cheyne-Stokes Respiration, Apnea, Paradoxical Breathing

(continued)

Table 1 (continued)

Physiological Parameters	Device used	Normal range	Symptom Identification	Pattern Recognition	Risk stratification	Disease Diagnosis
Oxygen Saturation (SpO_2) [10]	Smartwatches, Fitness Trackers, Smart Rings, Smart Glasses, Smart Clothing, few hearable devices	Healthy individual: 95–100%	Dyspnoea, Tachypnoea, Tachycardia, Cyanosis, Fatigue, Dizziness, headache, chest pain	SpO2 levels consistently fall below the normal range in association with shortness of breath, cyanosis, confusion, or dizziness	High	Hypoxemia, Acute Respiratory Distress Syndrome (ARDS), Chronic Obstructive Pulmonary Disease (COPD), Asthma, Sleep Apnea, Severe Anaemia Pulmonary Embolism
Cough Detection [11]	Smartwatches, Fitness Trackers, Smart Clothing, Wearable Health Monitors, Environmental Sensors	No quantitative range	Associated symptoms: Fever, Shortness of breath, Chest pain or discomfort, Sputum production, Weight loss, Night sweats, Runny nose, Sore throat	Cough Type, Cough Frequency, Cough Duration, Cough Characteristics (Barking Cough, Whooping Cough, Wheezing Cough, Staccato Cough), Nighttime Cough	Moderate	Chronic obstructive pulmonary disease (COPD), gastroesophageal reflux disease (GERD)
Geolocation and Contact Tracing [12, 13]	Smartphones, Smartwatches, Fitness Trackers, Wearable Tags and Badges, Wearable Safety Wearables, Wearable Social Distancing Devices, Wearable GPS Trackers, Wearable Panic Buttons	No quantitative range	Not associated with specific symptoms	Location Data Analysis, Interaction Analysis, Temporal Analysis, Geographic Analysis, Anomaly Detection, Contact Tracing Efficiency	High	Infectious Disease Control, Outbreak Investigation, Monitoring Quarantine and Isolation Epidemiological Studies

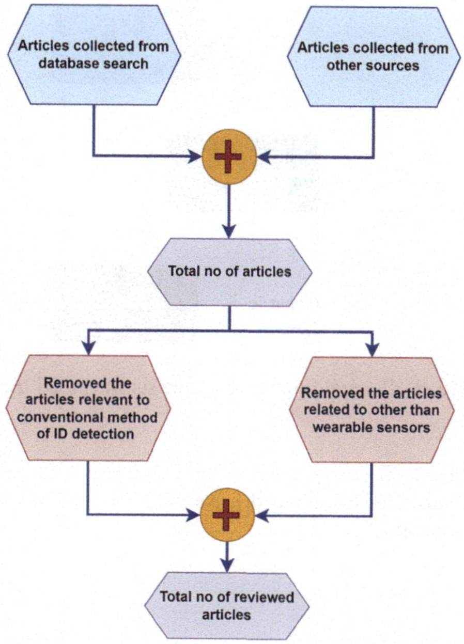

Fig. 2 Collection of research articles related to Infectious Disease (ID) detection

2 Methodology

Most of the existing literature related to ID detection follows the five different stages such as data acquisition, preprocessing, feature extraction, feature selection, and classification/diagnosis. This section will review the earlier works based on the individual section. Figure 3 shows the overview of the research methodology used for Infectious disease (ID) detection using wearable sensors.

(a) **Data acquisition**

Data acquisition is an essential part of wearable data processing because it makes it possible to gather, store, analyze, and utilize the data produced by wearable devices. It is fundamental in transforming sensor data from raw measurements into knowledge that may be applied to improve user quality of life, personalized healthcare, and research. Physionet [18] is a web-based repository that contains physiological and biomedical data widely used by academicians, researchers, students, and clinicians for their projects. It was created and managed by the PhysioNet Research Resource for Complex Physiologic Signals, a unit of the Physiological Measurement Laboratory at Beth Israel Deaconess Medical Center and Harvard Medical School. There are many different types of physiological data available in the database, such as time series data of physiological indicators including the Electrocardiogram (ECG), Electroencephalogram (EEG), blood pressure, respiration signals, etc. The details are useful for research and assessment since they are often collected from patients in medical settings. PhysioNet offers datasets so that academics can carry

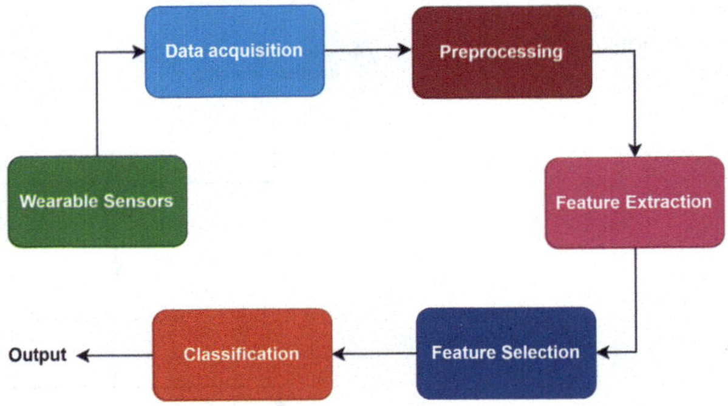

Fig. 3 General flow of wearable sensor-based Infectious disease (ID) detection

Fig. 4 Most useful wearable sensors for Infectious disease detection

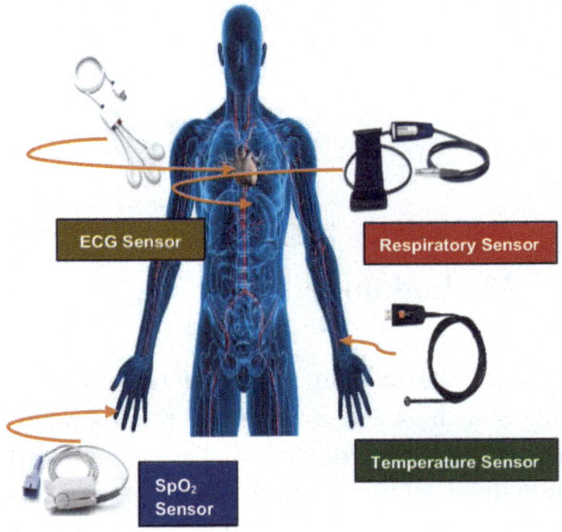

out experiments, generate and test newly developed algorithms, and enhance the study of physiological signal interpretation and analysis. Additionally, educational institutions can use it to educate students on biomedical statistical analysis as well as signal processing techniques. Following the proliferation of more datasets and new advanced technologies over time, PhysioNet keeps growing. It has significantly contributed to the development of investigations in the fields of cardiac monitoring, physiological signal analysis, and numerous other healthcare-related fields. The most promising and useful type of wearable sensor used for infectious disease detection is shown in Fig. 4.

(b) **Preprocessing**

A wearable sensor for detecting or monitoring infectious diseases is often affected by external noise signals (baseline wandering, powerline interference, muscular movement, etc.) generated by the body or by other external factors. Therefore, it is necessary to preprocess the acquired data to achieve high accuracy in ID detection. In general, preprocessing techniques have three major stages such as (1) data cleaning, (2) transforming the data into different dimensions or formats, and (3) preparing the data for analysis.

(i) **Noise removal**

Preprocessing noise from wearable devices is an important part of preparing a dataset for analysis. This increases the data's accuracy and quality, making it more suitable for analysis and interpretation. A wearable physiological monitoring system for real-time healthcare monitoring was proposed in [19]. They used Electrocardiogram (ECG)/Electromyogram (EMG) signals for monitoring cardiac patients in both indoor and outdoor environments. Adaptive digital filtering was used during data acquisition to eliminate noise caused by the indoor environment. A second-order low pass filter was used to eliminate power supply noise for ECG signals, while a twin-T notch filter was employed to minimize power line interference. A review of wearable sensors in chronic diseases was presented in [20]. Motion artifacts and contact noise are likely to occur during data acquisition from the sensors. Moreover, they mentioned that a high-pass filter has been used by many researchers to remove motion artifacts and low-impedance electrodes to reduce contact noise.

Consumer-grade wearables were employed [21] to detect the presence of infections in the population, specifically COVID-19. Heartbeat and respiration dynamics, walking cadence, and cough frequency spectrum have been used as physiological features. The authors used a 2nd order Butterworth low-pass filter with a cutoff frequency of 1 Hz to remove the noise in respiration rates and cough signals, as well as a wavelet denoising filter to remove the noise in cough signal features. They have also used a multi-tier signal filtering approach and a Discrete Wavelet Transform (DWT) approach to extract the R-R interval from sensor data. According to [22], authors discuss different methods for filtering ECG and Photoplethysmography (PPG) signals. The most common filters are wavelet transforms or Digital Signal Processing (DSP) filters such as low-pass, high-pass, band-pass, adaptive, Chebyshev, Kalman, and notch. Additionally, they mentioned that many studies are focused on removing motion artifacts during data acquisition using DSP methods.

Pulse oximeters, ECG, and temperature sensors were used to collect the body's temperature, blood pressure (BP), HR, respiration rate (RR), and pulse [23]. Cloud services were used to record and store sensor-managed data for analysis through Internet of Things (IoT) technology. Meanwhile, features are generated from a smartwatch dataset collected from 25 participants wearing Amazfit GTS 2 Band watches. Data collected from smartwatches was used to train the Ensemble Deep Learning-based AI-assisted diagnostic model, and results were predicted from the smartwatch-based dataset. Noise filtering methods are used to eliminate noise from the dataset.

Wearable biosensors such as smartwatches and fitness bands were used [24] to collect physiological information such as sleep rate, fluctuations in sleeping patterns, heart rate, and activity related to physical movement. Wearable sensors provide physiological data that can be used to identify anomalies. Researchers developed a technique to identify abnormalities based on physiological information. Using data from wearable devices, a prediction model was developed for the COVID-19 outbreak pattern in several nations. However, the authors have pointed out that the data could be affected due to different types of noises since the data has been collected from different hospitals in different cities. Therefore, a filtering technique or noise reduction method was required to solve the problem. However, the report does not describe the method used to reduce noise.

The method proposed in [25] involves collecting physiological data from wearable sensors, particularly PPG and ECG readings, which may be gained early in the treatment process by using a triage procedure. The authors also include pictures of wearable gadgets that could be used to collect ECG and PPG data. Wearable sensors that capture physiological data are frequently subject to noise and motion distortions, the authors note. This problem is addressed by employing a high pass filter followed by using a Gaussian filter for normalization. Texas Instruments (TI) Sensor Tag device was used in [26] to capture relevant physiological features. Data was collected using the infrared thermometer, gyroscope, and dynamic accelerometer on the Sensor Tag gadget. A chest-worn device, consisting of gyroscope sensors and accelerometers, was used to measure fluctuations in inertial activity during coughing and breathing periods, as well as temperature over a 10-minute period. Data is transferred in real-time to a computing device (computer) for analysis and abnormality detection. The Single Vector Activity Index (SVAI) is typically determined by the Standard Deviation of accelerometer data. Breathing and coughing patterns are monitored using the SVAI variable, and the. Density-Based Spatial Clustering of Applications with Noise (DBSCAN) algorithm is used to detect outliers as noise. The early signs of COVID-19 were determined by analysing physiological data obtained from chest-worn equipment. In [27] the authors proposed a healthcare framework using wearable sensors to collect the temperature, heartbeat, pulse, oxygen saturation, etc. to monitor and analyse health metrics. In the data rectification process, the Kalman filter, an unsupervised screening and filtering technique, is employed as a preprocessing tool to remove noise from data.

There are three main categories of preprocessing methods for wearable data collected from sensors: (1) data cleaning, (2) data transformation into new dimensions, and (3) data preparation for analysis. A significant part of the preprocessing of a wearable technology dataset is the removal of noise. To reduce power line interference and to remove power supply noise from ECG signals, several studies used a second-order low pass filter and a second-order twin-T notches filter. Moreover, they used low-impedance electrodes to eliminate contact noise and a high-pass filter to eliminate motion artifacts. Furthermore, the authors suggested using wearable sensors for physiological monitoring of medical conditions. A digital filtering process was applied to remove noise caused by the indoor environment during data collection. Among the most commonly used data preprocessing filters are wavelet transforms or DSP filters, such as notch, band-pass, adaptive, low-pass, high-pass, Chebyshev, and Kalman filters.

(ii) **Missing Data Handling**

Missing data is a crucial factor in the data analysis process, especially for data collected from wearable devices, or preserving data completeness, maintaining data quality, and facilitating data integration. Data acquired without values should be removed before being used and deployed in operation. Missing values are handled by replacing them with mean/median or zeros, moving averages, regression, correlation, k-nearest Neighbors (kNN), multivariate imputation, exclusion, and pixel gap filling in [28].

In [29], the authors confirmed the presence of COVID-19 by observing RR, HR, and HRV. An accelerometer and PPG sensor are used to collect data. The time between successive heartbeats is cleaned to remove noise due to missed heartbeats, motion artifacts, and electronic noise. The authors of [30] used heart rates and steps to detect COVID-19 disease. Resting Heart Rate (RHR) signals were mostly used, which are the heart rate recordings where steps are zero. They used resampling and windowing methods to locate the missing values in RHR signals.

With the help of wearable devices, the authors extricate data pertaining to pulse rate, temperature, oxygen saturation level, and temperature for health monitoring [27]. The proposed healthcare monitoring system collects health monitoring signals periodically from the patient's body and maintains them in dispersed edge devices by means of a network of wearable sensors. Correlation metrics were also employed to identify missing values from the incoming sensory data.

In [31], the research used a variety of commercially available (COTS) wearable devices to enable real-time inference about infection risk among US military personnel operating during the COVID-19 pandemic. Several wearable technologies were tested in the study, including Oura smart rings and Garmin smartwatches. An algorithmic technique used in this study extracts physical activity and hypnogram data during resting periods. After that, missing information was adjusted using an ensemble technique. Data from raw wearables were only collected during sleep time to minimize the effect of daily activities and other environmental factors on physiological movement. Several plausibility filters were used to eliminate measured values that were considered unreasonable or exceeded physiological limits. The process produced segmented time-series data for each physiological measurement (such as body temperature and heart rate), where each segment denoted a different sleep session. Based on the physiological data collected during sleep, three primary characteristics are identified: (1) sleep period analytics; (2) trend analytics; and (3) deviations from the individual baseline. The three feature types attempt to represent anomalous physiological characteristics in different ways. Statistics about the sleep period features, which included derived features such as maximum duration, minimum duration, median value, mean value, standard deviation, and interquartile range, were used to determine the distributional characteristics of physiological parameters from the most recent accessible sleep period. The authors stated that appropriate plausibility filters were applied to the raw wearables dataset to remove illogical values.

It is crucial to deal with missing data as part of the data analysis process, especially when dealing with data collected through wearable devices, to maintain the quality of the data, maintain the completeness of the data, and reduce the integration time. Missing values during data collection are considered noise that must be eliminated for practical application and implementation. The mean, median, moving average, pixel gap filling, zeros, correlation, regression, kNN, exclusion, and multivariate inference are used to replace missing values. Researchers examined physiological signs including heart rate variability, respiration rates, and variations in heart rate to evaluate COVID-19. A respiration rate periodic data is processed to eliminate noise caused by missed heartbeats, electronic noise, and movement possessions.

(iii) **Data Augmentation**

Before a machine learning model can be trained, numerous transformations and variations may be carried out to the original data during a preprocessing step called "data augmentation". This is an optional step in preprocessing and is used to limit the dataset to avoid overfitting and enhance the generalization capacity of the deep learning model. As a sample study, the authors developed a deep learning method for predicting COVID-19 infection using steps, time interval data, and heart rate collected from Fitbit devices [32]. By using various data augmentation approaches, the training data given by each user was roughly transformed eight times.

During the preprocessing stage, data enrichment or augmentation and feature engineering are crucial steps to extract significant features from the collected data. An approach that uses data augmentation makes it possible to overcome the difficulty of insufficient data availability and to enhance the model's efficiency. The feature engineering process involves determining the most pertinent features, removing extraneous features, and converting the data into an analysis-ready format. By utilizing wearable devices, it is essential to demonstrate outstanding performance when analyzing infectious diseases. In the workflow between data preprocessing and classification by machine learning, feature extraction, and feature selection play an important role. In feature extraction, a subset of new features or characteristics is extracted from the original primary features using various functional mapping techniques. The objective of this process is to convert large quantities of input data into low-dimensional characteristic vectors that can be used as inputs for machine learning models to perform classification.

The next section will discuss finding and extracting informative features from the processed data following the discussion of data preprocessing.

(c) **Feature Extraction and Feature Selection**

Feature extraction is one of the key processes in the pipeline between data preprocessing and machine learning techniques However, this step is not always mandatory for Deep Learning models, as these models are designed to handle this process autonomously. To enhance the functionality and accessibility of data by machine learning models, the raw data must undergo three steps namely: (1) create—creating a dataset in a specific structure, (2) transform—transform a data into a machine-readable format, i.e. numerical data, and (3) select relevant features—changing the dimension of data. The feature extraction process takes in-depth knowledge about the data, creativity in transforming the data to represent it in different dimensions, and a domain-specific understanding of the problem to be solved. The extraction and selection of features are crucial steps in the analysis of data collected from wearable devices because they reduce dimensionality, reduce overfitting, and improve interpretability. Additionally, it makes it possible to predict and classify infectious diseases more effectively based on data obtained from wearable devices.

Feature extraction involves extracting a set of features from input data by using functional mapping techniques. It involves transforming large input data into a low-dimensional feature vector that is used as input to a classification algorithm or a machine learning algorithm. Assuming there are n features (or attributes) $A1$, $A2$, $\ldots$, An, after feature extraction, a new set of features is generated which is represented as $B1$, $B2$, $\ldots$, Bn, $Bi = Fi$ ($A1$; $A2$;:::; An), and Fi is a mapping function. To find good transformations, it is generally necessary to conduct an intensive search. A feature extraction algorithm aims to find a minimum set of new features based on some performance measure such as prediction accuracy improvement or minimizing error functions such as Root Mean Square Error. The empirical mean, for example, can be inaccurate even if it is a simple feature. A feature plays an important role in making predictions based on a model. A task of classification requires class labels, so predictive accuracy can be used to evaluate the quality of features extracted. In the case of clustering, the data do not have class labels, so other measures must be used such as inter-cluster and intra-cluster similarity, variance, etc. Features that are uncorrelated or superfluous will be removed during feature extraction. In recent years, machine learning, deep learning, and optimization algorithms have been used to extract features.

Physiological features like respiratory rate, cough signals, heart rate (HR), heart rate variability (HRV), and walking cadence are estimated in [21], to predict COVID-19. The features are extracted in time-series and frequency domains. Four features were extracted from the respiratory rate signals, such as (1) Respiration Rate (RR), (2) RR during pre- and post-walk, (3) a number of peaks in the power spectrum derived by using Fast Fourier Transform (FFT), and (4) a number of peaks in the FFT spectrum during pre- and post-walk was collected. Both time and frequency domain features were extracted from the cough signals. In the time domain, the features include Root Mean Square (RMS), crest factor, maximum time duration, absolute difference, Inter-quartile Range, sample entropy, and Lempel-Ziv complexity. In the case of frequency domain features, dominant frequency, spectral entropy, spectral centroid, and spectral spread were analyzed. The walking portion of the sensor recording was manually extracted to estimate walking cadence. Next, the L2 norm of acceleration was computed, and the stepping frequency (cadence) was calculated as the dominant frequency of the FFT.

According to [33], COVID is predicted by considering 24 factors, including age, shortness of breath, fever temperature, cough, body ache, and eye pain. The authors of [34] predict COVID-19 using multimodal features such as images, audio, video, and text. A long touch of the head by one hand from the right side and a long touch of the head by one hand from the left side are considered image features. Text features analyse headaches, diarrhea, etc. A video and audio feature of coughing and sneezing were extracted. According to [26], the authors extracted breathing signals and cough signals at different time intervals while doing different activities. The Principal Component Analysis (PCA) method reduces feature dimensions and selects the most prominent features. In the next step, Receiver Operating Characteristics (ROC) are used to reduce the dimensionality of the data. ROCs were used to calculate the likelihood of events reflecting the degree of separability between features.

To normalize the dataset in [32], the authors adopt data splitting techniques. Seven days before and 21 days after symptom onset were considered infectious, 10–20 days before and after were considered non-infectious, and days after were considered recovery days. This labeling allows the data to be divided into training data using the days before the non-infectious period and test data using the days during the non-infectious period, infectious period, and recovery period. After that, a Long Short-Term Memory Network (LSTMN)-based autoencoder analysed the resting heart rate (RHR) in a fixed window size. Data is augmented to change the magnitude of the signals in a time series. The original data was further scaled by window wrapping—a random selection of 10% of the original data was speeded up by 2 or slowed down by 0:5, as well as window slicing—a random selection of 90% of the original data series was slowed down by 0:5. As a result of scaling the baseline data and rotating the scaled data, eight times the baseline data was created.

To improve prediction quality, the authors of [27] extracted four features. The features are: (1) mean value, which can be used to determine the central tendency of the transmitted signal to identify a key characteristic, (2) Min and Max values, used to specify the lower and upper bounds of a window with size that slides through the symptoms, (3) Standard Deviation, which determines how much the symptoms vary over a given time frame, and (4) Correlation: determining how unique the characteristics are. As in [23], the authors eliminated unnecessary features one at a time until the model was fine-tuned. Several processes such as filtering and normalization were then performed on the model.

According to [35], four features such as Heart Rate Variability acrophase, HRV MESOR (M: the mean HRV during the day), age and Body Mass Index (BMI) have high significance, while Resting Heart Rate metrics (maximum, minimum, SD, mean) are the most important/influential factor. HRV amplitude is less influential. The physiological signals of RHR, activity, and sleep length are used for anomaly detection in [24]. Moreover, temperature, geographical regions, and festival seasons are considered to determine disease spread. Based on the Pearson correlation coefficient, geographical conditions, and features influence COVID-19's spread. Using Apple Watch data and signs of heart rate fluctuations, the study examined [35] data to forecast SARS-CoV-2 infections. To prevent minor and ephemeral fluctuations in the Heart Rate Variability (HRV) pattern from having a significant impact on daily HRV measures, this research employed a smoothed technique,

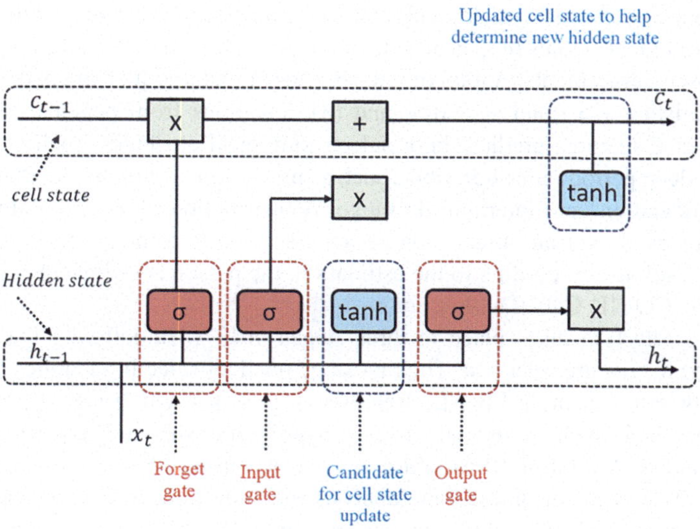

Fig. 5 Long-short-term memory (LSTM) networks

and by employing feature engineering, significant and sustained alterations were identified from the respondents' COVID-negative background.

In [36], the authors used a FLUVEY dataset consisting of 48 features collected from wearable devices to identify COVID-19 daily. FFT was used in [25] to predict the spectrogram levels of ECG signals for disease prediction. In the next step, information fusion (concatenation of different spectrogram features) is performed using Convolutional Neural Network (CNN) models. The recurrent neural network (RNN) models the longitudinal dependency among subsequent samples taken from a patient to determine severity based on individual body condition. Long-short-term memory (LSTM) networks as in Fig. 5 are used to prevent vanishing and exploding gradients in recurrent networks. During the on-site triage process, the RNN-based longitudinal model is fed the output of the input feature vector. In the absence of feature fusion, longitudinal modeling would be applied to the decision fusion of triage outputs from different modalities. Decision fusion addresses the limitations of feature-level fusion when the feature dimension of each modality is high. Furthermore, each modality is exploited separately during the triage step, which is advantageous when the modalities are less correlated, and each has different discriminatory characteristics. In decision fusion, triage outputs from multiple modalities can either be concatenated (DC) or accumulated (DA). A DC concatenates the class probability vectors of different modalities, while a DA sums the prediction vectors per class across modalities. Autonomic nervous system dysfunction was predicted by using SoftMax normalization on the current hidden state of the longitudinal model.

Physiological data were extracted from raw wearables data only during sleep periods in [31], to predict COVID COVID-19. The unrealistic measured values outside of a very broad physiological range were discarded using plausibility filters. The physiological signals (e.g. heart rate or temperature) are collected as segmented time-series measurements. A total of three groups of features are extracted: (1) sleep period statistics; (2) trend statistics; and (3) deviations from personal baselines. The extracted features predict abnormal physiological attributes, such as the last available sleep period range durations, such as maximum, minimum, median, mean, standard deviation, and interquartile range. A distribution of z-score values for a feature observed over an observation period was used to estimate deviations from personal baselines. According to the estimation, the person is estimated either to be affected by COVID COVID-19 or not.

Feature selection takes place in three stages in [37]. Initially, 21 features are considered for feature selection. The first stage involves selecting features based on probability values using a Logistic Regression. Features with a higher probability value than 0.05, such as mental disease, hypothyroidism, and hyperthyroidism, were excluded. A total of 18 variables are selected from the first round of feature selection. Two types of multivariate analysis methods were utilized in the second stage. These methods were the Decision Trees-based multivariate analysis method, the Least Absolute Shrinkage and Selection Operator (LASSO)-based multivariate analysis method, and the Minimum redundancy maximum relevance (mRMRe)-method multivariate analysis method. According to the delivered sensitivity values, 6 levels are selected at 85%, 90%, and 95%. Based on the selected three 6-variable feature sets, decision tree (DT) models, logistic regression (LR) models, and DNN models are used to predict prediction accuracy. A conditional probability criterion is used by the authors of [23] to select the features.

A framework of infectious disease prediction commonly extracts heartbeat rate signals, cough signals, respiration rate, and walking rhythm. Time-series data on respiratory rate were collected as a feature such as a number of FFT spikes, breathing rate, and walk cadence before and after walking. A time-series analysis of cough signals has been conducted, including the root mean square, interquartile range, absolute difference, maximum duration, crest factor, average entropy, and Lempel-Ziv complexity. Furthermore, other features that are collected for prediction include heart rate variability, skin temperature, and electrodermal activity. However, the specific features will differ based on the application and the physiological signals observed.

Frequency domain modeling is commonly used to extract features such as power spectral density, frequency, and spectrum bands, while time-series modeling is typically used to extract empirical and statistical moments. In many applications, either a frequency-domain or time-series evaluation technique is employed, but the appropriate method depends on the specific situation. In order to ensure quality treatment and data protection, machine learning in medical fields requires precise validation, ethical considerations, and compliance with data privacy rules. A transdisciplinary partnership between healthcare professionals, data analysts, and domain experts is crucial to the successful application of machine learning to the classification of illness.

As a result of the above discussion on feature selection and extraction methods, features such as HR, Activity, Motion, ST, RR, BP, Electroencephalogram (EEG), Gait, and Posture were extracted for the classification of infectious diseases. This step will ultimately result in higher classification performance and more insightful analyses of wearable device data by improving the classification process' effectiveness, reliability, and interpretability.

(d) **Classification for ID Detection and Diagnosis**

To automatically classify infectious diseases from wearable device data, the classification process is essential. This section discusses the most promising works on ID detection using Artificial Intelligence (AI) methods such as Machine Learning and Deep Learning.

(i) **Classifier Models**

Based on Susceptible, Exposed, Infectious, Removed (SEIR) framework, the authors of [38] examined wearable sensor-based pandemic mitigation solutions. The researchers developed a compartmental model of Canada's second COVID-19 wave based on SARS-CoV-2, tested counterfactual deployment scenarios for wearable sensors, and evaluated algorithm accuracy, uptake, and adherence. Presymptomatic, asymptomatic, and symptomatic are the three sub-states into which they have divided the infectious state. They have considered Physiological Biomarkers such as Resting Heart Rate, Sleep Duration, Steps, Heart Rate Variability and Cough Audio for the detection system. Moreover, they concluded that wearable sensors capable of detecting asymptomatic or pre-symptomatic infections could reduce the burden of disease during pandemics. Health care can be transformed in numerous ways using machine learning, and diseases can be classified more accurately. Logistic regression is a commonly used statistical model for binary classification problems. It is a special type of regression analysis that can be useful for forecasting the likelihood of a binary event, such as "yes/no," "1/0," or "true/false." With logistic regression, the dependent variable is binary, and the algorithm determines whether the input in question belongs to one of two classes based on its likelihood.

Based on physiological responses collected during brief periods of activity, or "snapshots," the authors of [21] examined COVID-19 symptoms. Wearable sensors were used to record cough noises, cardio-respiratory function, and physical activity using a soft body-conforming sensor positioned on the uprasternal notch. A statistical learning model was built using the features of cough signals from Respiration Rate (R) intervals, steps, respiration, and frequency spectrum (Logistic Regression with Elastic Net regularization). By comparing models trained on the Pre/Post cardiac and cadence, PrePost respiration, and cough feature sets with those trained on the combined feature sets, they were able to determine the relative importance of particular physiological parameters. Using the label of each snapshot (COVID-positive vs. Healthy), a (Logistic Regression with Elastic Net regularization) model was created to classify the likelihood of COVID-19 infection. Applying a leave-one-subject-out cross-validation, we tested the model by training on snapshots from a cohort with a known diagnosis along with assessing on snapshots of a fresh participant with an unknown diagnosis, mimicking the use-case of the framework.

Using symptoms and age, sex, and Body Mass Index (BMI) as input characteristics, the authors created a Logistic Regression classifier with four-fold cross-validation to predict the need for hospitalization of COVID-19 patients [29]. In addition, they developed a neural network classifier to determine if an individual is ill. This is done using data on their respiration, heart rate, and variability in heart rate that day and the 4 days before. As suggested in [19], the authors suggested using an algorithm that uses machine learning to determine R-peaks and atrial fibrillation (AFAF) whenever ECG data is updated on the server. In addition to HRV and BPM calculation, they also provided a set of data analysis methods based on R-peak detection. The raw real-time EMG data were rectified and combined for EMG analysis to measure muscle activity for the computation of patients' average activities.

A Decision Tree Model (DTN) and a Deep Neural Network Model (DNN) are two distinct categories of machine learning-based prediction models developed by the authors for Infectious Disease detection [37]. These models perform well because they are based on DT algorithms that use univariate analysis and linear transformations to derive decision rules. In general, advanced DNN models have higher prediction performance than other kinds of prediction models.

A review of [22] highlighted how biometric information can be applied to close current discrepancies in the recognition and treatment of viral diseases based on existing knowledge. Additionally, they highlighted new developments in data processing algorithms, clinical insights related to the diagnosis of influenza-like diseases (ILIs), and biometric monitoring technology (BioMeTs). This paper focuses in particular on data quality, machine learning (ML) methods, standards, and unresolved clinical problems.

An analysis of patient physiological data anomalies was conducted [26] to diagnose early COVID-19 symptoms. To analyze fever and cough, two of the most common symptoms, in combination, an unsupervised machine learning model was employed. An analysis of physiological characteristics from a chest-worn device was conducted to study abnormalities in patient data for early diagnosis of COVID-19 symptoms. Coughing and breathing patterns can be tracked using a metric called the Single Vector Activity Index (SVAI). Second, the variance of the dataset is analyzed using the DBSCAN segmentation and outlier detection method. The model's accuracy is lastly assessed to find anomalies in real-time data using feature dissimilarities.

Based on heart rate and sleep data acquired from wearable devices, the authors proposed a system for forecasting COVID-19 epidemic trends in a variety of nations and cities. In conjunction with a biological abnormality detection algorithm developed using data from wearable devices, an online neural network forecasting methodology that combines the rate of observed physiological anomalies and the past COVID-19 infection rate is evaluated. Due to the expansion of patient data availability and improvements in machine learning algorithms, the disease prediction will become increasingly important in the fight against diseases.

(ii) **Deep Convolution Neural Network (CNN) Models for ID Diagnosis**

Deep learning is a subclass of machine learning that has improved disease categorization and can increase productivity and accuracy in a variety of healthcare applications. Thakur et al. [39] provides a prediction and forecast of infectious disorders such as COVID-19, lung transparency, Middle East respiratory syndrome, normal pneumonia, SARS, tuberculosis, and viral pneumonia. Several deep learning models have also been demonstrated, including EfcientNetB0, EfcientNetB1, EfcientNet2, EfcientNet3, NASResNetLarge, DenseNet169, ResNet152V2, and InceptionNetV2. The model was trained with following datasets assembled from several sources: covid 19 (3616 images), lung opacity (6012 images), MERS (540 images), pneumonia (3875 images), tuberculosis (2530 images), SARS (1134 images), normal lung imaging (10,200 images), and viral pneumonia (1345 images). Exploratory Data Analysis and preprocessing (a horizontal flip and a vertical flip) were applied on these images. The efficiency of the models were evaluated based on parameters like accuracy, loss recall, precision, F1 score, root mean error square (RMSE).During the testing phase, the InceptionResNetV2 model had the best loss ratio of 0.399, a root means square error of 0.63 and a peak accuracy of 88% when compared to the models discussed above.

In [40] the authors developed the Multiple Infectious Disease Diagnostic Model (MIDDM),, which performs multi-classifications of infectious disorders to aid clinical infectious disease decision-making. The data such as Patient information, Physical examination, Symptom, Medical history, medical laboratory examination and Examination reports were extracted from the medical records of the patients. Bidirectional Long Short-Term Memory—Conditional Random Field (BiLSTM-CRF) was used to realize the information extraction from the original EMRs. The addition of residual networks and attention mechanisms improved the performance of the MIDDM model. They predicted and confirmed seven infectious diseases, including viral hepatitis, infectious diarrhea, influenza, measles, hand, foot, and mouth disease, tuberculosis, and syphilis. With the identical input data, taking viral hepatitis as an example for infectious disease, the MIDDM's accuracy of 99.44% is significantly greater than the accuracy results of XGBoost (96.19%), Decision tree (90.13%), logistic regression (91.26%) and Bayesian technique (85.19%). Significantly, better predictions of other diseases were made by MIDDM than by the models listed above.

Said [34] presents a people-monitoring system based on people's behavior using the Internet of Things (IoT). By tracking the movements of those who are afflicted, their method can predict the spread of sickness. The proposed deep-learning (CNN) model is based on a five-layer neural network with input layers, General Futures (GF) Layer, Core Futures (CF) Layer, Adapted Futures (AF) Layer and Output layer. Results showed that their proposed method can predict sickness symptoms and their spread accurately. Additionally, they offered a variety of computer techniques and resources. A revolutionary edge-centric healthcare system was developed by the authors of [27], which incorporates wearable sensors and a cutting-edge machine learning (ML) model for quick judgments. Deep Transfer Learning (DTL), a cutting-edge machine learning technique, was introduced for data processing at edge networks. In DTL, the well-trained model's information is converted into a lightweight ML model able to handle the resource constraints of distributed edge devices. To implement the DTL technique for data analytics of COVID-19 disease prediction, they suggested using the Bag-of-neural-networks (BoNN) model in edge networks.

A method that predicts the likelihood of COVID-19 infection was developed by combining biometric data from smartwatches like Fitbit with electronic symptom reports [41]. As a result, the researchers hope to enhance the effectiveness of test distribution when monitoring disease spread in resource-constrained environments. They provided examples of models like CovIdentify that could be applied to already-existing exposure notification programs. CovIdentify may be used to guide the distribution of diagnostics for infectious diseases soon. Multimodal AI-driven risk prediction in health care has implications for clinical decision-making, diagnostics, and prognostics. A deep learning architecture based on entity embedding networks, long-short term memory, and convolutional neural networks was suggested in [42] to accurately learn diverse medical data to diagnose disease infections. In addition, they combined a multi-agent system that allows each agent within the system to readily communicate its learning results with other agents, enhancing the autonomy of the framework. They also incorporated bee swarm optimization and memetic algorithms to explore the hyper-optimization parameter space of their framework.

By identifying abnormal rest heart rates in test results relative to the user's baseline, the authors of [32] developed a deep learning system that used a Long Short-Term Memory Networks-based autoencoder called LAAD to predict COVID-19 infection. According to this study, deep learning may be is able to distinguish COVID-19 periods more accurately than previous techniques that have been used. Furthermore, they suggested that wearable sensors could be used as an early indicator of COVID-19 based on the results of their experiment. To predict verified numbers and cases of death, the authors used Holt-trend and Long-Short Term Memory (LSTM) [43]. With regard to Saudi Arabia, Italy, and Spain specifically, the LSTM model's predictions for the number of Covid-19 mortality are 99.86%, 98.876%, and 99.16%, respectively. In Holt-Trend model, the values of the trend (beta) parameter was 0.20, and the level (alpha) parameter was 0.1, 0.5, and 0.15. The optimal values were determined by measuring the mean square error (MSE) of alpha = 0.15 and beta = 0.20, which corresponded to the lowest prediction errors as determined by the conventional evaluation metrics. The Holt-Trend model's predictions for the number of mortality cases in Saudi Arabia, Italy, and Spain are 99.80%, 99.96%, and 99.94%, respectively. Based on various performance indicators such as mean error, correlation, root mean square error, and mean square error, the LSTM and Holt-Trend models demonstrated effective performance. Furthermore, for Covid-19 case prediction, the LSTM and Holt-Trend models are more acceptable.

(iii) **Ensemble Models for ID Diagnosis**

A key benefit of ensemble methods in illness classification is that they strengthen the resilience of machine-learning models, prevent overfitting, and improve predicted accuracy. As a result, these techniques combine many base models' predictions-often called "weak learners"-to create a more precise and reliable prediction. To create and build a diagnostic model that analyzes medical Big Data and detects diseases by identifying irregularities in the early stages. This is done by utilizing medical data provided as input. Wearable sensors and Electronic Medical Records (EMRs) are the two main data sources that the framework rely on. The user's smart wearable gathers essential metrics for monitoring, including location, heart rate, glucose level, respiration rate, oxygen saturation, and other internal and external physiological data. EMRs are a vital resource for information on patients' medical histories, physical and radiological tests, lab results, diabetes, and other past conditions. The authors of [23] focused on integrating ensemble deep learning algorithms with IoT devices. Their Ensemble Deep Learning-based AI-assisted diagnostic model aims to be a useful application for medical service systems and patients by being able to identify diseases in the early stages and provide insightful information to support individualized treatment by combining the predictions from each base model and producing a final prediction that will support individualized treatment.

An Ensemble framework was developed in [44] to retrieve biomedical data from widespread and homogeneous sensors. Several deep learning architectures, including VGG16, RESNET, and DenseNet, along with (detectioN Using enseMble dEep leaRning And aTtention mEchanism)(NUMERATE), were used to identify and classify diseases. In addition, they thoroughly examined the biological data. In terms of training time, they observe that NUMERATE performs better than Xception and SqueezeNet methods. The fact that NUMERATE uses both ensemble and attention mechanisms, rapidly converges on ground truth, explains this performance.

To improve the accuracy of disease identification predictions for human and animal diseases, the authors conducted a PRISMA systematic review in [28]. They reviewed the different types of IDs modelled, ML and DL models applied, geographical distribution, prediction tasks conducted, input features, spatial and temporal scales, error metrics, computational effectiveness, uncertainty quantification, and strategies for managing missing data. Furthermore, they identified patterns and weaknesses in ML and DL for ID estimation and offered recommendations for future research to improve biopreparedness.

To classify chronic disease identification or surveillance via wearable technology, several algorithms were used, including deep learning algorithms like LSTM, machine learning algorithms like ensemble models, and InceptionNetV2. A recurrent neural network called an LSTM is frequently employed for time-series statistical analysis and has proven to be effective for disease classification. InceptionNetV2 is a deep learning model that has proven successful in image-based disease classification problems, as well as ensemble models combined with other models demonstrating enhanced performance. In addition to decision trees,

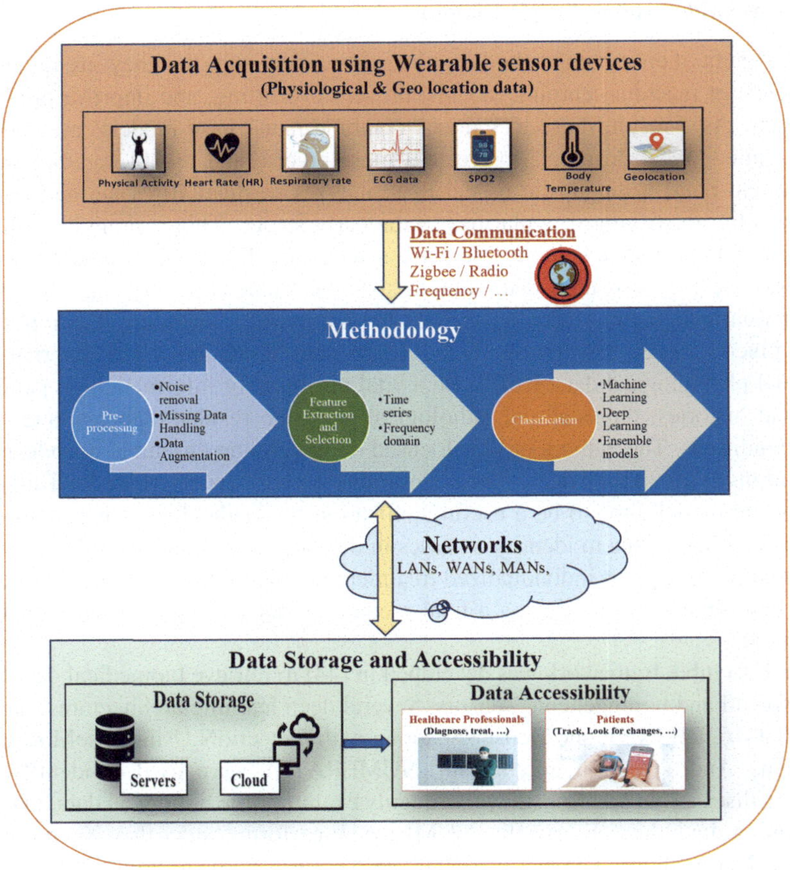

Fig. 6 Overall flow of disease monitoring using wearables

support vector machines, and random forests, other machine-learning techniques are effective at predicting diseases. A classification model must be able to precisely categorize data and provide useful information for detecting and evaluating infectious diseases. Machine learning models, such as support vector machines and logistic regression, are frequently applied to binary classification problems, in contrast to deep learning computational models like LSTM and InceptionNetV2, which are capable of automatically identifying and representing complex patterns from data. In addition to integrating multiple models, ensemble approaches are also popular for enhancing performance.

A brief overview of adapted preprocessing approaches, feature extraction followed by feature selection, and the different types of machine learning and deep learning classification models used by current researchers is presented and shown in Fig. 6.

3 Conclusion

The chapter discusses the challenges and constraints associated with using wearable sensors to support the preliminary detection of infectious diseases. In particular, the chapter discusses the importance of wearable sensors for early diagnosis and observation of infectious disorders, such as COVID-19, influenza, and various respiratory infections. Physiological signals such as heart rate, cough, breathing rate, and skin temperature were mainly used as the signals or features for classification. An important observation is that dimensionality reduction and feature selection may improve the effectiveness of classification models. For binary classification problems, machine learning models such as logistic regression and SVM were widely used, whereas deep learning models such as RNN-LSTM and Inception-NetV2 are useful for disease diagnosis since they can automatically recognize and characterize complex patterns among data. As a result of integrating many models, ensemble models improve classification performance. According to the application and physiological signals acquired, the best ML model can differ. It is generally true that the best results are achieved by adopting a combination of good strategies. During the adoption of machine learning in patient care and data protection, it is essential to remember that precise validation, ethical guidelines, and following data privacy policies are extremely significant. Machine learning for disease classification will also require a transdisciplinary partnership between healthcare professionals, data analysts, and domain experts. According to the review, continuous physiological signal surveillance along with wearable sensor devices have the potential to revolutionize early diagnosis and surveillance of infectious diseases. Finally, medical practitioners, healthcare professionals, domain experts, and data scientists should collaborate to enhance patient care and public health.

References

1. https://apps.who.int/iris/rest/bitstreams/1435584/retrieve. Accessed on 9 Aug 2023
2. P. Makam, R. Matsa, "Big Three" infectious diseases: Tuberculosis, malaria and HIV/AIDS. Curr. Top. Med. Chem. **21**(31), 2779–2799 (2021). https://doi.org/10.2174/1568026621666210916170417
3. E. Grzesiak, B. Bent, M.T. McClain, et al., Assessment of the feasibility of using non-invasive wearable biometric monitoring sensors to detect influenza and the common cold before symptom onset. JAMA Netw. Open **4**(9), e2128534 (2021). https://doi.org/10.1001/jamanetworkopen.2021.28534
4. D.S. Temple, M. Hegarty-Craver, R.D. Furberg, E.A. Preble, E. Bergstrom, Z. Gardener, P. Dayananda, L. Taylor, N.M. Lemm, L. Papargyris, M.T. McClain, B.P. Nicholson, A. Bowie, M. Miggs, E. Petzold, C.W. Woods, C. Chiu, K.H. Gilchrist, Wearable sensor-based detection of influenza in presymptomatic and asymptomatic individuals. J. Infect. Dis. **227**(7), 864–872 (2023). https://doi.org/10.1093/infdis/jiac262
5. C.J. Goergen, M.J. Tweardy, S.R. Steinhubl, S.W. Wegerich, K. Singh, R.J. Mieloszyk, J. Dunn, Detection and monitoring of viral infections via wearable devices and biometric data. Ann. Rev. Biomed. Eng. **24**, 1–27 (2022). https://doi.org/10.1146/annurev-bioeng-103020-040136

6. H.C. Ates, A.K. Yetisen, F. Güder, et al., Wearable devices for the detection of COVID-19. Nat. Electron **4**, 13–14 (2021). https://doi.org/10.1038/s41928-020-00533-1
7. S. Agrebi, A. Larbi, Use of artificial intelligence in infectious diseases. Artif. Intell. Precis. Health., 415–438 (2020). https://doi.org/10.1016/B978-0-12-817133-2.00018-5
8. M.B.A. Mol, M.T.A. Strous, F.H.M. van Osch, F.J. Vogelaar, D.G. Barten, M. Farchi, et al., Heart-rate-variability (HRV), predicts outcomes in COVID-19. PLoS One **16**(10), e0258841 (2021). https://doi.org/10.1371/journal.pone.0258841
9. A. Natarajan, H.W. Su, C. Heneghan, et al., Measurement of respiratory rate using wearable devices and applications to COVID-19 detection. npj Digit. Med. **4**, 136 (2021). https://doi.org/10.1038/s41746-021-00493-6
10. https://www.ncbi.nlm.nih.gov/books/NBK525974/. Accessed on 9 Aug 2023
11. K.S. Alqudaihi, N. Aslam, I.U. Khan, Cough sound detection and diagnosis using artificial intelligence techniques: Challenges and opportunities. IEEE Access **9**, 102327–102344. Published 2021 Jul 15 (2021). https://doi.org/10.1109/ACCESS.2021.3097559
12. J. González-Cabañas, Á. Cuevas, R. Cuevas, M. Maier, Digital contact tracing: Large-scale geolocation data as an alternative to Bluetooth-based apps failure. Electronics **10**(9), 1093 (2021). https://doi.org/10.3390/electronics10091093
13. P.O. Ugwoke, F.S. Bakpo, C.N. Udanor, M.C. Okoronkwo, A framework for monitoring movements of pandemic disease patients based on GPS trajectory datasets. Wirel. Netw **28**(1), 1–28 (2022). https://doi.org/10.1007/s11276-021-02819-4
14. Z. Tafferner, I. Balázs, O. Krammer, A. Géczy, Can ChatGPT help in electronics research and development? A case study with applied sensors. Sensors **23**(10), 4879 (2023). https://doi.org/10.3390/s23104879
15. N. Peiffer-Smadja, T.M. Rawson, R. Ahmad, A. Buchard, P. Georgiou, F.X. Lescure, G. Birgand, A.H. Holmes, Machine learning for clinical decision support in infectious diseases: A narrative review of current applications. Clin. Microbiol. Infect. **26**(5), 584–595 (2020). https://doi.org/10.1016/j.cmi.2019.09.009
16. H. Li, J. Yuan, G. Fennell, V. Abdulla, R. Nistala, D. Dandachi, D.K.C. Ho, Y. Zhang, Recent advances in wearable sensors and data analytics for continuous monitoring and analysis of biomarkers and symptoms related to COVID-19. Biophys. Rev. **4**(3), 031302 (2023). https://doi.org/10.1063/5.0140900
17. T. Mishra, M. Wang, A.A. Metwally, Pre-symptomatic detection of COVID-19 from smartwatch data. Nat. Biomed. Eng. **4**, 1208–1220 (2020). https://doi.org/10.1038/s41551-020-00640-6
18. https://physionet.org/about/database/. Accessed on 9 Aug 2023
19. J.W. Jeong, W. Lee, Y.J. Kim, A real-time wearable physiological monitoring system for home-based healthcare applications. Sensors (Basel) **22**(1), 104. Published 2021 Dec 24 (2021). https://doi.org/10.3390/s22010104
20. G. Yang, G. Pang, Z. Pang, G. Ying, M. Mäntysalo, H. Yang, Non-invasive flexible and stretchable wearable sensors with nano-based enhancement for chronic disease care. IEEE Rev. Biomed. Eng. **12**, 34–71 (2018). https://doi.org/10.1109/RBME.2018.2887301
21. L. Lonini, N. Shawen, O. Botonis, M. Fanton, C. Jayaraman, C.K. Mummidisetty, S.Y. Shin, C. Rushin, S. Jenz, S. Xu, J.A. Rogers, A. Jayaraman, Rapid screening of physiological changes associated with COVID-19 using soft-wearables and structured activities: A pilot study. IEEE J. Transl. Eng. Health Med. **9**, 4900311 (2021)
22. C.J. Goergen, M.K.J. Tweardy, S.R. Steinhubl, S.W. Wegerich, K. Singh, R.J. Mieloszyk, J. Dunn, Detection and monitoring of viral infections via wearable devices and biometric data. Annu. Rev. Biomed. Eng. **24**, 1–27 (2022). https://doi.org/10.1146/annurev-bioeng-103020-040136
23. M. Venkatachala Appa Swamy, J. Periyasamy, M. Thangavel, Design and development of IoT and deep ensemble learning based model for disease monitoring and prediction. Diagnostics (Basel). **13**(11), 1942. Published 2023 Jun 1 (2023). https://doi.org/10.3390/diagnostics13111942

24. G. Zhu, J. Li, Z. Meng, Y. Yi, Y. Li, X. Tang, Y. Dong, G. Sun, R. Zhou, H. Wang, K. Wang, W. Huan, Cognitive modeling of multimodal data intensive systems for applications in nature and society (COMDICS). Hindawi (2020). https://doi.org/10.1155/2020/6152041
25. G.A. Tadesse, H. Javed, N. Le Nguyen, H.D. Thanh, H. Thi, L. Van Tan, L. Thwaites, D.A. Clifton, T. Zhu, Multi-modal diagnosis of infectious diseases in the developing world. IEEE J. Biomed. Health Inform. **24**, 2131 (2020)
26. O. Ali, M.K. Ishak, M.K.L. Bhatti, A machine learning approach for early COVID-19 symptoms identification. Comput. Mater. Contin. **70**, 3803–3820 (2022). https://doi.org/10.32604/cmc.2022.019797
27. M. Adhikari, A. Hazra, S. Nandy, Deep transfer learning for communicable disease detection and recommendation in edge networks. IEEE/ACM Trans. Comput. Biol. Bioinform. **20**(4), 2468–2479 (2023)
28. R. Keshavamurthy, S. Dixon, K.T. Pazdernik, L.E. Charles, Predicting infectious disease for biopreparedness and response: A systematic review of machine learning and deep learning approaches. One Health, 15 (2022). https://doi.org/10.1016/j.onehlt.2022.100439
29. A. Natarajan, S. Hao-Wei, C. Heneghan, Assessment of physiological signs associated with COVID-19 measured using wearable devices. MedRxiv preprint. https://doi.org/10.1101/2020.08.14.20175265
30. A. Alavi, G.K. Bogu, M. Wang, E.S. Rangan, A.W. Brooks, Q. Wang, E. Higgs, A. Celli, T. Mishra, A.A. Metwally, K. Cha, P. Knowles, A.A. Alavi, R. Bhasin, S. Panchamukhi, D. Celis, T. Aditya, A. Honkala, B. Rolnik, E. Hunting, O. Dagan-Rosenfeld, A. Chauhan, J.W. Li, C. Bejikian, V. Krishnan, L. McGuire, X. Li, A. Bahmani, M.P. Snyder, Real-time alerting system for COVID-19 and other stress events using wearable data. Nat. Med. **28**, 175–184 (2022). https://doi.org/10.1038/s41591-021-01593-2
31. B. Conroy, I. Silva, G. Mehraei, R. Damiano, E.S. BrianGross, T. Feng, J. Schneider, N. Olson, A.G. Rizzo, C.M. Curtin, J. Frassica, D.C. Mc Farlane, Real-time infection prediction with wearable physiological monitoring and AI to aid military workforce readiness during COVID-19. Sci. Rep. **22**, 3797 (2022). https://doi.org/10.1038/s41598-022-07764-6
32. G.K. Bogu, M.P. Snyder, Deep learning-based detection of COVID-19 using wearables data. medRxiv preprint. https://doi.org/10.1101/2021.01.08.21249474
33. W. Ju-Yu, Y. Wang, C.T.S. Ching, H.-M.D. Wang, L.-D. Liao, IoT-based wearable health monitoring device and its validation for potential critical and emergency applications. Front. Public Health **11**, 1188304 (2023). https://doi.org/10.3389/fpubh.2023.1188304
34. O. Said, A large-scale IoT-based scheme for real-time prediction of infectious disease symptoms. Mobile Netw. Appl. (2022). https://doi.org/10.1007/s11036-023-02111-z
35. R.P. Hirten, L. Tomalin, M. Danieletto, E. Golden, M. Zweig, S. Kaur, D. Helmus, A. Biello, R. Pyzik, E.P. Bottinger, L. Keefer, D. Charney, G.N. Nadkarni, M. Suarez-Farinas, Z.A. Fayad, Evaluation of a machine learning approach utilizing wearable data for prediction of SARS-CoV-2 infection in healthcare workers. JAMIA Open. **5**(2), 1–9 (2022). https://doi.org/10.1093/jamiaopen/ooac041
36. B. Nestor, J. Hunter, R. Kainkaryam, E. Drysdale, J.B. Inglis, A. Shapiro, Machine learning COVID-19 detection from wearables. Lancet Digit. Health **5**(4) (2023). https://doi.org/10.1016/S2589-7500(23)00045-6
37. H.-Y.R. Chiu, C.-K. Hwang, S.-Y. Chen, F.-Y. Shih, H.-C. Han, C.-C. King, J. ReubenGilbert, C.-C. Fang, Y.-J. Oyang, Machine learning for emerging infectious disease feld responses. Sci. Rep., 22 (2022). https://doi.org/10.1038/s41598-021-03687-w
38. N. Duarte, Deploying wearable sensors for pandemic mitigation. A thesis submitted to McGill University (2022)
39. K. Thakur, M. Kaur, Y. Kumar, A comprehensive analysis of deep learning-based approaches for prediction and prognosis of infectious diseases. Arch. Comput. Methods Eng. **30**, 4477–4497 (2023). https://doi.org/10.1007/s11831-023-09952-7
40. M. Wang, Z. Wei, M. Jia, L. Chen, H. Ji, Deep learning model for multi-classifcation of infectious diseases from unstructured electronic medical records. BMC Med. Inform. Decis. Mak. **22**(41) (2022). https://doi.org/10.1186/s12911-022-01776-y

41. Intelligent risk prediction in public health using wearable device data. Digit. Med. **5**(153) (2022). https://doi.org/10.1038/s41746-022-00701-x
42. Y. Djenouri, G. Srivastava, A. Yazidi, J.C.-W. Lin, An edge-driven multi-agent optimization model for infectious disease detection. Appl. Intell. **52**, 14362–14373 (2022). https://doi.org/10.1007/s10489-021-03145-0
43. T.H.H. Aldhyani, M. Alrasheed, M.H. Al-Adaileh, A.A. Alqarni, M.Y. Alzahrani, A.H. Alahmadi, Deep learning and Holt-Trend algorithms for predicting Covid-19 pandemic. Comput. Mater. Contin. **67**(2), 2141–2160 (2021). https://doi.org/10.32604/cmc.2021.014498
44. Y. Djenouri, A. Belhadi, A. Yazidi, G. Srivastava, J.C.-W. Lin, Artificial intelligence of medical things for disease detection using ensemble deep learning and attention mechanism. Exp. Syst., 1–13 (2022). https://doi.org/10.1111/exsy.13093

Use of Artificial Intelligence in the Surveillance of Seasonal Respiratory Infections

Adiba Tabassum Chowdhury, Mehrin Newaz, Purnata Saha, Shona Pedersen, Muhammad Salman Khan, and Muhammad E. H. Chowdhury

1 Introduction

Flu and the respiratory syncytial virus (RSV), cause significant global morbidity and mortality and pose a continuous public health threat. Each year, influenza and respiratory syncytial virus (RSV) together cause millions of serious respiratory diseases, up to 650,000 influenza-related deaths, and over 200,000 RSV-related deaths globally [11]. Traditional surveillance methods, reliant on manual data collecting lack speed, accuracy, and scalability hindering our ability to swiftly detect epidemics and implement effective responses [20]. Consequently, the incorporation of AI into the healthcare sector offers a promising solution to enhance our ability to detect, monitor and manage seasonal respiratory diseases in the face of the evolving landscape of infectious diseases in the twenty-first century [26].

The potential contributions of AI to this field are vast and varied, from precise outbreak predictions using machine learning to early symptom detection via natural language processing on social media [24]. With infectious diseases continually evolving, there is a pressing need for surveillance systems that are dynamic and adaptable, attributes AI can deliver [27]. The complications arising from the COVID-19 pandemic further accentuates the urgency to improve our monitoring of respiratory diseases, reinforcing the relevance of AI solutions in this domain [21].

A. T. Chowdhury · M. Newaz · P. Saha
Department of Electrical and Electronic Engineering, University of Dhaka, Dhaka, Bangladesh

S. Pedersen
Department of Basic Medical Sciences, College of Medicine, Qatar University, Doha, Qatar
e-mail: spedersen@qu.edu.qa

M. S. Khan · M. E. H. Chowdhury (✉)
Department of Electrical Engineering, Qatar University, Doha, Qatar
e-mail: salman@qu.edu.qa; mchowdhury@qu.edu.qa

M. E. H. Chowdhury, S. Kiranyaz (eds.), *Surveillance, Prevention, and Control of Infectious Diseases*, https://doi.org/10.1007/978-3-031-59967-5_10

This narrative review encourages readers to explore the intriguing nexus of AI and respiratory infection surveillance, offering insights into the current landscape, potential advancements, and hurdles that will define the future of this crucial healthcare segment.

In the subsequent sections, we analyze conventional surveillance techniques with AI-driven methods. We discuss data sources, diseases in focus, and data collection strategies. We then provide an overview of the epidemiology of seasonal respiratory infections and delve into the role of mobile networks and mobile applications. The efficacy of government-mandated interventions is assessed, and the inherent limitations of these strategies are highlighted. Lastly, we examine the future trajectory and prospects in this field.

2 Traditional vs AI Surveillance in Seasonal Respiratory Infections

The mainstay of tracking infectious diseases has historically been traditional surveillance, which relies on manual data collection, reporting, and retrospective analysis. The inherent delay in this manual approach can hinder timely interventions, sometimes allowing outbreaks to escalate before containment actions are initiated [25]. The effectiveness of these methods often hinges on the alertness of healthcare professionals and the accessibility of resources, leading to variability and gaps in data quality [27]. In contrast, AI surveillance heralds a new era marked by real-time data processing, predictive modeling, early warning systems, etc. as shown in Fig. 1. AI algorithms can swiftly sift through vast datasets, identifying anomalies and nuanced patterns often overlooked by human scrutiny [20]. Such capabilities empower public health organizations to pinpoint outbreaks at inception, facilitating swift and targeted interventions [36]. AI surveillance transcends traditional medical data boundaries, offering a holistic view of infection trends by amalgamating diverse data streams including social media, wearable technologies, and environmental data [25]. With unparalleled forecasting accuracy, artificial intelligence (AI) has rev-

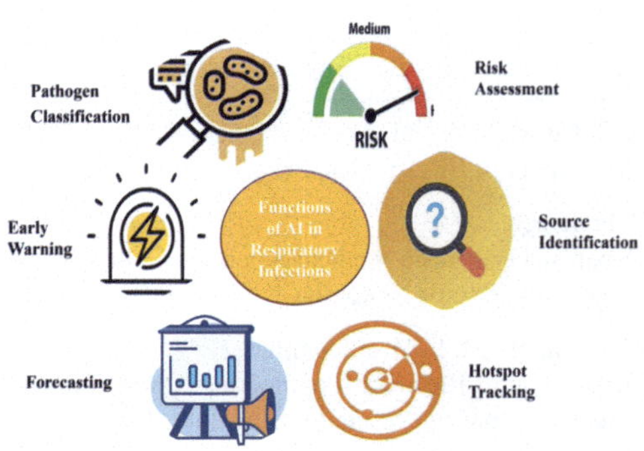

Fig. 1 Functions of AI in respiratory seasonal infections

olutionized respiratory seasonal infection surveillance, surmounting conventional approaches. Its real-time processing ability, coupled with the integration of diverse datasets such as clinical, social, and climatic data ensures prompt outbreak detection and accurate progression forecasts [35].

Unlike traditional surveillance, AI's dynamism ensures continual refinement of its predictive prowess, fostering timely interventions and efficient resource management. By attaining up to a 40% improvement in early detection rates, AI can objectively beat conventional systems in respiratory seasonal infection surveillance, resulting in earlier interventions. Additionally, it can process and analyze large datasets at 100 times faster rates, improving public health response and possibly saving thousands of lives annually [14].

3 Data Sources, Collection and Processing

For AI surveillance of Seasonal Respiratory Infections, data is aggregated from various sources such as healthcare records [22], laboratory tests [5], symptom trackers [4], and primarily hospital patients [42]. AI data collection in this study rigorously adheres to ethical and privacy standards to ensure the utmost confidentiality. Figure 2 gives a visual depiction of the data sources utilized across various research papers in this study. This visualization vividly illustrates that the primary data pertaining to patients has been sourced predominantly from hospitals and various surveillance websites, underscoring the reliability and diversity of our data inputs.

Hospitals usually collect patient demographic information, clinical and diagnostic data, treatment details, complications, epidemiological information, vaccination status, and research data to monitor, diagnose, treat, and study seasonal respiratory diseases, supporting patient care, public health surveillance, and research efforts. For the study by Agca et al. [1], nasopharyngeal swab samples from a Turkish hospital (March 2020–February 2021) were analyzed, identifying flu and rhinovirus/enterovirus. After preprocessing for accuracy, the data revealed a notable drop in influenza cases during the COVID-19 pandemic (from 17.3%

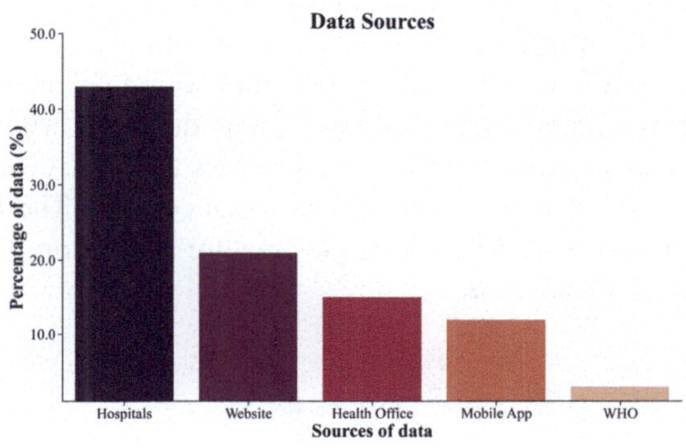

Fig. 2 Sources of data of seasonal respiratory infections

to 2.3%) with rhinovirus and enterovirus remaining prevalent. In another study examining ICU admissions in the Netherlands over a decade [42], hospital data analysis revealed significant variations in severe acute respiratory infection (SARI) incidence, mortality, and severity during the influenza seasons. This emphasizes the importance of prospective ICU SARI and acute respiratory distress syndrome (ARDS) surveillance for monitoring evolving influenza epidemics. Surveillance of seasonal respiratory diseases utilizes clinical symptoms like fever, cough, or epidemiological data, demographics, and environmental factors to monitor and understand disease spread and trends, aiding in public health decision-making [16].

For AI-driven surveillance in respiratory diseases, key parameters like hospitalization, oxygen usage, difficulty in breathing, mortality, (P)ICU admission, dehydration, feeding challenges, abnormal respiratory sounds, fever, vomiting, and wheezing are crucial [29]. These factors processed by AI algorithms provide an in-depth perspective of a patient's health, facilitating early detection and assessment of disease severity. Time series studies are also used for predicting illness. A particular study proposed by [33] presents an ANN-based system for predicting seasonal influenza epidemics in Tehran, incorporating climatic factors and influenza-like illness cases with satisfactory accuracy while proposing potential enhancements involving air pollution data integration. To comprehensively analyze the data related to respiratory diseases, a combination of descriptive and analytical epidemiological methods is employed, encompassing techniques such as time series analysis, age-specific incidence rates, and correlation analysis [31].

4 Covered Diseases with Different Statistical and Machine Learning Models

AI has revolutionized disease monitoring, especially in the realm of seasonal respiratory infections. This section examines the various statistical and machine learning models employed and critically assesses the role of AI in tracking respiratory diseases, such as influenza and COVID-19. Table 1 elucidates the intricate interplay between AI techniques and epidemiological challenges, highlighting the profound influence of AI on public health surveillance.

In the realm of using AI for the surveillance of seasonal respiratory infections, the period from 2014 to 2023 has witnessed remarkable advancements in understanding, predicting, and controlling various diseases. From early attempts to more recent sophisticated models, a broader spectrum of diseases, including influenza, RSV, and more recently COVID-19, has been covered. The future holds even more exciting prospects as AI technologies mature and become more integrated into the public health landscape.

Table 1 Statistical and mathematical models for infectious diseases using big data discussed in papers

Author	Model	Disease	Approach	Key findings
[33]	Artificial neural networks (ANNs)	♦Seasonal influenza	Utilizes ANN with multi-layer perceptron (MLP) structure.	Developed a forecasting system to predict seasonal influenza epidemics in Tehran.
	Time series analysis		Employed to predict future behavior based on past experiences.	
[44]	Multiple regression model	♦Influenza	The genetic algorithm-based backpropagation neural network (GA-BP) method is used to optimize the model.	Proposes a new method for estimating influenza-like illness (ILI) activity levels using search-engine query data.
[20]	Pearson correlation coefficient	♦Influenza like illnesses (ILI)	For correlation analysis	Contributes to the field of influenza prediction by combining various data sources and using the LSTM algorithm
	Long short-term memory		The input gate regulates input activations and the output gate controls the flow of cell activations.	
[14]	Non-negative matrix factorization (NMF)	♦Influenza	Employs non-negative matrix factorization (NMF) to extract latent features, revealing hidden characteristics	Presents a flexible and near-real-time surveillance tool that can complement traditional surveillance systems

(continued)

Table 1 (continued)

Author	Model	Disease	Approach	Key findings
[7]	Binary logistic regression classifiers	♦Influenza ♦Cholera ♦Dengue ♦Malaria	Used to predict if a report contains at least one symptom	Authors could not discern compelling proof that one's health status concerning cold and flu-like illnesses can be foretold based on the content or actions observed in tweets.
	Linear regression models		Predict the number of symptoms reported	
[39]	ANOVA, chi-square test, nonparametric Kruskal Wallis test	♦Viral respiratory infections	Assess the impact of different virus categories on hospital length of stay and ICU admission	Identifies the specific viruses causing respiratory illness in hospitalized pediatric patients
[27]	AI model	♦Influenza	The ILI-only data for the nine provinces in the area monitored take the historic ILI rates as input and forecast future ILI rates	Develops AI-based predictive model for forecasting at the national and provincial levels
[6]	SIR model	♦Influenza A/B ♦RSV ♦Rhinovirus ♦Adenovirus ♦Parainfluenza	Population is divided into three compartments by the model, with transitions determined by the proportionate rates and quantity of infectious individuals.	Proposes a novel TCM strategy to dynamically adjust the control measures against respiratory infectious diseases
[13]	XGBoost, CForest, RF, RANGER, SVM, ANN	♦Influenza	Predicts influenza based on clinical features, algorithms were assessed using sensitivity, specificity, and AUROC.	Developed ML algorithms to predict influenza in patients with ILIs.
[22]	LightGBM	♦RSV infection ♦Pertussis (whooping cough)	Develops two sets of models, one for predicting pertussis infection and another for predicting RSV infection	Emphasizes that ML-based clinical decision support systems may be developed in large networks to create accurate tools for public health surveillance.

5 Epidemiology of Seasonal Respiratory Infections

This epidemiology of seasonal respiratory infections is influenced by factors like temperature, humidity, and indoor crowding [33]. It primarily spreads through respiratory droplets from infected individuals when they cough, sneeze, or talk. Close contact in crowded settings facilitates transmission. Community-based investigations have played a pivotal role in identifying the causes of seasonal respiratory illnesses. Specialized studies have further refined our understanding. For example, a recent study by Agca et al. [1] explored the epidemiology shifts of respiratory viruses, including influenza, during the first year of the COVID-19 pandemic. This study analyzed nasopharyngeal swab samples from a Turkish hospital between March 2020 and February 2021, and revealed a marked decline in influenza cases during the pandemic (17.3% to 2.3%), while rhinovirus/enterovirus prevalence persisted. Given the symptomatic similarities to COVID-19, the importance of using multiplex kits that contain SARS-CoV-2, rhinovirus/enterovirus, and human metapneumovirus (MPV), is emphasized [38]. The positive rate of seasonal viruses during the pandemic is shown in Fig. 3 below.

Despite robust influenza-like illness (ILI) monitoring in European primary care levels, a study highlighted the data gap concerning SARI in intensive care units (ICUs), particularly during influenza epidemics [14]. This research assessed WHO (World Health Organization)-established metrics on the ICU impact of SARI during influenza epidemics, using Dutch ICUs between 2007 and 2016. Given the varied influenza seasonality across China, our findings have significant implications for healthcare planning and vaccination program improvement [8]. Another study [17] evaluated the impact of China's COVID-19 lockdown on the influenza peak in January 2020, showing a significant drop in flu cases and related hospitalizations due to non-pharmaceutical interventions, nearly eradicating influenza within 5 weeks [12]. Seasonal infections often exhibit seasonal patterns, with higher transmission rates during specific times of the year, typically in colder months.

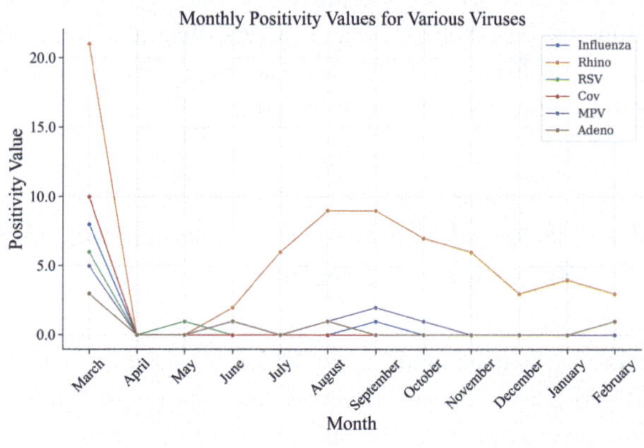

Fig. 3 Number of patients in hospital tested positive with seasonal respiratory infection in pandemic period (March 2020–February 2021)

6 Worldwide Networks for Surveillance

AI advancements have significantly bolstered our capacity to monitor and manage infectious diseases, introducing tools like early warning systems and enhanced pathogen classification. Brownstein et al. [4] cite instances of AI-powered tools that have been effective in disease surveillance, such as HealthMap, a web-based system that searches text for indicators of infectious disease events, and the Enhanced Detection System for Healthcare-Associated Transmission (EDS-HAT), which combines whole-genome surveillance sequencing and machine learning to automatically analyze patient records for outbreak clues. The authors pinpoint significant drawbacks in using AI for public health surveillance, while discussing ways to optimize its future use. Given the swift nature of disease outbreaks, they emphasize the pressing need for advanced AI tools in timely disease detection and intervention. For efficient response to respiratory diseases, including understanding their causes and transmission patterns, robust local and global surveillance systems are vital, as outlined by Al-Tawfiq et al. [2]. Table 2 provides a snapshot of a website focusing on tracking emerging respiratory illnesses.

7 Efficacy of Government-Imposed Nonpharmaceutical Interventions

Nonpharmaceutical interventions (NPIs) are crucial steps in epidemiology and public health because they serve to lower the disease's fundamental reproduction number (R0), prevent overburdening the healthcare system, and protect vulnerable populations. To combat the COVID-19 pandemic caused by the severe acute respiratory syndrome coronavirus 2 (SARS-CoV-2), many nations implemented stringent NPIs. Given that influenza shares transmission modes with COVID-19, these NPIs may be successful in limiting seasonal influenza virus epidemics [23]. This section assesses the impact of various NPIs on managing seasonal respiratory ailments, based on Qiu et al. [28]. As illustrated in Fig. 4, Qiu et al. found significant synergies between NPI pairs. The most effective pair was mask requirements with gathering restrictions, as shown in Fig. 5.

7.1 Value of Vaccination in Prevention of Seasonal Respiratory Infection Outbreaks

AI can enhance our ability to detect and address epidemics, but vaccines have proven effective in reducing infection rates [20]. Since the effectiveness of the seasonal influenza vaccine is typically between 40% and 70% and the national vaccination coverage is below 50%, it is unlikely that the widespread influenza vaccination had

Table 2 Worldwide monitoring networks and their websites [2, 41]

Name of website	URL	Characteristics
Global Influenza Surveillance and Response System	https://www.who.int/health-topics	Observes the development of influenza viruses and provides a worldwide alert
Influenzanet	https://influenzanet.info/	ILI surveillance is voluntary with leven various European countries' volunteers
FluTracking	https://info.flutracking.net/	Provides participants with tools to collect flu samples and asks them to report any symptoms they may be experiencing
HealthMap	http://healthmap.org/	Provides informal sources for disease outbreak monitoring and real-time surveillance of emerging public health threats
ProMED	http://promedmail.org/	Early warning of outbreaks
FluSurvey	https://flusurvey.net/	Sends weekly emails to participants to report any flu or COVID-19 symptoms.
Google search queries	https://trends.google.com/trends/fullscreen/m/IN	Analyzes COVID-19 symptoms in search queries, prioritizing based on symptom frequency from other data, and contrasting with historical daily data.
FluDetector	https://fludetector.cs.ucl.ac.uk/	Creates instantaneous ILI estimations
Syndromic surveillance systems	https://health.alaska.gov/dph/Epi/id/Pages/synd_surv/default.a	Gives early notice of potential dangers to human or veterinary public health

a significant impact on the disappearance of influenza outbreaks in South Korea [3]. However, vaccination campaigns targeting community immunity are crucial in preventing the spread of viruses like respiratory syncytial virus (RSV) and influenza.

Vaccinations reduce the risk of contracting and transmitting seasonal respiratory viruses, serving as a preventive barrier against infection. Beyond individual protection, widespread vaccination also supports the idea of "herd immunity," where a large portion of the population develops immunity, limiting the virus from propagating successfully within the society [10]. AI can effectively disseminate knowledge about vaccination by offering personalized advice and instructional content tailored to specific concerns and preferences. It motivates individuals to get vaccinated by emphasizing its benefits and sharing success stories [27]. AI-driven models can predict the timing and severity of seasonal respiratory outbreaks, enabling timely vaccine resource allocation. By identifying high-risk locations for outbreaks, tailoring vaccination regimens based on individual health data, and optimizing logistics for vaccine distribution, AI can support vaccination efforts, ultimately increasing immunization coverage and efficacy. Such proactive approaches enhance

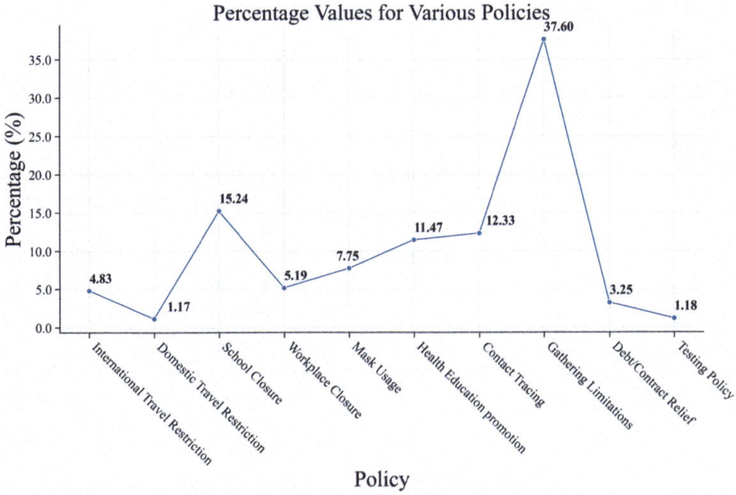

Fig. 4 Estimation of the non-pharmaceutical interventions' (NPIs') contributions to reducing influenza transmission throughout the season's decline in 2019–2020

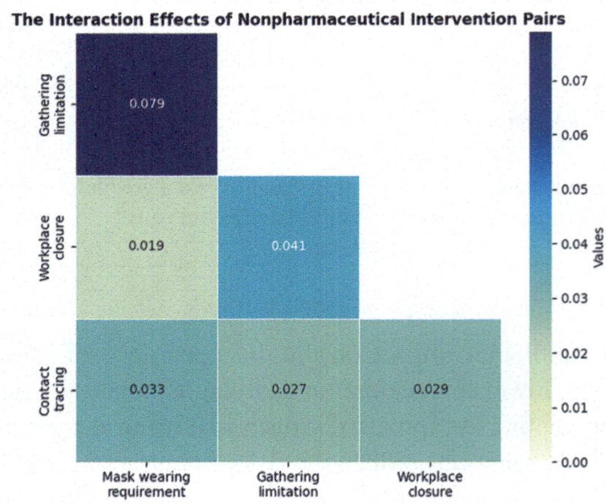

Fig. 5 The interaction effects of non-pharmaceutical intervention (NPI) pairs

immunization program efficacy by targeting high-risk individuals during prime transmission times [32].

In a nutshell, while AI enhances early diagnosis and treatment of seasonal respiratory diseases, the importance of vaccination remains paramount. A holistic strategy against these viruses combines AI-driven surveillance with immunization, safeguarding public health throughout every season [19]. It is vital to recognize how AI and vaccination work together in our collective mission to mitigate the global impact of seasonal respiratory illnesses [43].

7.2 *Value of Quarantine and International Travel Bans in the Prevention of Seasonal Respiratory Infection Outbreaks*

Quarantine measures and travel restrictions play a crucial role in public health initiatives and strategies to combat seasonal respiratory virus outbreaks. Supported by data from AI surveillance systems, these methods are vital for preventing the spread of illnesses, especially during high-risk periods [28].

Quarantining those exposed to infectious agents can halt the spread of seasonal respiratory diseases. AI-driven surveillance helps identify individuals who may have had contact with infected people or the people with high risk. By promptly quarantining these individuals, public health officials can efficiently interrupt the chain of transmission by quickly placing these people in quarantine, hence reducing the severity of outbreaks [18]. However, false negatives in AI diagnosis may lead to the inadvertent spread of infections, as individuals who are wrongly cleared may unknowingly carry and transmit the disease, potentially undermining containment efforts and public health.

AI analytics can help monitor quarantine adherence and detect breaches, enabling prompt interventions and strengthening preventive steps. It can inform international travel bans, another key tactic in epidemic containment [41]. When AI systems detect infection surges in specific regions, travel restrictions can be enacted to prevent disease import from affected zones. This proactive approach proved particularly effective during the onset of new respiratory diseases, like the COVID-19 pandemic [15]. However, if misapplied, travel restrictions can heavily impact global trade, tourism, and diplomacy. Quarantine measures also pose ethical questions about personal freedoms and rights. Therefore, the benefits to public health must be weighed carefully against the ethical and practical issues surrounding these interventions [40].

AI-driven surveillance systems enhance the efficacy of quarantine regulations and international travel bans in combating seasonal respiratory disease outbreaks. The combination of swift decision-making, targeted interventions, and AI-driven surveillance highlights the value of a comprehensive public health strategy [15, 28]. The intelligent application of these techniques, guided by AI, plays a critical role in preserving global health during seasonal respiratory infection outbreaks.

7.3 *Value of Mask Usage, Workplace and School Closure in Prevention of Seasonal Respiratory Infection Outbreaks*

When correctly worn, masks serve as physical barriers, blocking respiratory droplets with infectious agents. In busy public areas, they are a straightforward yet incredibly effective precaution that can greatly reduce the danger of virus spread [28].

Closing workplace and school during outbreaks limits close contact between coworkers and classmates. This step is crucial in settings where individuals are closely spaced, such as open-office layouts or factories. Promoting remote work options and temporarily shutting down educational institutions and offices can significantly decrease infection risks [28]. AI analyzes big datasets for COVID-19 trends to assess masking and prevention strategies. Policy decisions are aided by simulation models, which forecast outcomes under various situations. Natural Language Processing analyzes textual data to determine public opinion and compliance. Analysis of images and videos evaluates compliance with mask-wearing guidelines in the real world. Taking immunization rates and population density into account, predictive analytics projects the effects of treatments. Health monitoring systems integrate data on preventive interventions and track health outcomes. AI's flexibility makes it possible to continuously learn from fresh data, which is essential in dynamic pandemic scenarios [28, 43].

8 Effect of Other Comorbid Diseases in Respiratory Infection

The prevalence and effects of various diseases are closely entwined with the landscape of seasonal respiratory infections, generating a complex web of interconnections that further emphasize the significance of good surveillance, especially when supported by artificial intelligence. Some effects of prevalent symptoms as diseases are illustrated in Table 3 which shows the percentage of patients with acute respiratory infections in India between 2016 and 2018 who tested positive for respiratory viruses based on clinical-epidemiological characteristics [5]. From the table, the percentage of patients having positive respiratory virus testing based on clinical factors is shown in Fig. 6. When respiratory infections coincide with existing health conditions, the consequences can be more severe, leading to increased hospitalizations and higher fatality rates. For example, individuals with diabetes often have compromised immune systems, making them more vulnerable to respiratory illnesses like influenza. Likewise, those with heart diseases face elevated risks due to the additional strain respiratory pathogens place on their cardiovascular and respiratory systems [5].

AI can also help monitor the incidence and prevalence of comorbidities within populations, deepening our understanding of the interplay between chronic conditions and seasonal respiratory infections. With the help of this knowledge, healthcare systems can prioritize vaccination campaigns and other preventative actions for individuals with specific risk factors, ultimately lowering the prevalence of respiratory disease rates and their associated complications [41]. AI-driven surveillance improves our ability to understand the dynamics of respiratory infections and the unique challenges presented by concurrent health issues [9]. Understanding these intricate relationships is crucial for refining prevention and treatment strategies, leading to improved public health outcomes, as we continue to explore the rapidly changing environment of healthcare.

Table 3 Clinical-epidemiological characteristic-based percentage of patients with acute respiratory infections who tested positive for respiratory viruses, India, 2016–2018

Disease	Tested number	Any respiratory virus		Influenza		RSV	
		Numbers	Percentage (%)	Numbers	Percentage (%)	Numbers	Percentage (%)
Fever	14,636	5055	34.5	2227	15.2	982	6.7
Cough	14,896	5063	34	2158	14.5	975	6.5
Diarrhea	4858	1795	37	824	17	309	6.4
Nasal discharge	10,472	3815	36.4	1589	15.2	703	6.7
Asthmatic	8116	2639	32.5	1105	13.6	541	6.7
Fatigue	5273	1785	33.8	1024	19.4	237	4.5
Wheeze	2925	1030	35.2	324	11.1	309	10.6
Vomiting	4858	1795	37	824	17	309	6.4
Sore throat	8134	4232	52	1258	15.5	382	4.7

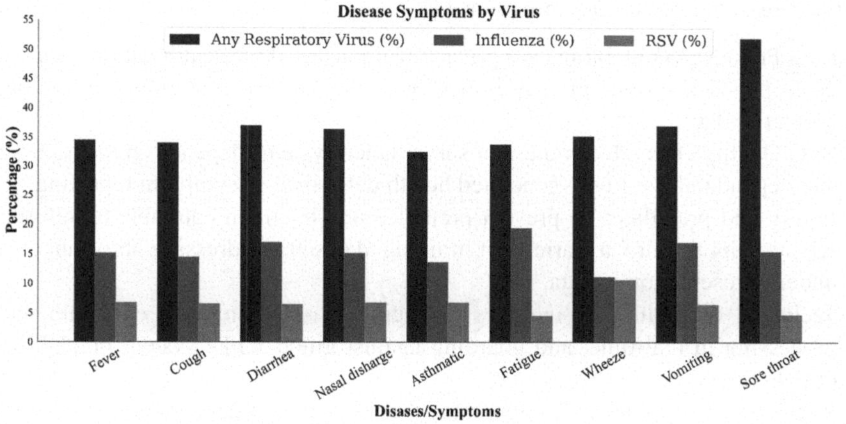

Fig. 6 Percentage of clinical and epidemiological characteristics used in calculating the patients with positive respiratory virus tests, India, 2016–2018

9 Use of Mobile Applications and Internet Data in the Surveillance of Seasonal Respiratory Infections

In our digitally connected era, harnessing internet data and mobile applications has become a potent addition to traditional surveillance techniques for tracking and monitoring seasonal respiratory diseases [14]. Mobile applications that log symptoms and health data have been instrumental in detecting the early stages of respiratory infection outbreaks. These mobile apps allow users to self-report their symptoms, generating a wealth of data that AI can consolidate and scrutinize to

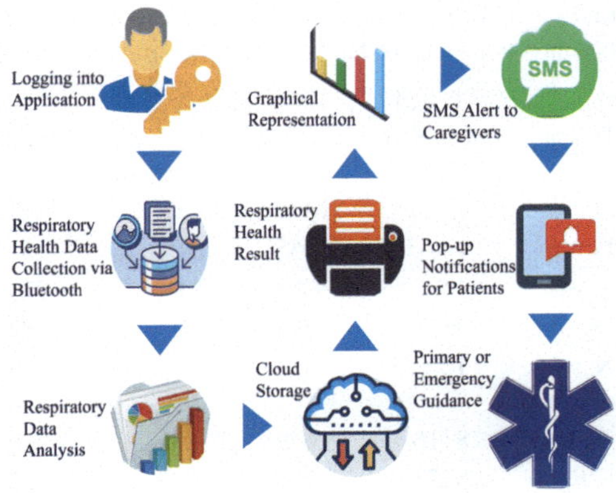

Fig. 7 A sample mobile application that uses AI surveillance to monitor respiratory infections

identify emerging patterns and localized epidemics [4]. An illustration of a mobile application using AI to monitor seasonal respiratory infections is shown in Fig. 7. The following are some difficulties with deploying an AI-powered smartphone app to track seasonal respiratory infections [4]:

- Data Privacy: Maintaining user privacy while using their health data for surveillance presents serious privacy issues and calls for stringent adherence to data protection laws.
- Data Quality: The effectiveness of surveillance systems depends on the accuracy and dependability of user-generated health data, such as symptom reporting.
- Equity and prejudice: To prevent prejudice and maintain equitable monitoring, AI systems require a variety of training datasets, addressing the danger of underrepresentation in data.
- Technical difficulties: It includes managing massive amounts of health data, processing in real-time, and guarding against glitches like system breakdowns or data leaks.
- Regulatory Compliance: To guarantee the security and dependability of healthcare, compliance with regulations and standards is essential.

In addition, Internet data, including news articles, search engine queries, and social media posts, provides a wealth of information for AI-driven surveillance systems. By employing AI and NLP methodologies, these systems can sift through enormous amount of unstructured data to detect signals of respiratory illness outbreaks in real-time [7]. Particularly on social media platforms, users can share their health-related experiences, creating a useful data stream for tracking symptoms and assessing public opinion. However, it is crucial to strike a balance between public health monitoring and individual privacy, necessitating strong data protection procedures [27].

10 Limitations and Future Direction

AI, with ongoing research, refinement, and a commitment to ethical principles, can strengthen our defenses against respiratory illnesses, leading to healthier, more proactive, and informed communities [22]. Future joint efforts involving AI researchers, healthcare practitioners, and legislators are needed to improve AI surveillance for respiratory infections. The goal of this program is to create standardized data-sharing protocols and moral AI practices, which could save the time it takes to respond to new threats by up to 25%. Additionally, the potential to save thousands of lives a year through the accelerated development and dissemination of customized therapies and vaccinations is offered by smart partnerships with pharmaceutical companies [20]. For responsible AI adoption, it is imperative to establish precise norms and criteria for AI-driven surveillance, uphold privacy protection, and tackle biases and fairness concerns [34].

Combining AI with cutting-edge innovations like the Internet of Things (IoT) and 5G networks can pave the way for a unified healthcare ecosystem. This integration could significantly improve our ability to manage seasonal respiratory infections through real-time data collecting, remote patient monitoring, and swift response mechanisms [43]. Despite the clear promise of AI in respiratory infection surveillance, it is important to recognize the current constraints and difficulties. For training and validation, AI models need large amounts of high-quality data, which may not always be available, especially in areas with limited resources [6]. To ensure that AI systems are fair and efficient, it is essential to address data biases and gaps. There are difficulties in interpreting insights generated by AI [37]. Although AI can identify patterns and anomalies, it cannot substitute the expertise and situational understanding of healthcare professionals. Therefore, a synergistic approach is essential, where AI aids rather than replacing human judgment [30]. Continuous research and development is crucial to guarantee the robustness and generalizability of AI algorithms across many geographic locations and seasons, representing a formidable challenge [29].

11 Conclusion

A significant step toward improving our capacity to manage the intricate problems presented by these enduring health hazards is the incorporation of AI into the surveillance of seasonal respiratory infections. The chapter emphasizes the rising significance of AI in improving the management of seasonal respiratory diseases. It elaborates on AI's transformative role in monitoring, predicting, and preventing diseases like the flu and RSV, offering benefits such as early epidemic detection, improved immunization techniques, and individualized treatment regimens. To ensure the effectiveness and public trust of AI, collaboration among data scientists, medical practitioners, politicians, and the public is vital. The preservation of public confidence in the revolutionary role of AI in respiratory infection treatment depends heavily on ethical considerations in AI-based surveillance systems, including privacy protection and bias reduction. To improve accuracy and equity in respiratory disease prevention and treatment, future attention should be focused on model improvement and interdisciplinary collaboration that demonstrate human ingenuity and adaptability, presenting an opportunity to strengthen community resilience, health, and awareness throughout the year.

Funding and Acknowledgment This work was made possible by High Impact grant# QUHI-CENG-23/24-216 from Qatar University. The statements made herein are solely the responsibility of the authors.

References

1. H. Agca, H. Akalin, I. Saglik, M. Hacimustafaoglu, S. Celebi, B. Ener, Changing epidemiology of influenza and other respiratory viruses in the first year of COVID-19 pandemic. J. Infect. Public Health **14**(9), 1186–1190 (2021). https://doi.org/10.1016/j.jiph.2021.08.004
2. J.A. Al-Tawfiq, A. Zumla, P. Gautret, G.C. Gray, D.S. Hui, A.A. Al-Rabeeah, Z.A. Memish, Surveillance for emerging respiratory viruses. Lancet Infect. Dis. **14**(10), 992–1000 (2014). https://doi.org/10.1016/S1473-3099(14)70840-0
3. E.A. Belongia, M.D. Simpson, J.P. King, M.E. Sundaram, N.S. Kelley, M.T. Osterholm, H.Q. McLean, Variable influenza vaccine effectiveness by subtype: A systematic review and meta-analysis of test-negative design studies. Lancet Infect. Dis. **16**(8), 942–951 (2016). https://doi.org/10.1016/S1473-3099(16)00129-8
4. J.S. Brownstein, B. Rader, C.M. Astley, H. Tian, Advances in artificial intelligence for infectious-disease surveillance. N. Engl. J. Med. **388**(17), 1597–1607 (2023). https://doi.org/10.1056/NEJMra2119215
5. M. Chadha, A.O. Prabhakaran, M.L. Choudhary, D. Biswas, P. Koul, K. Kaveri, L. Dar, C.S. Mamta, S. Jadhav, S.D. Bhardwaj, K. Laserson, S. Saha, V. Potdar, Multisite surveillance for influenza and other respiratory viruses in India: 2016–2018. PLOS Glob. Public Health **2**(11), e0001001 (2022). https://doi.org/10.1371/journal.pgph.0001001
6. W. Cheng, H. Zhou, Y. Ye, Y. Chen, F. Jing, Z. Cao, D.D. Zeng, Q. Zhang, Future trajectory of respiratory infections following the COVID-19 pandemic in Hong Kong. Chaos (Woodbury, N.Y.) **33**(1), 013124 (2023). https://doi.org/10.1063/5.0123870
7. A.R. Daughton, R. Chunara, M.J. Paul, Comparison of social media, syndromic surveillance, and microbiologic acute respiratory infection data: Observational study. JMIR Public Health Surveill. **6**(2), e14986 (2020). https://doi.org/10.2196/14986
8. C. Diamond, H. Gong, F.Y. Sun, Y. Liu, B.J. Quilty, M. Jit, J. Yang, H. Yu, W.J. Edmunds, M. Baguelin, Regional-based within-year seasonal variations in influenza-related health outcomes across mainland China: A systematic review and spatio-temporal analysis. BMC Med. **20**(1), 58 (2022). https://doi.org/10.1186/s12916-022-02269-5
9. J.D. Diaz-Decaro, B. Launer, J.A. Mckinnell, R. Singh, T.D. Dutciuc, N.M. Green, M. Bolaris, S.S. Huang, L.G. Miller, Bayesian evidence and epidemiological implications of environmental contamination from acute respiratory infection in long-term care facilities. Epidemiol. Infect. **146**(7), 832–838 (2018). https://doi.org/10.1017/S0950268818000729
10. J. Dong, H.-Q. Wu, D. Zhou, K. Li, Y. Zhang, H. Ji, Z. Tong, S. Lou, Z. Liu, Application of big data and artificial intelligence in COVID-19 prevention, diagnosis, treatment and management decisions in China. J. Med. Syst. **45** (2021). https://doi.org/10.1007/s10916-021-01757-0

11. E. Farfour, T. Pascreau, E. Jolly, S. Zia-Chahabi, L. Mazaux, M. Vasse, Spring is coming, where are the respiratory syncytial virus and influenza viruses? J. Clin. Virol. **139**, 104824 (2021). https://doi.org/10.1016/j.jcv.2021.104824
12. J.L. Hadler, Will severe acute respiratory syndrome coronavirus 2 prevention efforts affect the coming influenza season in the United States and northern hemisphere? J. Infect. Dis. **222**(11), 1759–1761 (2020). https://doi.org/10.1093/infdis/jiaa571
13. S.-K. Hung, C.-C. Wu, A. Singh, J.-H. Li, C. Lee, E.H. Chou, A. Pekosz, R. Rothman, K.-F. Chen, Developing and validating clinical features-based machine learning algorithms to predict influenza infection in influenza-like illness patients. Biom. J. **46**(5), 100561 (2023). https://doi.org/10.1016/j.bj.2022.09.002
14. K. Kalimeri, M. Delfino, C. Cattuto, D. Perrotta, V. Colizza, C. Guerrisi, C. Turbelin, J. Duggan, J. Edmunds, C. Obi, R. Pebody, A.O. Franco, Y. Moreno, S. Meloni, C. Koppeschaar, C. Kjelsø, R. Mexia, D. Paolotti, Unsupervised extraction of epidemic syndromes from participatory influenza surveillance self-reported symptoms. PLoS Comput. Biol. **15**(4), e1006173 (2019). https://doi.org/10.1371/journal.pcbi.1006173
15. J.-H. Kim, H.Y. Kim, M. Lee, J.G. Ahn, J.Y. Baek, M.Y. Kim, K. Huh, J. Jung, J.-M. Kang, Respiratory syncytial virus outbreak without influenza in the second year of the coronavirus disease 2019 pandemic: A national sentinel surveillance in Korea, 2021-2022 season. J. Korean Med. Sci. **37**(34), e258 (2022). https://doi.org/10.3346/jkms.2022.37.e258
16. K. Kurahashi, Epidemiology and risk factors of ARDS: How many is the real incidence of ARDS? in *Acute Respiratory Distress Syndrome: Advances in Diagnostic Tools and Disease Management*, ed. by S. Tasaka, (Springer, 2022), pp. 19–32. https://doi.org/10.1007/978-981-16-8371-8_2
17. H. Lei, M. Xu, X. Wang, Y. Xie, X. Du, T. Chen, L. Yang, D. Wang, Y. Shu, Nonpharmaceutical interventions used to control COVID-19 reduced seasonal influenza transmission in China. J. Infect. Dis. **222**(11), 1780–1783 (2020). https://doi.org/10.1093/infdis/jiaa570
18. G.S. Leite, A.B. Albuquerque, P.R. Pinheiro, Applications of technological solutions in primary ways of preventing transmission of respiratory infectious diseases—A systematic literature review. Int. J. Environ. Res. Public Health **18**(20), 10765 (2021). https://doi.org/10.3390/ijerph182010765
19. A.J. Lepak, L.N. Taylor, C.A. Stone, L.T. Schulz, M.C. Anderson, B.C. Fox, J.L. Temte, Association of changes in seasonal respiratory virus activity and ambulatory antibiotic prescriptions with the COVID-19 pandemic. JAMA Intern. Med. **181**(10), 1399–1402 (2021). https://doi.org/10.1001/jamainternmed.2021.2621
20. L. Liu, M. Han, Y. Zhou, Y. Wang, LSTM recurrent neural networks for influenza trends prediction, in *Bioinformatics Research and Applications*, ed. by F. Zhang, Z. Cai, P. Skums, S. Zhang, (Springer, 2018), pp. 259–264. https://doi.org/10.1007/978-3-319-94968-0_25
21. A. Maharaj, J. Parker, J. Hopkins, E. Gournis, I. Bogoch, B. Rader, C. Astley, N. Ivers, J. Hawkins, N. Slipp, A. Tuite, D. Fisman, J. Brownstein, L. Lapointe-Shaw, The effect of seasonal respiratory virus transmission on syndromic surveillance for COVID-19 in Ontario, Canada. Lancet Infect. Dis. **21** (2021). https://doi.org/10.1016/S1473-3099(21)00151-1
22. K.A. Mc Cord-De Iaco, F. Gesualdo, E. Pandolfi, I. Croci, A.E. Tozzi, Machine learning clinical decision support systems for surveillance: A case study on pertussis and RSV in children. Front. Pediatr. **11**, 1112074 (2023). https://doi.org/10.3389/fped.2023.1112074
23. S. Mekruksavanich, Forecasting the spread of seasonal influenza epidemics by neural networks with spatial data. Int. J. Geoinform. **13**(1), 69–77 (2017)
24. R.A. Morbey, D. Todkill, C. Watson, A.J. Elliot, Machine learning forecasts for seasonal epidemic peaks: Lessons learnt from an atypical respiratory syncytial virus season. PLoS One **18**(9), e0291932 (2023). https://doi.org/10.1371/journal.pone.0291932
25. P.E. Obermeier, A. Heim, B. Biere, E. Hage, M. Alchikh, T. Conrad, B. Schweiger, B.A. Rath, Linking digital surveillance and in-depth virology to study clinical patterns of viral respiratory infections in vulnerable patient populations. iScience **25**(5), 104276 (2022). https://doi.org/10.1016/j.isci.2022.104276

26. S. Okiyama, M. Fukuda, M. Sode, W. Takahashi, M. Ikeda, H. Kato, Y. Tsugawa, M. Iwagami, *Diagnosing Influenza Infection from Pharyngeal Images Using Deep Learning: Machine Learning Approach* (medRxiv, 2022), p. 2022.07.19.22276126. https://doi.org/10.1101/2022.07.19.22276126
27. S.O. Olukanmi, *Artificial Intelligence-Based Influenza Forecasting Using Google Search Data: A South African Case Study—University of Johannesburg* (Doctor of Philosophy (PHD), University of Johannesburg, 2022) https://hdl.handle.net/10210/503503
28. Z. Qiu, Z. Cao, M. Zou, K. Tang, C. Zhang, J. Tang, J. Zeng, Y. Wang, Q. Sun, D. Wang, X. Du, The effectiveness of governmental nonpharmaceutical interventions against COVID-19 at controlling seasonal influenza transmission: An ecological study. BMC Infect. Dis. **22**(1), 331 (2022). https://doi.org/10.1186/s12879-022-07317-2
29. B. Rath, T. Conrad, P. Myles, M. Alchikh, X. Ma, C. Hoppe, F. Tief, X. Chen, P. Obermeier, B. Kisler, B. Schweiger, Influenza and other respiratory viruses: Standardizing disease severity in surveillance and clinical trials. Expert Rev. Anti-Infect. Ther. **15**(6), 545–568 (2017). https://doi.org/10.1080/14787210.2017.1295847
30. H.D. Ravkin, E. Yom-Tov, L. Nesher, The effect of nonpharmaceutical interventions implemented in response to the COVID-19 pandemic on seasonal respiratory syncytial virus: Analysis of Google trends data. J. Med. Internet Res. **24**(12), e42781 (2022). https://doi.org/10.2196/42781
31. P. Roche, S. Lambert, J. Spencer, Surveillance of viral pathogens in Australia: Respiratory syncytial virus. Commun. Dis. Intell. Q. Rep. **27**(1), 117–122 (2003)
32. C. Rodrigues, S. Plotkin, Impact of vaccines; health, economic and social perspectives. Front. Microbiol. **11** (2020). https://doi.org/10.3389/fmicb.2020.01526
33. F. Saberian, A. Zamani, M.M. Gooya, P. Hemmati, M.A. Shoorehdeli, M. Teshnehlab, Prediction of seasonal influenza epidemics in Tehran using artificial neural networks, in *2014 22nd Iranian Conference on Electrical Engineering (ICEE)*, (2014), pp. 1921–1923. https://doi.org/10.1109/IranianCEE.2014.6999855
34. A.D. da Silva, A.B.G. da Veiga, O.G. da Cruz, L.S. Bastos, M.F.C. da Gomes, Severe acute respiratory infection surveillance in Brazil: The role of public, private and philanthropic healthcare units. Health Policy Plan. **37**(9), 1075–1085 (2022). https://doi.org/10.1093/heapol/czac050
35. R.B. Simpson, J. Gottlieb, B. Zhou, S. Liang, X. Jiang, M.A. Hartwick, E.N. Naumova, Navigating global public influenza surveillance systems for reliable forecasting, in *Integrated Science of Global Epidemics*, ed. by N. Rezaei, (Springer, 2023), pp. 111–137. https://doi.org/10.1007/978-3-031-17778-1_6
36. S. Soudani, A. Mafi, Z. Al Mayahi, S. Al Balushi, G. Dbaibo, S. Al Awaidy, A. Amiche, A systematic review of influenza epidemiology and surveillance in the Eastern Mediterranean and North African region. Infect. Dis. Ther. **11**(1), 15–52 (2022). https://doi.org/10.1007/s40121-021-00534-3
37. V. Srivastava, B. Srivastava, Towards timely public health decisions to tackle seasonal diseases with open government data, in *AAAI Workshops*, (2014) https://www.aaai.org/ocs/index.php/WS/AAAIW14/paper/view/8728/8221
38. L. Tapak, O. Hamidi, M. Fathian, M. Karami, Comparative evaluation of time series models for predicting influenza outbreaks: Application of influenza-like illness data from sentinel sites of healthcare centers in Iran. BMC. Res. Notes **12**(1), 353 (2019). https://doi.org/10.1186/s13104-019-4393-y
39. S. Tripathi, B. Al-Sayyed, T.R. Gladfelter, Comparative epidemiology, hospital course, and outcomes of viral respiratory infections in hospitalized pediatric patients. Indian J. Med. Microbiol. **39**(1), 24–29 (2021). https://doi.org/10.1016/j.ijmmb.2020.10.011
40. K. Trujillo, *The impact of permanent travel restrictions on global tourism | QuartzMountain*. (2023, October 4). https://quartzmountain.org/article/perm-travel-restrictions

41. UK Health Security Agency, *Sources of surveillance data for influenza, COVID-19 and other respiratory viruses*. GOV.UK. (2023, June 8). https://www.gov.uk/government/publications/sources-of-surveillance-data-for-influenza-covid-19-and-other-respiratory-viruses/sources-of-surveillance-data-for-influenza-covid-19-and-other-respiratory-viruses
42. L. Van Asten, A. Luna Pinzon, D.W. De Lange, E. De Jonge, F. Dijkstra, S. Marbus, G.A. Donker, W. Van Der Hoek, N.F. De Keizer, Estimating severity of influenza epidemics from severe acute respiratory infections (SARI) in intensive care units. Crit. Care **22**(1), 351 (2018). https://doi.org/10.1186/s13054-018-2274-8
43. Q. Wang, M. Jia, M. Jiang, W. Liu, J. Yang, P. Dai, Y. Sun, J. Qian, W. Yang, L. Feng, Seesaw effect between COVID-19 and influenza from 2020 to 2023 in World Health Organization regions: Correlation analysis. JMIR Public Health Surveill. **9**, e44970 (2023). https://doi.org/10.2196/44970
44. H. Xue, Y. Bai, H. Hu, H. Ldfs, Influenza activity surveillance based on multiple regression model and artificial neural network. IEEE Access, 1 (2017). https://doi.org/10.1109/ACCESS.2017.2771798

Index

M. E. H. Chowdhury, S. Kiranyaz (eds.), *Surveillance, Prevention, and Control of Infectious Diseases*, https://doi.org/10.1007/978-3-031-59967-5

SPRINGER NATURE

GPSR Compliance

The European Union's (EU) General Product Safety Regulation (GPSR) is a set of rules that requires consumer products to be safe and our obligations to ensure this.

If you have any concerns about our products, you can contact us on ProductSafety@springernature.com

In case Publisher is established outside the EU, the EU authorized representative is:

Springer Nature Customer Service Center GmbH
Europaplatz 3
69115 Heidelberg, Germany

The manufacturer's authorised representative in the EU is Springer Nature Customer Service Centre GmbH, Europaplatz 3, 69115 Heidelberg, Germany. If you have any concerns regarding our products, please contact ProductSafety@springernature.com

Printed and bound by CPI Group (UK) Ltd, Croydon, CR0 4YY
05/10/2026
02228130-0005